CARDIAC ARRHYTHMIAS AND DEVICE THERAPY:

RESULTS AND PROSPECTIVES FOR THE NEW CENTURY

Edited by

I.Eli Ovsyshcher, MD, PhD, FESC, FACC
*Professor of Medicine/Cardiology, Director, Arrhythmia Service
& Research Electrophysiology Laboratory, Cardiology
Department, Soroka University Medical Center & Faculty of
Health Sciences, Ben Gurion University of the Negev, Beer-
Sheva, Israel*

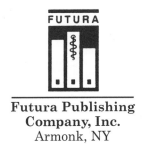

Futura Publishing
Company, Inc.
Armonk, NY

FOREWORD

This book brings together an impressive faculty to present state-of-the art data on a wide range of basic and clinical topics relating to cardiac arrhythmias and device therapy.

Much research has gone into identifying non-invasive methods to determine patients at risk for sudden death. T-wave alternans is a promising new technique to accomplish this goal, and both the electrophysiology underlying T-wave alternans and its clinical applicability are discussed. Impulse propagation, including the effects of subthreshold stimulation, an area dear to my own heart, is discussed. Doctors Moss and Scheinman review the genetics and clinical evaluation of patients with Long QT syndrome. Issues concerning ablation of left-sided accessory pathways as well as the use of adenosine triphosphate to diagnose mechanisms of supraventricular tachycardia are reviewed.

Atrial fibrillation has been the "arrhythmia of the 1990s," and investigation of its mechanisms and treatment proceeds boldly into the new millennium. As such, multiple chapters concerning atrial fibrillation are included. These range from pathophysiologic aspects to pharmacologic and nonpharmacologic treatment. New data on ablation, pacing, and implantable defibrillators are discussed. Sudden cardiac death remains a major worldwide epidemiologic problem. Several chapters are dedicated to this important area including genetics, pathology, clinical manifestations, risk stratification, results of ICD trials, and newer aspects of ICD technology. Future ICD indications are also covered.

Cardiac pacing has become such a routine form of therapy that we often take for granted the major technological advances that have occurred in this area over the past decades. In addition to a review of indications for various forms of pacing, cutting-edge advances in both lead technology and stimulation techniques are discussed in detail. Further, newer indications for pacing such as in patients with hypertrophic cardiomyopathy or congestive heart failure are reviewed.

The editor is to be congratulated for assembling such an excellent array of authors to discuss topical issues of concern for clinicians.

ERIC N. PRYSTOWSKY, MD, FACC
Consulting Professor of Medicine
Duke University Medical Center
Durham, North Carolina,
Director, Clinical Electrophysiology Laboratory,
St. Vincent Hospital, Indianapolis, IN, USA

PREFACE

The final decades of the last century have been a period of expansive growth for the electrophysiological management of cardiac arrhythmias. Rapid application of technological advances within clinical practice has been the main focus of these extraordinary developments, rendering the communication and exchange of ideas in this field paramount.

The purpose of this book is to provide its readers with the latest knowledge. The book covers a wide variety of the topics: basic electrophysiology, including genetics and the molecular base of arrhythmias; invasive and noninvasive clinical electrophysiology, and most important of all the clinical aspects of cardiac pacing and defibrillation. It contains an overview of various methods in treatment of AF, including ablation and defibrillation, the role of pacing in prevention of AF and in treatment of congestive heart failure, dilated, hypertrophic obstructive and restrictive cardiomyopathies. The results of recent clinical trials in cardiac pacing and in prevention and treatment of malignant ventricular arrhythmias are also presented. Special sections have been dedicated to the various aspects of preventing sudden death including the use of internal and external defibrillation.

Most of the chapters of this book emphasize the more clinical aspects of pacing and electrophysiology, presenting the impressive contributions by experts in the field. The book also provides a current review of a variety of 'hot' topics, with personal experiences and critical evaluations by the authors, taking into perspective modern pacing and electrophysiology. We hope that this information will be beneficial to clinicians in selecting and providing appropriate treatment for patients with various cardiac arrhythmias.

I wish to express my gratitude to the authors, who are all leaders in their fields, for their willingness to contribute to the creation of this volume, despite the tight time schedule, which enabled us to achieve our goal - disseminating this knowledge and information to electrophysiologists, pacemaker specialists, bioengineers, technicians and nurses engaged in all aspects of the field. *I hope you all will find this enjoyable, useful and applicable!*

I also wish to express my indebtedness to the various companies for their generous support without which the publication of this book would not have been possible.

I. ELI OVSYSHCHER, MD, PhD, FESC, FACC

Professor of Medicine/Cardiology

CONTRIBUTORS

CHRISTINE ALONSO, MD
>Assistant, Department of Cardiology and Vascular Diseases, University Hospital, Rennes, France

HENNING RUD ANDERSEN, MD, DMSC
>Department of Cardiology, Skejby Sygehus, Aarhus University Hospital, Aarhus N, Denmark

BOAZ AVITALL, MD, PHD, FACC
>Professor of Medicine, Director of Clinical and Research Cardiac Electrophysiology, University of Illinois, Chicago, IL, USA

S. SERGE BAROLD, MD, FRACP, FACC, FACP, FESC
>Cardiac Electrophysiology Service, North Ridge Hospital, Fort Lauderdale, Florida, USA. Associate Editor, PACE.

M. KEMAL BATUR, MD
>Assistant Professor of Cardiology, Department of Cardiology, Hacettepe University, School of Medicine, Ankara,Turkey

BERNARD BELHASSEN, MD
>Professor of Cardiology, Director, Cardiac Electrophysiology Laboratory, Department of Cardiology, Tel-Aviv Sourasky Medical Center, Israel

CHARLES I. BERUL, MD
>Associate in Cardiology, Director of Pacing & Defibrillator Program, Children's Hospital, Boston, Harvard Medical School, MA, USA

SAROJA BHARATI, MD
>Director, Maurice Lev Congenital Heart & Conduction System Center, The Heart Institute for Children, Hope Children's Hospital, Christ Hospital & Medical Center, Oak Lawn, IL; Professor of Pathology, Rush Medical College, Rush University Rush-Presbyterian-St. Luke's Medical Center, Chicago, IL; Clinical Professor of Pathology, Finch University of Health Sciences Chicago Medical School, North Chicago, IL, and Visiting

Professor of Pathology University of Illinois at Chicago, Chicago, IL, USA

SERGE CAZEAU, MD

InParys, Saint-Cloud, France

STUART J. CONNOLLY, MD

Professor of Medicine, Faculty of Health Sciences, McMaster University, Hamilton, ON, Canada

EUGENE CRYSTAL, MD

Arrhythmia Service & Electrophysiology Research Laboratory, Cardiology Department, Soroka University Medical Center; Lecturer, Faculty of Health Sciences, Ben Gurion University of the Negev, Beer-Sheva, Israel

J. CLAUDE DAUBERT, MD

Professor of Cardiology, Chief, Department of Cardiology and Vascular Diseases, University Hospital, Rennes, France

BARBAROS DOCUMACI, MD

Associate Professor of Medicine, Cardiology, SSK Regional Hospital, Eskisehir, Turkey

HUGO ECTOR, MD, PhD

Professor of Medicine, Cardiology Department, UZ Gasthuisberg, University of Leuven, Belgium

NABIL EL-SHERIF, MD

Professor of Medicine & Physiology & Director, Clinical Cardiac Electrophysiology Program, State University of New York Health Science Center; Director, Cardiology Division, Veterans Affairs Medical Center, Brooklyn, New York, USA

ILYA FLEIDERVISH, MD, PhD

Electrophysiology Research Laboratory, Faculty of Health Sciences, Ben Gurion University of the Negev, Beer-Sheva; Koret School of Veterinary Medicine, The Hebrew University of Jerusalem, Israel

PAUL A. FRIEDMAN, MD, FACC

Assistant Professor of Medicine, Division of Internal Medicine & Cardiovascular Diseases, Mayo Clinic, Rochester, MN, USA

SEYMOUR FURMAN, MD, FACC, FACS
Professor of Medicine and Surgery, Albert Einstein College of Medicine, Attending, Cardiothoracic Surgery and Department of Medicine, Division of Cardiology, Montefiore Medical Center, Bronx, NY, USA

DAN GELVAN, PhD
Faculty of Agriculture, The Hebrew University of Jerusalem, Rehovot, Israel

LEON GLASS, PhD, FRSC
Professor of Physiology, McGill University, Montreal, Quebec, Canada

JAY N. GROSS, MD
Associate Professor of Medicine, Albert Einstein College of Medicine, Director, Inter-Campus Pacemaker Service, Department of Medicine, Division of Cardiology, Montefiore Medical Center, Bronx, NY, USA

MICHAEL GLIKSON, MD, FACC
Heart Institute, Chaim Sheba Medical Center, Tel Aviv University, Tel Hashomer, Israel

DAVID L. HAYES, MD
Vice-Chair, Cardiovascular Diseases, Mayo Clinic, Rochester, MN; Professor of Medicine, Mayo Medical School, Rochester, MN, USA.

SUSANNE HERWIG, MD
Department of Medicine - Cardiology, University of Bonn, Bonn, Germany

HEIN HEIDBUCHEL, MD, PhD
Professor, Cardiology–Electrophysiology, UZ Gasthuisberg, University of Leuven, Belgium

WERNER JUNG, MD, FESC
Associate Professor of Medicine, Department of Medicine - Cardiology, University of Bonn, Bonn, Germany

PRAPA KANAGARTNAM, MRCP
Imperial College of Science Technology and Medicine, London, UK

EMMANUEL M. KANOUPAKIS, MD
Senior Registrar of the Cardiology Department, Heraklion University, Crete, Greece

WLODZIMIERZ KARGUL, MD, PhD
Electrophysiology, Silesian Center of Cardiology, Katowice, Poland

LENE KRISTENSEN, MD
Department of Cardiology, Skejby Sygehus, Aarhus University Hospital, Aarhus N, Denmark

ANDRZEJ KUTARSKI, MD, PhD
Department of Cardiology, University Medical Academy, Lublin, Poland

JAIRO KUSNIEC, MD
Senior Physician, Arrhythmia Unit, Rabin Medical Center, Petah-Tikva, Israel

CHRISTOPHE LECLERCQ, MD
Assistant Professor, Department of Cardiology and Vascular Diseases, University Hospital, Rennes, France

PAUL A. LEVINE, MD
Vice President & Medical Director, St. Jude Medical-Cardiac Rhythm Management Division, Sylmar, CA; Clinical Professor of Medicine, Loma Linda University School of Medicine, Loma Linda, CA, USA

FRED W. LINDEMANS, PhD
Medtronic Bakken Research Center BV, Maastricht, The Netherlands

BERNDT LUDERITZ, MD, FACC, FESC
Professor of Medicine, Head, Department of Medicine - Cardiology, University of Bonn, Bonn, Germany

DAVID LURIA, MD
Division of Internal Medicine & Cardiovascular Diseases, Mayo Clinic, Rochester, MN, USA

PHILIPPE MABO, MD
Professor of Cardiology, Chief, Clinical Electrophysiology Unit, University Hospital, Rennes, France

MAREK MALIK, MD, PhD, DSc, FACC, FESC
St. George's Hospital Medical School, Department of Cardiological Sciences, London, UK

EMMANUEL G. MANIOS, MD
Lecturer in Cardiology, Cardiology Department, Heraklion University Hospital, Crete, Greece

HARRY G. MOND, MD, FRACP, FACC
Physician to the Pacemaker Clinic, The Royal Melbourne Hospital Victoria, Australia.

ARTHUR J. MOSS, MD
Professor of Medicine (Cardiology); Director, Heart Research Follow-up Program, University of Rochester Medical Center, Rochester, NY, USA

JAN NEMEC, MD
Division of Internal Medicine & Cardiovascular Diseases, Mayo Clinic, Rochester, MN, USA

JENS COSEDIS NIELSEN, MD
Department of Cardiology, Skejby Sygehus, Aarhus University Hospital, Aarhus N, Denmark

ALI OTO, MD, FESC, FACC
Professor of Medicine & Cardiology, Department of Cardiology, Hacettepe University School of Medicine, Ankara, Turkey

I. ELI OVSYSHCHER, MD, PhD, FESC, FACC
Professor of Medicine/Cardiology, Director, Arrhythmia Service & Research Electrophysiology Laboratory, Cardiology Department, Soroka University Medical Center & Faculty of Health Sciences, Ben Gurion University of the Negev, Beer-Sheva, Israel

NICHOLAS S. PETERS, MD, FRCP
Professor, Cardiac Electrophysiology & Honorary Consultant Cardilogist, Imperial College of Science Technology and Medicine, London, UK

AVINOAM RABINOVITCH, PhD
Professor of Physics, Department of Physics, Ben Gurion University of the Negev, Beer-Sheva, Israel

HINDRIK W.J. ROBBE, PhD
Manager Research & Outcomes Studies, Tachy/AF/EPS, Medtronic Bakken Research Center, Maastricht, The Netherlands

DAN M. RODEN, MD
Professor of Medicine & Pharmacology, William Stokes Professor of Experimental Therapeutics; Director, Division of Clinical Pharmacology, Vanderbilt University School of Medicine, Nashville, TN, USA

DAVID S. ROSENBAUM, MD
Associate Professor of Medicine, Biomedical Engineering, Physiology & Biophysics; Director, Heart & Vascular Research Center; Section Chief, Cardiac Electrophysiology Service Metro Health Campus, Case Western Reserve University, Cleveland, OH, USA

SHIMON ROSENHECK, MD, FACC, FESC
Director, Electrophysiology Laboratory, Cardiology Unit, Hadassah University Hospital, Mount Scopus, Jerusalem, Israel

MASSIMO SANTINI, MD
Professor of Medicine, Director, Department of Heart Diseases, San Filippo Neri Hospital, Rome, Italy

SANJEEV SAKSENA, MD, FACC, FESC
Clinical Professor of Medicine, UMD-RWJ Medical School; Director, Arrhythmia & Pacemaker Service, EHI-Atlantic Health System, NJ, USA

MAX SCHALDACH, MD, PhD
Professor of Physics, Chairman, Department of Biomedical Engineering, Friedrich-Alexander University, Erlangen, Germany

MELVIN M. SCHEINMAN, MD
Professor of Medicine, University of California, S.F. Medical Center, San Francisco, CA, USA

BORIS STRASBERG, MD
Professor of Cardiology, Sackler School of Medicine, Tel - Aviv University, Director of Arrhythmia Unit, Rabin Medical Center, Petah-Tikva, Israel

KAREL F.A.A. SMITS, MSc
Medtronic Bakken Research Center, Maastricht, The Netherlands.

PHILIP SPURRELL, MD, MRCP
Department of Cardiology, Eastbourne General Hospital, Eastbourne, UK.

MARSHALL S. STANTON, MD
Vice President, Medical Affairs, Cardiac Rhythm Management Division, Medtronic, Inc. Minneapolis, MN, USA

NEIL SULKE, MD, FACC
Department of Cardiology, Eastbourne General Hospital, Eastbourne, UK

GIOIA TURITTO, MD
Associate Professor of Medicine, Director Coronary Care Unit and Cardiac Electrophysiology Laboratory, State University of New York Health Science Center, Brooklyn, NY, USA

PANOS E. VARDAS, MD, PhD, FESC, FACC
Professor of Medicine, Head of the Cardiology Department, Heraklion University Hospital, Crete, Greece

RIK WILLEMS, MD
Research Assistant, Fund for Scientific Research, Flanders, UZ Gasthuisberg, University of Leuven, Belgium

JAMES E. WILLENBRING, BSEE
Cardiac Rhythm Management Division, Medtronic, Inc., Minneapolis, MN, USA

CONTENTS

Foreword
    Eric N. Prystowsky iii

Preface
    I. Eli Ovsyshcher v

Contributors vii

I. Basic and Clinical Electrophysiology

1. Morphological Determinants of Arrhythmogenesis
    Prapa Kanagartnam, Nicholas S. Peters 3

2. The Relationship Between T-wave Alternans and Cardiac
Arrhythmogenesis as Elucidated by Optical Mapping
    Joseph M. Pastore, David S. Rosenbaum 11

3. T-wave Alternans: A Link to Clinical Practice
    M. Kemal Batur, Ali Oto 23

4. Pulse Propagation in Excitability Changing Medium
    *Avinoam Rabinovitch, Ira Aviram, Menahem Friedman, Natalie
Gulko, Eugene Crystal, Ilya A. Fleidervish,I. Eli Ovsyshcher* 29

5. Modeling of Defibrillation Thresholds
    Marek Malik, Karel Faa. Smits, Fred W. Lindemans 35

6. Subthreshold Conditioning Stimuli Modulate Refractoriness in Murine
Ventricular Slices
    *Eugene Crystal, Ilya A. Fleidervish, Avinoam Rabinovitch, I. Eli
Ovsyshcher* 41

7. Adenosine Triphosphate in Cardiac Arrhythmias: From Therapeutic to
Bedside Diagnostic Use
    Bernard Belhassen 47

8. Long QT Syndrome: Phenotype-Genotype Considerations
    Arthur J. Moss, Wojciech Zareba, Jenifer L. Robinson 55

9. QT Syndrome: Electrophysiological and Clinical Aspects
   Melvin M. Scheinman 63

10. Left Atrial "Isthmus" Concept: Pitfalls in Lateral Accessory Pathway
Ablation
   David Luria, Jan Nemec, Paul A. Friedman 73

11. How Does Spontaneous Ventricular Tachycardia Initiate: Analysis of
Stored Intracardiac Electrograms?
   Maria Trusz-gluza, Wlodzimierz Kargul, Tadeusz Zajac, Artur
Filipecki, Ewa Konarska-kuszewska, Maciej Pruski, Zbigniew Michalak,
Krzysztof Szydlo 79

II. Atrial Fibrillation, Common Aspects

12. Control of Atrial Fibrillation: A Theoretical Perspective
   Leon Glass, Marc Courtemanche 87

13. Slow Development of Atrial Fibrillation in a Transvenously Paced Sheep
Model
   Rik Willems, Hugo Ector, Hein Heidbüchel 95

14. Catheter Mapping of Atrial Fibrillation in Patients with Spontaneous
Atrial Fibrillation
   Sanjeev Saksena, Atul Prakash, Ryszard B. Krol, Steven Kim, George
Philip 101

15. Quality of Life in Atrial Fibrillation
   Berndt Lüderitz, Susanne Herwig, Werner Jung 107

III. Atrial Fibrillation, Treatment

16. Combined Antiarrhythmic Therapy for the Prevention of Paroxysmal
Atrial Fibrillation
   Boris Strasberg, Jairo Kusniec, Ronit Zabarsky 115

17. Ablation of Atrial Fibrillation
   Boaz Avitall, Arvidas Urbonas, Scott C. Millard 119

18. Pathology of Atrial Fibrillation—Ultrasound versus Radiofrequency
Saroja Bharati 131

19. Temporary Internal Atrial Defibrillation in Patients with AF:
Conclusions from the Use of the Latest Technology
*Panos E. Vardas, Emmanuel M. Kanoupakis, Emmanuel G.
Manios* 137

20. The Implantable Atrial Defibrillator: Indications and Results
*Massimo Santini, Renato Ricci, Claudio Pandozi, Maria Carmela
Scianaro, Salvatore Toscano, Giuliano Altamura* 145

IV. Pacing for AF Prevention

21. Prevention of Atrial Fibrillation by Pacing
*J. Claude Daubert, Gilles Revault D'allonnes, Dominique Pavin,
Philippe Mabo* 155

22. Practical and Technical Aspects of Biatrial Pacing
Andrzej Kutarski 167

23. Multisite Atrial Pacing for the Prevention of Recurrence of Atrial
Fibrillation: Optimistic and Pessimistic Views.
*Panos E. Vardas, Emmanuel G. Manios, Emmanuel N.
Simantirakis* 175

24. Pacing and Defibrillation for the Prevention and Termination of Atrial
Fibrillation
Philip Spurrell, Neil Sulke 181

V. **Implantable Cardioverter Defibrillator**

25. Impact of ICD Studies on Their Use: A Critical Analysis
Seah Nisam 191

26. Dual Chamber Implantable Cardioverter Defibrillator Technology
Marshall S. Stanton, James E. Willenbring 201

27. Dual Chamber ICDs: Should This be the Standard of Care for all ICD Patients?
Jay N. Gross, Stanislav Weiner 211

28. Implantable Cardioverter-Defibrillators in Pediatrics
Charles I. Berul 217

29. Cost-effectiveness of Implantable Cardioverter-Defibrillator Therapy
Hindrik Wj. Robbe, Fred W. Lindemans 223

30. Predictors of Long-term Survival in Patients with Implantable Cardioverter Defibrillator
Shimon Rosenheck 229

31. Pacemaker – ICD Interactions: Are They Still Relevant? Past, Present and Future
Michael Glikson, Paul Friedman 241

VI. Sudden Death

32. The Genetics of Sudden Death
Dan M. Roden 249

33. Pathology of the Conduction System in Sudden Death in the Young, Athletes and Healthy
Saroja Bharati 257

34. Sudden Cardiac Death in the Young: Genetic Aspects
Melvin M. Scheinman 263

35. The Need for Powerful Risk Stratification of Sudden Cardiac Death in the Era of Prophylactic ICD
Nabil El-sherif, Gioia Turitto 273

36. MADIT and the Prevention of Sudden Cardiac Death
Arthur J. Moss 285

VII. Cardiac Pacing

37. The History of the Comprehension of AV Conduction, Heart Block and
Stokes - Adams Syndrome
    Seymour Furman 295

38. The 1998 ACC/AHA Guidelines for Pacemaker Implantation Should Be
Revised
    S. Serge Barold, Helen S. Barold, Robert S. Fishel 307

39. Therapy Concept and Clinical Relevance of Closed Loop Stimulation
    Max Schaldach, M. Schier, T. Christ, M. Hubman, K. Malinowski .. 315

40. Outcome of Patients with Sick Sinus Syndrome Treated by Different
Pacing Modalities
    Lene Kristensen, Jens Cosedis Nielsen, Henning Rud Andersen 323

41. Clinical Trials of Pacing Mode Selection
    Stuart J. Connolly 333

42 Clinical Experience with Dual Chamber Ventricular Autocapture
    Paul A. Levine 339

43. Diagnostic Value of the 12 Lead ECG during Cardiac Pacing
    S. Serge Barold, Helen S. Barold, Robert S. Fishel 349

44. Pacing Leads for the New Century
    Harry G. Mond 357

45. Electromagnetic Interference and Implantable Devices
    David L. Hayes 365

46. Influence of New Pacing Algorithms on Generator Longevity
    ***Dan Gelvan, Eugene Crystal, Barbaros Dokumaci, I. Eli
Ovsyshcher*** 373

VIII. New Indications for Cardiac Pacing: As We Approach The New Century.

47. Long-term Experience with Biventricular Pacing in Refractory Heart Failure
   J. Claude Daubert, Christophe Leclercq, Christine Alonso, Serge S. Cazeau 385

48. Implantable Device Therapy for Patients with Hypertrophic Cardiomyopathy
   David L. Hayes, Paul A. Friedman 393

49. Easy and Safe Permanent Left Atrial Pacing ñ Challenge for the Beginning of the New Century
   Andrzej Kutarski, Max Schaldach 401

50. Cardiac Pacing in Patients with Marked First-degree AV Block
   I. Eli Ovsyshcher, S. Serge Barold 409

Author Index 419

Part I.

Basic and Clinical Electrophysiology

1.
MORPHOLOGICAL DETERMINANTS OF ARRHYTHMOGENESIS

Prapa Kanagaratnam MRCP, Nicholas S Peters MD FRCP

Imperial College of Science Technology and Medicine, London, UK

Conduction of the cardiac impulse is dependent both on active membrane properties and the passive properties determined by architectural features of the myocardium. The influence of tissue architecture on conduction is principally determined by the size, shape and packing of individual myocytes, and by the quantity, three-dimensional distribution and physiological behavior of the specialized intercellular junctions responsible for impulse propagation from cell to cell, the gap junctions.[1] It has long been recognized that abnormalities in conduction of the cardiac impulse are an important cause of arrhythmias[2] by altering the relationships between conduction velocity, path length and recovery of excitability (the determinants of reentrant excitation). However, it was not until more recently that myocardial architecture was considered important in determining patterns of activation and conduction velocity [3,4] and therefore to have a central role in arrhythmogenesis.[5]

The Electrophysiological Architecture of Ventricular Myocardium

In ventricular myocardium, conduction is faster in the direction parallel to the myocardial fiber axis and this is principally due to the lower resistivity of myocardium in the longitudinal direction.[6] Gap-junctional channels create continuity between the cytoplasmic compartments of neighbouring myocytes, but act as resistive discontinuities to the cytoplasmic current flow between the intracellular compartments of the cells. Longitudinal resistivity is lower than transverse because this intracellular pathway encounters fewer cell boundaries per unit distance.

Gap junctions are specialized regions of the intercalated disk (for reviews see 1,7,8,9) clusters of gap-junctional channels, each formed by two connexons, each comprising of six constituent connexin proteins.[8] The connexons from each myocyte membrane align and the pair forms a complete channel linking the cytoplasmic compartments providing a relatively low resistance pathway for the passage of ions and small molecules (up to 1 kDa)[10], and for electrical propagation.[11] In the mammalian heart, a connexin with a molecular weight of 43,000 (connexin43) is the most abundant connexin, but connexin40 (also

From Ovsyshcher IE. *Cardiac Arrythmias and Device Therapy: Results and Perspectives for the New Century.* Armonk, NY: Futura Publishing Company, Inc., © 2000

abundant in the atria, specialized conducting tissues and subendocardial ventricular myocardium) and connexin45 are the other connexins expressed by cardiac myocytes.[12]

In normal adult ventricular myocardium gap junctions are confined almost exclusively to the intercalated disks[1,13,14], the sites of mechanical, metabolic and electrical cellular coupling[15,7] that facilitate coordinated interaction of the cells. In ventricular myocardium, large intercalated disks exist at the ends of the myocytes, with smaller disks along the length of the cell.[7] Therefore, with respect to gap-junctional coupling in ventricular myocardium, activation wavefronts may conduct readily between adjacent cells in the longitudinal or transverse directions. However, the resistivity of gap-junctional membrane, although several orders of magnitude lower than non-gap-junctional plasma membrane, is several orders of magnitude higher than the cytoplasmic intracellular resistivity. The result is that over a given distance, a wavefront will encounter more gap junctions in the transverse direction than in the longitudinal direction, resulting slower conduction transversely.

A further level of complexity in the relationship between myocardial architecture and electrical propagation, is the properties of the extracellular space. In the papillary muscles, connective tissue septa subdivide the myocardium into unit bundles composed of 2-30 cells surrounded by a connective tissue sheath.[16] This septation would be expected to contribute further to the anisotropy of conduction, but the relevance of this observation to other regions of ventricular myocardium is unknown.[4]

Morphological changes in ventricular myocardium leading to ventricular tachycardia after myocardial infarction

Healing Phase

In a canine model studied 4 days after left anterior descending (LAD) coronary artery ligation, conduction disturbances are demonstrated in the myocardium of the healing infarct border, despite a normal action potential indicating these disturbances are likely to be due to remodeling of intercellular coupling.[17] The changing microscopic architecture of the surviving subepicardial myocardial fibers of the canine infarct border zone has important time-dependent influences on impulse conduction that cause arrhythmias in the experimental model.[18,19] The subepicardial fiber orientation, perpendicular to the LAD, forms an anisotropic structure that is maintained during the first week after coronary occlusion, when the fibers may remain tightly packed together or become partially separated by edema.[17-19] Although the surviving myocytes in the border zone adjacent to necrotic cells have normal histological features, they have varying degrees of disruption of connexin43 gap junction distribution[18], similar to that which has also been described in healed human infarcts[20]. In contrast with normal, the healing canine epicardial border zone reveals immunolabeled connexin43 distributed around the entire cell surface with a large amount located along the lateral membrane. The disturbed gap-junctional pattern is most prominent adjacent to the necrotic tissue, and extends through the border zone toward the epicardial surface[18] where the subepicardial myocytes distant from the necrotic tissue almost universally show the normal transversely oriented pattern describing the locations of the normal intercalated disks . However, in thinner regions of the epicardial border zone, the layer of disturbed gap-junctional distribution extends throughout the entire thickness of the surviving epicardial border zone, all the way to the epicardial surface.

These profound alterations in the organization of intercellular connections occur in the healing experimental canine epicardial border zone that exhibits non-uniformity of anisotropic conduction, fractionated electrograms and ready inducibility stable monomorphic ventricular tachycardia but no evidence of any fibrotic scarring.[17-19] Reentrant circuits in these epicardial border zones are functional, in that they are not formed by fixed anatomical block to conduction, but are induced by programmed stimulation when a sufficiently premature impulse encounters a refractory region and deviate around to form a complete circuit of continuous reentrant excitation dependent on the functional properties of the tissue.[19-21] The mechanism for block may involve anisotropic properties of this region, with preferential longitudinal conduction block[22], or a prolonged refractory period at the site of block.[21]

Although the mechanisms for the formation of the stable functional lines of block in canine anisotropic reentrant circuits 4 days after infarction remains uncertain, there is a relationship between their location and the microscopic anatomy of these regions.[18] A stable reentrant circuit causing sustained, monomorphic ventricular tachycardia appears to occur only if the altered distribution of connexin43 extends throughout the full thickness of a region of the infarct border zone, and this region defines the location and dimensions of the lines of functional block, and of the central common pathway between them. Boundaries between the region of full-thickness abnormalities and adjacent regions that have abnormal connexin43 distribution extending only part way through the epicardial border zone, are the locations of the functional lines of block in the reentrant circuits.[18]

The mechanism by which the change in gap-junctional distribution influences the location and characteristics of the reentrant circuit has yet to be determined.

Healed Phase

Remodeling of experimental and human infarct structure continues as the infarct heals, leading to further changes with time.[17,20] Although a human infarct may be described as transmural, there may be surviving subepicardial muscle supporting reentry as in the canine infarct model[17-23], and surviving muscle and Purkinje fibers on the subendocardial surface.[24] The reentrant pathway in most clinical reentrant circuits causing ventricular tachycardia principally involves this surviving subendocardial tissue, but deeper myocardial and epicardial involvement may be critical to maintaining the circuit.

The deposition of the connective tissue scar distorts the normal relationship of the surviving myocardial fiber bundles.[25] In some regions myocardial fibers become markedly separated from each other along their length.[17,25,26] In the myocardium associated with healed canine infarcts there is a concomitant reduction in the number of cells to which each myocyte is connected associated with a greater reduction of predominantly side-to-side cell interconnections (by 75%) than end-to-end (22%), with smaller and fewer gap junctions.[26] In the border zone of healed human infarcts, altered connexin43 gap junction distribution occurs in surviving myocytes up to 700um from the interface with the fibrotic infarcted tissue.[20] Within this border zone region, comparatively few labeled gap junctions are organized into discrete, transversely-orientated intercalated disks, and many are spread longitudinally over the cell surface, apparently similar to the disturbance in the canine epicardial border zone 4 days after infarction.[20] Some of these junctions are apparently isolated and distant from any of the other components, such as the anchoring junctions, of the intercalated disk. In addition, a small proportion of junctional contacts are entirely disrupted and internalized. [2]

Consistent with such observations, detailed measurements in isolated superfused preparations of the epicardial border zone from healed canine infarcts have shown that very slow conduction displaying non-uniformity of anisotropy occurs despite normal transmembrane potentials recorded at most sites. Rather than abnormalities in action potential generation, therefore, the slow and deranged activation appears to be dependent on the underlying derangement of cellular connections among and between disarrayed myocardial fiber bundles.[17,18,28]

The Electrophysiological Architecture of Atrial Myocardium

A role of atrial architecture in determining arrhythmogenic substrate is also beginning to emerge. The activation sequence of atrial flutter has been described and in common atrial flutter a component of the re-entrant circuit is a line of functional block along the crista terminalis, a thick muscular ridge into which the pectinate muscles insert.[29] The mechanism by which this line of conduction block occurs is not understood. It has been shown that small number of muscle fibres connect with a larger myocardial mass it is possible to develop block as predicted by the *sink/source hypothesis*.[30] It has also been suggested that this interface can be very sensitive to the level of gap-junctional intercellular coupling and paradoxically reduced coupling can lead to improved conduction.[31] The degree of transverse conduction of the crista terminalis has been suggested to determine whether patients develop atrial fibrillation or atrial flutter with futter patients developing transverse conduction block at longer coupling interval than patients with fibrillation.[32] In atrial fibrillation, the potential architectural features, which lead to arrhythmogenesis are multiple. Various studies have looked at the frequency of activation and local re-entry in different regions of the right and left atria. The septum and the crista terminalis both display a higher degree of local re-entry. In the crista terminalis this may be due to re-entry between the pectinate muscles and the crista terminalis. Studies using in-vitro high density mapping of atrial tissue have demonstrated that such re-enry is feasible, however, it is unclear if this type of re-entry occurs in vivo. [33]

Conclusion

Due to the complex topology of the cellular interactions, it has proven difficult to generate experimental data linking morphological characteristics directly to conduction properties and to an arrhythmogenic substrate in whole myocardium. These morphological determinants of arrhythmias may provide an alternative approach to anti-arrhythmic therapy,

References:

1. Page, E. Cardiac Gap Junctions. In: The Heart and Cardiovascular System. H.A. Fozzard, E. Haber, R.B. Jennings, A.M. Katz, and H.E. Morgan (eds). New York: Raven Press Ltd. 1992;1003-1048.

2. Mines GR. On circulating excitations in heart muscles and their possible relation to tachycardia and fibrillation. *Trans Roy Soc Can IV.* 1914;43-52.

3. Spach MS, Miller WT III, Dolber PC et al. The functional role of structural complexities in the propagation of depolarization in the atrium of the dog. *Circ Res.* 1982;50:175-191.

4. Spach MS, Dolber PC. Relating extracellular potentials and their derivatives to anisotropic propagation at a microscopic level in human cardiac muscle.*Circ Res.*1986;58:356-371.

5. Spach MS, Dolber PC. The relation between discontinuous propagation in anisotropic cardiac muscle and the "vulnerable period" of reentry. In: Cardiac Electrophysiology and Arrhythmias. D.P. Zipes and J. Jalife (eds). Grune and Stratton, Orlando. 1985;241-252.

6.Sano T, Takayama N, Shimamoto T. Directional difference of conduction velocity in the cardiac ventricular syncytium studied by microelectrodes. *Circ Res.* 1959;7:262-267.

7. Severs NJ. The cardiac gap junction and intercalated disc. *Int J Cardiol.* 1990;26:137-173.

8. Beyer EC. Gap junctions. *Int Rev Cytol.* 1993;137C:1-37.

9. Bruzzone R, White TW, Paul DL. Connections with connexins: the molecular basis of direct intercellular signaling. *Eur J Biochem.* 1996;238:1-27.

10. Imanaga I, Kameyama M, Irisawa H. Cell-to-cell diffusion of fluorescent dyes in ventricular paired cells isolated from guinea-pig heart. *Am J Physiol (Heart Circ Physiol).* 1987;252:H223-H232.

11. Spray DC, Burt JM. Structure-activity relations of the cardiac gap junction channel. *Am J Physiol.* 1990;258:C195-C205.

12. Davis LM, Rodefeld ME, Green K et al. Gap junction protein phenotypes of the human heart and conduction system. *J Cardiovasc Electrophysiol.* 1995;6:813-822.

13. Peters NS, Green CR, Poole-Wilson PA, Severs NJ. Reduced content of connexin43 gap junctions in ventricular myocardium from hypertrophied and ischaemic human hearts. *Circulation.* 1993;88:864-875.

14. Peters NS, Severs NJ, Rothery SM et al. Spatiotemporal relation between gap junctions and fascia adherens junctions during postnatal development of human ventricular myocardium. *Circulation.* 1994;90:713-725.

15. Sjöstrand FS, Andersson-Cedergren E. Intercalated disks of heart muscle. In The Structure and Function of Heart Muscle   vol.1. G.H. Bourne, ed. (New York: Academic Press). 1960;421-445.

16. Sommer JR, Dolber PC. Cardiac muscle: Ultrastructure of its cells and bundles. In: <u>Normal and Abnormal Conduction in the Heart</u>. A. Paes de Carvalho, B.F. Hoffman, M. Lieberman (eds). Futura Publishing Co., Mt. Kisco, New York. 1982:1-27.

17. Gardner PI, Ursell PC, Fenoglio JJ Jr., Wit AL. Electrophysiologic and anatomic basis for fractionated electrograms recorded from healed myocardial infarcts. *Circulation.* 1985;72:596-611.

18. Peters NS, Severs NJ, Coromilas J, Wit AL. Disturbed connexin43 gap junctional distribution correlates with the location of reentrant circuits in the epicardial border zone of healing canine infarcts that cause ventricular tachycardia. *Circulation. 1997 95;988-996*

19. Dillon SM, Allessie MA, Ursell PC, Wit AL. Influences of anisotropic tissue structure on reentrant circuits in the epicardial border zone of subacute canine infarcts. *Circ Res.* 1988;63: 182-206.

20. Smith JH, Green CR, Peters NS et al. Altered patterns of gap junction distribution in ischemic heart disease. An immunohistochemical study of human myocardium using laser scanning confocal microscopy. *Am J Pathol.* 1991;139:801-821.

21. El-Sherif N. The figure 8 model of reentrant excitation in the canine postinfarction heart. In: <u>Cardiac Electrophysiology and Arrhythmias</u>. D.P. Zipes, and J. Jalife (eds). Grune & Stratton, New York. 1985;363-378.

22. Spach MS, Dolber PC, et al. Influence of the passive anisotropic properties on directional differences in propagation following modification of the sodium conductance in human atrial muscle. A model of reentry based on anisotropic discontinuous propagation. *Circ Res.* 1988; 62:811-832.

23. Littmann L, Svenson RH, Gallagher JJ et al. Functional role of the epicardium in postinfarction ventricular tachycardia. Observations derived from computerized epicardial activation mapping, entrainment, and epicardial laser photoablation. *Circulation.* 1991;83:1577-1591.

24. Fenoglio JJ Jr, Pham TD, Harken AH et al. Recurrent sustained ventricular tachycardia: structure and ultrastructure of subendocardial regions in which tachycardia originates.*Circulation.* 1983; 68:518-533.

25. Ursell PC, Gardner PI, Albala A et al. Structural and electrophysiological changes in the epicardial border zone of canine myocardial infarcts during infarct healing.*Circ Res.*1985;56:436-451.

26. Luke RA, Saffitz JE. Remodeling of ventricular conduction pathways in healed canine infarct border zones. *J Clin Invest.* 1991;87:1594-1602.

27 Buja LM, Ferrans VJ, Maron BJ. Intracytoplasmic junctions in cardiac muscle cells. *Am J Pathol.* 1974;74:613-648.

28. de Bakker JMT, van Capelle FJL, Janse MJJ et al. Slow conduction in the infarcted human heart. "Zigzag" course of activation. *Circulation.* 1993;88:915-926.

29. Olgin JE, Kalman JM, Fitzpatrick AP, Lesh MD: Role of right atrial endocardial structures as barriers to conduction during type I atrial flutter. *Circulation* 1995;92:1839-1848

30. Cabo C, Pertsov AM, Baxter WT et al: Wave-front curvature as a cause of slow conduction and block in isolated cardiac muscle. *Circ Res.*
1994; 75:1014-1028

31. Kucera JP, Kléber AG, Rohr S. Slow Conduction in Cardiac Tissue, II : Effects of Branching Tissue Geometry. *Circ.Res.* 1998 83: 795-805

32. Schumacher B, Jung W, Schmidt H et al: Transverse conduction capabilities of the crista terminalis in patients with atrial flutter and atrial fibrillation. *JACC* 1999; 34:2:363-373

33. Wu TJ, Yashima M, Xie F et al. Role of pectinate muscle bundles in the generation and maintenance of intra-atrial reentry. *Circ Res.* 1998; 83:448-462

2.
THE RELATIONSHIP BETWEEN T-WAVE ALTERNANS AND CARDIAC ARRHYTHMOGENESIS AS ELUCIDATED BY OPTICAL MAPPING

Joseph M. Pastore, Ph.D. and David S. Rosenbaum, M.D.

The Heart & Vascular Research Center, MetroHealth Campus, Case Western Reserve University, and the Department of Biomedical Engineering, Case Western Reserve University, Cleveland, OH, USA.

Electrical alternans is defined as a beat-to-beat change in the amplitude of the electrocardiogram (ECG) that repeats once every other beat. Shortly after the ECG was introduced to clinical medicine, electrical alternans of the T-wave was recognized as a precursor to ventricular arrhythmias[1]. T-wave alternans was subsequently observed immediately preceding ventricular arrhythmias in many pathological conditions such as Prinzmetal's angina[2,3], acute myocardial infarction[4,5], catecholamine excess[6,7], electrolyte imbalances[8,9], and long QT syndrome[10,11]. Recently, we have used sensitive ECG processing techniques to establish a relationship between microvolt-level, visually-inapparent T-wave alternans and vulnerability to ventricular arrhythmias in humans[12]. Despite substantial evidence that T-wave alternans is closely associated with the development of reentrant ventricular arrhythmias and sudden cardiac death, it was not known if a mechanistic link exists between T-wave alternans and cardiac arrhythmogenesis.

There are two prevailing hypotheses on the cellular mechanisms underlying T-wave alternans. One states that a spatial dispersion of refractoriness gives rise to alternations in propagation and repolarization. According to this hypothesis, repolarization alternans is secondary to propagation alternans which occurs when the activating wavefront propagates into an area of refractory tissue on an every other beat basis. This hypothesis was supported by an experimental study in which ECG alternans elicited during regional ischemia was generated by alternating conduction block into the ischemic zone[13]. However, such alternating conduction block has not been observed in the absence of regional ischemia. The second hypothesis states that T-wave alternans is caused primarily by alternations in the repolarization phase of the action potential [14-19]. These primary repolarization alternans may give rise to secondary propagation alternans. However, which of these two hypotheses explains the development of T-wave alternans in the intact heart, and the possible role cellular alternations play in the mechanism of ventricular arrhythmias

From Ovsyshcher IE. *Cardiac Arrythmias and Device Therapy: Results and Perspectives for the New Century.* Armonk, NY: Futura Publishing Company, Inc., © 2000

are poorly understood because: 1. Conventional recording techniques can not be used to monitor cellular membrane potential with sufficient spatial resolution during the development of electrocardiographic T-wave alternans, and 2. Experimental studies have focused on transient alternans during an abrupt change in cycle length (CL)[20-22] or alternans during myocardial ischemia[17,18,23-25]; whereas, the majority of patients at risk for sudden cardiac death exhibit T-wave alternans at a relatively constant heart rate (HR) and in the absence of acute ischemia[12]. Therefore, we applied the technique of high-resolution optical action potential mapping to a Langendorff perfused guinea pig model of T-wave alternans as a new approach to investigate the cellular mechanisms underlying T-wave alternans, and to establish a mechanism linking T-wave alternans to the initiation of reentry.

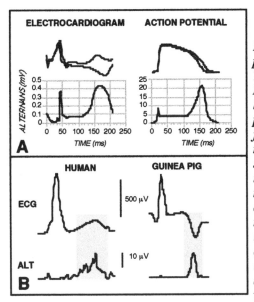

A

B

Figure 1: Changes in transmembrane potential of the guinea pig that underlie T-wave alternans on the surface ECG. In Panel A, the top row shows an ECG lead (left) and representative action potential (right) recorded simultaneously from one of 128 mapping sites. Tracing recorded from two consecutive beats are superimposed for the purposes of illustrating electrical alternans. The magnitude of electrical alternans during each time point of the cardiac cycle is represented by the difference between the amplitudes of the signals recorded on consecutive beats. T-wave alternans in the range of 100 - 430 _V was distributed symmetrically around the T-wave (Panel A, bottom left). Electrocardiographic T-wave alternans was explained by beat-to-beat alternation in the onset of phase 3 of the action potential. The magnitude of alternation of transmembrane potential amplitude (21 mV, Panel A, bottom right) was more than an order of magnitude larger than the magnitude of T-wave alternans on the surface ECG (0.43 mV, Panel A, bottom left). Panel B shows one lead of an ECG (top row) and corresponding distribution of alternans (bottom row) recorded from a patient (left) and guinea pig (right). Notice that the distribution of T-wave alternans recorded from the guinea pig closely corresponds to that recorded from a patient at high risk for ventricular arrhythmias.

Cellular Basis for Electrocardiographic T-wave Alternans: To investigate the cellular basis for electrocardiographic T-wave alternans, action potentials were recorded simultaneously from 128 epicardial sites encompassing the majority of the anterior left ventricular surface at a time when T-wave alternans was induced by steady state pacing[26]. Panel A of Figure 1 compares an ECG and an optical action potential recorded simultaneously from a representative ventricular site during two sequential beats of T-wave alternans. The tracings recorded during each beat are superimposed, and the difference between them indicate the magnitude of alternation of each point of the ECG and action potential, respectively. T-wave alternans of the surface ECG coincided with and was explained by alternation of phases 2 and 3 of the action potential; i.e., T-wave alternans arises from alternation of repolarization occurring at the cellular level. Note that the magnitude of cellular alternans (i.e., 20 mV) is nearly two orders of magnitude greater than the magnitude of T-wave alternans recorded simultaneously from the ECG (i.e. 400 μV). This finding may be highly relevant to T-wave alternans measured in patients, which is typically in the microvolt-level, and may therefore correspond to much more substantial alternations occurring on the cellular level.

Spatial Heterogeneity of Action Potential Alternans Parallels Heterogeneity of Intrinsic Repolarization Kinetics: Electrocardiographic T-wave alternans has been shown to occur above a critical heart rate in patients whose heart rate was modulated by exercise[28]. Alternans in APD recorded from single ventricular myocytes are similarly elicited above a critical threshold heart rate[19]. Consequently, it is not surprising that an alternans heart rate threshold is present in action potentials recorded from cells in the intact heart. Using multi-site optical action potential recordings, we found that the heart rate threshold for repolarization alternans varied between cells across the epicardial surface of the heart[26]. The distribution of local repolarization time alternans are plotted in Figure 2. Repolarization time alternans was calculated from the difference in cellular repolarization time measured during sequential beats. Therefore, positive and negative values indicate relative prolongation and abbreviation of local repolarization on a particular beat, respectively. Note that during the same beat, repolarization is prolonging near the base of the heart while shortening near the apex, indicating regional differences in the phase of alternation between epicardial cells. Such disruption of the phase relationship between cells has been referred to as discordant alternans[24,25,29]. Discordant alternans was consistently observed above a critical threshold heart rate, was always preceded by concordant alternans (action potential alternations having the same phase), and, in contrast to concordant alternans, produced marked changes in the pattern and sequence of ventricular depolarization and repolarization (next section).

Discordant alternans occurred between regions of epicardial cells despite the presence of normal inter-cellular coupling which suggested that the ionic currents which determine repolarization differ substantially between these regions so as to overcome electrotonic forces which ordinarily act to synchronize repolarization. Interestingly, the spatial pattern of discordant alternans was not random. Instead, cells typically alternated with opposite phase on the base and apex of the heart (Figure 2, left panel). Notice that the spatial pattern of discordant alternans closely follows regional differences in APD restitution (Figure 2, right panel) which is an index of cellular repolarization kinetics. This further supports a role of ion channel heterogeneity between cells in the development of discordant alternans. One would predict, therefore, that pathological conditions which increase spatial heterogeneity of membrane ionic properties or impair coupling between cells may facilitate the development of discordant alternans.

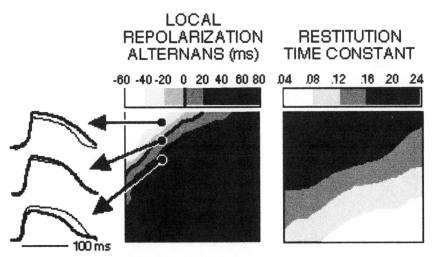

Figure 2: Distribution of action potential alternans and local repolarization kinetics in the intact ventricle. Shown on the left is a plot of local repolarization alternans measured as the difference in repolarization time between consecutive beats at each ventricular recording site. Notice the change in phase of repolarization alternans denoted by the thick black line, and demonstrated by action potential recordings shown for selected sites. The alternation of action potentials with opposite phase is termed discordant alternans. Local repolarization alternans varies from apex to base, similar to the variation in restitution time constant (right panel) which is a measure of intrinsic repolarization kinetics.

Role of Discordant Alternans in the InitßIation of Reentry

The initiation of T-wave alternans during steady-state pacing caused a reproducible cascade of events leading to reentrant ventricular fibrillation. As stated earlier, alternation of cellular repolarization is a property which is intrinsic to each cell and its initiation does not require any spatial dispersion of repolarization. Alternation of repolarization that occurs with the same phase between all cells (i.e. concordant alternans) was easily induced and typically manifested as microvolt-level T-wave alternans on the surface ECG. As shown in Figure 3, concordant alternans was associated with only subtle beat-to-beat alternation in the pattern of repolarization, and produced essentially no changes in beat-to-beat propagation patterns.

As pacing rate was further increased, a critical heart rate was achieved at which cells within neighboring regions of myocardium alternated with opposite phase (i.e., discordant alternans). As shown in Figure 3, discordant alternans produced several key changes in the pattern and sequence of propagation and repolarization of the heart. First, it is apparent that steep gradients of repolarization formed as evidenced by marked crowding of repolarization isochrone lines. Differences in the phase of action potential alternations across the epicardium directly accounted for the magnitude of these gradients. Second, the orientation of repolarization gradients undergoes nearly a complete reversal in direction from beat to beat. Although repolarization patterns are complex, they are highly reproducible on alternate beats (Figure 3, compare repolarization maps on beat 1 versus beat 3). Finally, because of steep gradients of repolarization present during discordant alternans, conduction begins to alternate as impulses slow when propagating against gradients of excitability. Under these conditions, a small reduction of stimulus cycle length (10 ms in Figure 3, beat 4) caused conduction block into a region

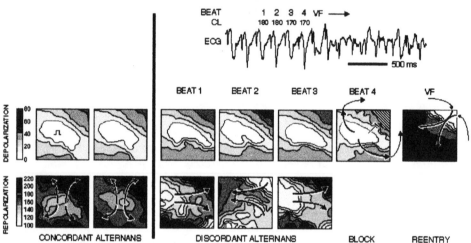

Figure 3: Mechanism linking action potential alternans to the initiation of ventricular fibrillation. Left panel shows 10 ms isochrone plots of depolarization and repolarization during concordant alternans.. Right panel shows 10 ms isochrone plots for 4 beats of discordant alternans preceding ventricular fibrillation. The boxed area shows one lead of the ECG recorded prior to and after the initiation of ventricular fibrillation. The upper right panel contains optical recordings from three ventricular sites marked on the depolarization isochrone map of beat 1. The ventricle was stimulated in the center of the mapping array. All depolarization and repolarization times during beats 1 through 4 have been referenced to the stimulus artifact, and the times during the first beat of ventricular fibrillation are referenced to the earliest activation time. The first beat of ventricular fibrillation occurred 120 ms after the pacing artifact of beat 4. On beats 1 through 3, the depolarizing wavefront propagated as expected from the site of stimulation. However, the patterns of repolarization differed substantially on consecutive beats, but were stable (compare beats 1 and 3). The pacing cycle length was decreased by 10 ms during beat 3. During beat 4, block occurred as represented by the hatched area in the depolarization map. Notice also the large increase in dispersion of repolarization during discordant alternans (601 ms^2) versus concordant alternans (263 ms^2).

having most delayed repolarization from the previous beat (beat 3 of repolarization map of Figure 3, upper right corner). The impulse then propagated around either side of the line of functional block (hatched area), and 90 ms later the zone of block regained excitability and the impulse reentered it from the opposite direction, forming the first spontaneous beat of reentrant ventricular fibrillation. In these experiments, discordant alternans was closely linked to the mechanism of reentry as the initiation of ventricular fibrillation was always first preceded by discordant alternans.

Therefore, in the presence of regional heterogeneities of cellular repolarization kinetics, discordant repolarization alternans could transform relatively minor spatial dispersions of repolarization into critical repolarization gradients which were directly responsible for the development of unidirectional block and reentrant ventricular fibrillation. This concept was supported by elegant studies in isolated myocytes which showed that the timing of membrane depolarization relative to the kinetics of membrane repolarization determined the phase of alternation[19]. One would predict, therefore, that pathological conditions that either increase spatial heterogeneity of repolarization or that impair coupling between cells may facilitate the development of discordant alternans. Therefore, it is not surprising that discordant alternans has been observed in clinical conditions associated with marked spatial dispersion of repolarization properties such as the congenital Long QT Syndrome[30]. Similarly, discordant alternans was also observed during interventions that reduce cell-to-cell coupling such as ischemia[25] and hypoxia[29].

Clearly, many questions remain unanswered regarding the role of T-wave alternans in the mechanism of sudden cardiac death. Based on currently available data, we propose one possible mechanism in Figure 4. First, it is apparent that patients with structural heart disease who are at risk for life-threatening ventricular arrhythmias develop microvolt-

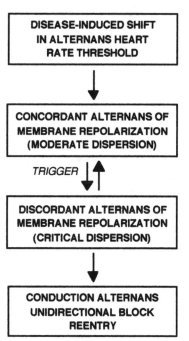

Figure 4: Central hypothesis relating electrical alternans to cardiac arrhythmogenesis.

level T-wave alternans at significantly lower heart rates (typically 90 - 100 bpm) than patients in lower risk groups[12,27,28]. Whether this downward shift in the alternans threshold heart rate is caused by disease-induced alterations in the expression of ion currents is unknown, but remains an interesting point of speculation. Microvolt-level T-wave alternans is most likely associated with concordant patterns of repolarization alternans (i.e. alternations that occur with the same phase) of cells within the heart. A critical step in the formation of a suitable substrate for reentry was the transformation of concordant to discordant alternans. Although we can not determine from our data what mechanisms might be responsible for triggering discordant alternans in patients, physiological perturbations such as transient ischemia, premature ventricular beats, or sympathetic stimulation are known to affect the phase and magnitude of repolarization alternans, and may potentially trigger discordant alternans in patients. Further studies aimed at delineating these mechanisms are expected to improve our ability to understand and potentially prevent the complex sequence of events which precipitate sudden cardiac death episodes in patients.

Summary

Spatial heterogeneities of repolarization properties appear to play a critical role in the development of arrhythmogenic substrates during T-wave alternans. Heterogeneous ion channel function and composition, as manifest by regional variation in cellular repolarization kinetics, create a situation where cellular repolarization within separate regions of myocardium alternate with differing magnitude and phase. Regional differences in the phase of alternans (i.e. discordant alternans) produce critical gradients of repolarization which form a suitable substrate for unidirectional block and reentrant ventricular tachycardia and fibrillation. These findings demonstrate the complexity of arrhythmogenic substrates that are dependent on dynamic and heterogeneous processes such as repolarization. It is possible that certain pathological conditions that alter the spatial heterogeneity of repolarization properties may also facilitate the development of discordant alternans. It is obvious that the factors which determine dispersion of repolarization in the heart are dependent on the specific pathophysiological substrate involved. Further studies are required to improve our understanding of how heterogeneities of repolarization and alternans, in the presence and absence of cardiac pathology, influence the electrophysiological substrate for reentry.

Acknowledgements
This study was supported by National Institutes of Health grant HL-54807, the Medical Research Service of the Department of Veterans Affairs, and the American Heart Association

References
1. Lewis T: Notes upon alternation of the heart. *Quart.J.Med.* 1910;4:141-144
2. Cheng TC: Electrical alternans: An association with coronary artery spasm. *Arch.Inter.Med* 1983;143:1052-1053
3. Kleinfeld MJ, Rozanski JJ: Alternans of the ST-segment in Prenzmetal's angina. *Circulation* 1977;55:574-577
4. Puletti M, Curione M, Righetti G, Jacobellis G: Alternans of the ST-segment and T-wave in acute myocardial infarction. *J.Electrocardiology* 1980;13:297-300
5. Salerno JA, Previtali M, Panciroli C, Klerbsy C, Chimienti M, Regazzi Bonora M, Marangoni E, Falcone C, Guasti L, Campana C, Rondanelli R: Ventricular arrhythmias during acute myocardial ischemia in man. The role and significance of R-ST-T alternans and the prevention of ischemic sudden death by medical treatment. *Europ.Heart.J.* 1986;7:63-75
6. Lepeschkin E: Electrocardiographic observations on the mechanism of electrical alternans of the heart. *Cardiologia* 1959;16:278-287
7. Wayne VS, Bishop RL, Spodick DH: Exercise-induced ST segment alternans. *Chest* 1983;83:824-825
8. Reddy CVR, Kiok JP, Khan RG, El-Sherif N: Repolarization alternans associated with alcoholism and hypomagnesemia. *Am.J.Cardiol.* 1984;53:390-391
9. Shimoni Z, Flateau E, Schiller D, Barzilay E, Kohn D: Electrical alternans of giant U waves with multiple electrolyte abnormalities. *Am.J.Cardiol.* 1984;54:920-921
10. Schwartz PJ, Malliani A: Electrical alternation of the T-wave: clinical and experiemntal evidence of its relationship with the sympathetic nervous system and with the long QT syndrome. *Am.Heart J.* 1975;89:45-50
11. Platt SB, Vijgen JM, Albrecht P, Van Hare GF, Carlson MD, Rosenbaum DS: Occult T wave alternans in long QT syndrome. *J.Cardiovasc.Electrophysiol.* 1996;7:144-148

12. Rosenbaum DS, Jackson LE, Smith JM, Garan H, Ruskin JN, Cohen RJ: Electrical alternans and vulnerability to ventricular arrhythmias. *N.Engl.J.Med.* 1994;330:235-241

13. Downar E, Janse M, Durrer D: The effect of acute coronary artery occlusion on subepicardial transmembrane potentials in the intact heart. *Circulation* 1977;56:217-224

14. Hoffman BF, Suckling EE: Effect of heart rate on cardiac membrane potentials and unipolar electrogram. *Am.J.Physiol.* 1954;179:123-130

15. Kleinfeld M, Stein E: Electrical alternans of components of the action potential. *Am.Heart J.* 1968;75:528-530

16. Murphy CF, Lab MJ, Horner SM, Dick DJ, Harrison FG: Regional electromechanical alternans in anesthetized pig hearts: modulation by mechanoelectric feedback. *Am.J.Physiol.* 1994;267:H1726-H1735

17. Kurz RW, Ren XL, Franz MR: Dispersion and delay of electrical restitution in the globally ischaemic heart. *Europ.Heart.J.* 1994;15:547-554

18. Dilly SG, Lab MJ: Electrophysiological alternans and restitution during acute regional ischemia in myocardium of anesthetized pig. *J.Physiol.(Lond.)* 1988;402:315-333

19. Rubenstein DS, Lipsius SL: Premature beats elicit a phase reversal of mechanoelectrical alternans in cat ventricular myocytes: A possible mechanism for reentrant arrhythmias. *Circulation* 1995;91:201-214

20. Saitoh H, Bailey J, Surawicz B: Alternans of action potential duration after abrupt shortening of cycle length: Differences between dog purkinje and ventricular muscle fibers. *Circ.Res.* 1988;62:1027-1040

21. Rosenbaum DS, Kaplan DT, Kanai A, Jackson L, Garan H, Cohen RJ, Salama G: Repolarization inhomogeneities in ventricular myocardium change dynamically with abrupt cycle length shortening. *Circulation* 1991;84:1333-1345

22. Hirayama Y, Saitoh H, Atarashi H, Hayakawa H: Electrical and mechanical alternans in canine myocardium in vivo: Dependence on intracellular calcium cycling. *Circulation* 1993;88:2894-2902

23. Smith JM, Clancy EA, Valeri R, Ruskin JN, Cohen RJ: Electrical alternans and cardiac electrical instability. *Circulation* 1988;77:110-121

24. Kurz RW, Mohabir R, Ren X-L, Franz MR: Ischaemia induced alternans of action potential duration in the intact heart: dependence on coronary flow, preload, and cycle length. *Europ.Heart.J.* 1993;14:1410-1420

25. Konta T, Ikeda K, Yamaki M, Nakamura K, Honma K, Kubota I, Yasui S: Significance of discordant ST alternans in ventricular fibrillation. *Circulation* 1990;82:2185-2189

26. Pastore JM, Girouard SD, Laurita KR, Akar FG, Rosenbaum DS: Mechanism linking T wave alternans to the genesis of cardiac fibrillation. *Circulation* 1999;99:1385-1394

27. Rosenbaum DS, Albrecht P, Cohen RJ: Predicting sudden cardiac death from T wave alternans of the surface electrocardiogram: Promise and pitfalls. *J.Cardiovasc.Electrophysiol.* 1996;7:1095-1111

28. Hohnloser SH, Klingenheben T, Zabel M, Li Y-G, Albrecht P, Cohen RJ: T wave alternans during exercise and atrial pacing in humans. *J.Cardiovasc.Electrophysiol.* 1997;8:987-993

29. Hirata Y, Toyama J, Yamada K: Effects of hypoxia or low pH on the alteration of canine ventricular action potentials following an abrupt increase in driving rate. *Cardiovasc.Res.* 1980;14:108-115

30. Shimizu W, Yamada K, Arakaki Y, Kamiya T, Shimomura K: Monophasic action potential recordings during T-wave alternans in congenital long QT syndrome. *Am.Heart J.* 1996;132:699-701

3

T WAVE ALTERNANS: A LINK TO CLINICAL PRACTICE

Mustafa Kemal Batur, MD, Ali Oto, MD, FESC, FACC

Hacettepe Medical School, Department of Cardiology, Ankara, Turkey

Introduction

Identification of patients at high risk of life-threatening ventricular tachyarrhythmias represents one of the most challenging issues in cardiology especially after myocardial infarction[1]. Programmed electrical stimulation has been used to assess vulnerability to life-threatening ventricular arrhythmias . However, this invasive technique has appeared to be of limited prognostic value in these patients[2]. Noninvasive methods to identify increased risk for ventricular arrhythmias include assessment of heart rate variability[3], baroreflex sensitivity testing[4], QT dispersion[5], and the signal-averaged ECG (SAECG)[6]. Poor sensitivity and low positive predictive value are common limitations of these noninvasive indexes, that is why new markers are necessary to idendify patient who susceptible to major cardiac arrhythmias.

T-wave Alternans as a new risk strafication marker

T-Wave alternans (TWA) can be defined as beat to beat changes in T-wave morphology (Figure 1), that occur during regular rhythm[7]. The clinical observations and experiments on the animals show that TWA is usually associated with a risk of ventricular fibrillation[8,9]. Thus it may be used as a noninvasive marker of susceptibility to life-threatening ventricular arrhythmias[9,10].

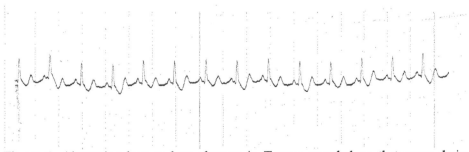

Figure 1. Alternating beat to beat changes in T-wave morphology that occur during balloon inflation of left anterior descending coronary artery in one of our patients.

Mechanisms of TWA

Many investigators have reported that transmembrane or intracellular calcium movement plays an important role in the mechanism of TWA[11].

From Ovsyshcher IE. *Cardiac Arrythmias and Device Therapy: Results and Perspectives for the New Century.* Armonk, NY: Futura Publishing Company, Inc., © 2000

Other ions such as potassium and sodium may also interact with calcium. According to Hashimoto[12] and his co-workers, the alternans corresponds to the alternation of phase 'phase 2' of a membrane action potential (MAP). In Hirayama's study[13], it is suggested that the square shaped MAP is associated with a small amount of free intracellular calcium and this decreased calcium may contribute to a positive shift and lengthening of 'plateau' in phase 2, by increasing the driving force for calcium, by slowing the inactivation of the calcium current or by decreasing the calcium sensitive transient outward current. Large amount of calcium can enter the cell during a prolonged MAP and can be stored in the cell until the following contraction is stronger. This time, the higher intracellular calcium concentration associated with stronger tension may contribute to shortening of 'plateau' by opposite actions. Therefore, it seems that the alternation of the calcium flow during 'phase 2' may be the cause of repolarization and propagation alternans.

Determination of TWA

The first clinical observation was made in 1913 by George R. Mines during a study on the influence of electrolytes on the electrical activity of the heart[14]. He observed a visible TWA on the ECG signal obtained from a frog's myocardium. Since then, there have been some case reports of visible alternans[14-16]. The clinical observation of TWA, however, is not so easy, and so common, because alternans occurs due to cells that were affected by a disease process. If the affected area is large, the corresponding alternans magnitude becomes high, thus it can be visually detected. But in most cases, the alternans magnitude is in microvolt level, and visual detection becomes impossible[8].

Is it possible to detect microvolt level TWA?

In order to detect non-visible TWA, novel signal processing techniques have been used: autocorrelation method[17], Fast Fourier Transformation analysis[9,18], complex demodulation[8,19], and autoregression technique[20]. These studies, either on laboratory animals or on human subjects, are in general carried during atrial pacing. Only in a few studies[8] human subjects are used and the ECG recordings were acquired during spontaneous heart rhythm.

Although very important developments have been made in detecting TWA, there are many aspects that need further investigation. There are some problems encountered during analysis of the data; phase reversals in TWA magnitude, QT length changes due to variable heart rate, amplitude changes of TWA time series, and the effects of EMG interference on the performance of the analysis. Thus, the algorithms for investigating the TWA should be examined carefully considering the mentioned problems so that the optimal method of analysis could be found. Also there is the problem of missing data, which is due to abnormalities in the ECG signal and lead disconnection during data acquisition.

Clinical Applications of TWA

TWA, visible or at microvolt level, occurs consistently in association with arrhythmias under different conditions, including coronary artery occlusion and release-reperfusion[8], variant angina pectoris[7], dilated[21], and hypertrophic cardiomyopathy[22]. There is a substantial evidence indicating that TWA is an intrinsic property of ischemic myocardium since ischemia induced alternans has been observed during balloon angioplasty[9,23-24], coronary artery bypass graft occlusion[25], and also in patients with stable coronary disease[26].

There have been numerous reports of the occurrence of visible TWA during attacks of acute ischemia[8,12,23-27]. Some investigators found a statistically significant association between the occurrence of visible TWA and ventricular arhythmias during ischemic attacks in a group of patients with variant angina[7,27-28]. Sutton and co-workers[25] investigated the monophasic action potentials from the left ventricular epicardium in 36 patients undergoing cardiopulmonary bypass surgery. They observed the electrical alternans in 14 cases (39%). Several case reports and studies which include small number of patients have indicated that acute coronary occlusion during angioplasty may produce T wave alternans[16,24,29,30]. Ian C. Gilchrist[29] evaluated the 407 consecutive patients undergoing PTCA, with continuous electrocardiographic monitoring and recording of ≥ 2 standard leads during balloon inflations. He observed the ST-segment alternans in 5 patients. Four of these cases occurred during angioplasty of the left anterior descending artery (LAD), and 1 of angioplasty of left circumflex (Cx) artery. In four patients, alternans was observed before 100 seconds. All patients were pre-treated with both nitrates and calcium channel blockers (nifedipine or diltiazem). Okamato et al[16] encountered a patient with typical electrical alternans of the ST segment in leads V_4 through V_6, which developed during PTCA of the proximal left anterior descending artery. Hemodynamic pulsus alternans of the aortic pressure tracing was not observed during electrical alternans, and a calcium blocker could not prevent this phenomenon during PTCA. Sochanski et al[30] reported the ST segment alternans that occurred in 4 patients during PTCA for LAD artery. Neither mechanical alternans nor increased ventricular ectopy were noted. Joyal et al[24] observed the ST segment alternans within 30 seconds during

PTCA for LAD artery in one patient. Recently, computer analysis techniques have made it possible to measure TWA at a microvolt level in patients in whom no TWA can be detected by visual inspection of the ECG[8-10].

Microvolt level TWA has been demonstrated to be a sensitive and specific marker of susceptibility to ventricular arrhythmias[8]. There is only one report related to ischemia induced TWA during PTCA in human using computer analysis techniques. Verrier and Nearing[8] observed that mid-LAD occlusion, in 7 patients, for 3 minutes resulted in significant increases in alternans that follow precisely the time course of changes observed in their studies. In another study, Verrier and his co-workers found that TWA magnitude nearly tripled from 0.27 ± 0.02 mVx ms before ischemia onset to 0.77 ± 0.08 mVx ms during ischemic episodes with Holter monitoring[12]. Recently we have shown that TWA at microvolt levels may also occur during right coronary artery (RCA) and Cx coronary artery balloon inflations[31,32]. However, calculated magnitude of TWA during LAD coronary artery inflations were greater than the other coronary artery balloon inflations ($p<0.05$). There were also further decrease in TWA values 24 hours after successful PTCA in patients undergoing LAD angioplasty0 as compared to angioplasty of other coronary arteries ($p<0.05$). The amplitude of the TWA probably is correlated with the amount of influenced myocardial tissue. Our observation and previous experience described above supports this concept. We have also observed a decrease in TWA after revascularisation. It might also be an explanation for the protective effect of revascularization on sudden cardiac death in patients with coronary artery disease.

Some investigators have shown the TWA might be useful as a marker of ventricular tachyarrhythmias and sudden cardiac death even in the absence of acute myocardial ischemia[9,21,22,33,34]. Likewise TWA has been found to be a powerful tool for predicting recurrence of ventricular tachyarrhythmias in ICD recipients and arrhythmia-free survival for high-risk population[9,33,34].

Conclusion

In conclusion, TWA analysis appears to be a promising new method to risk-stratify patients for future arrhythmic events. However, more data is needed to establish its definite role in patient who susceptible to major cardiac arrhythmias.

References

1. Roberts WC. Sudden cardiac death: definitions and causes. Am J Cardiol 1986;57:1410 3.
2. Freedman RA, Swerdlow CD, Soderholm-Difatte V, Mason JW. Prognostic significance of arrhythmia inducibility or noninducibility at initial electro-physiologic study in survivors of cardiac arrest. Am J Cardiol 1988;61:578-82.
3. Campbell RWF: Can anlysis of heart rate variability predict arrhythmias and antiarrhythmic effects? In Oto MA (ed): Practice and Progress in Cardiac Pacing and Electrophysiology. AA Dordrecht, The Netherlands, Kluwer Academic Publishers, 1996, pp. 63-70.
4. Billman GE, Schwartz PJ, Stone HL. Baroreceptor reflex control of heart rate: a predictor of sudden cardiac death. Circulation 1982;66:874 80.
5. Day CP, McComb JM, Campbell RWF. QT dispersion: an indication of arrhythmia risk in patients with long QT intervals. Br Heart J 1990;63:342 4.
6. Faber TS, Malik M. Signal averaged electrocardiogram. Current applications and limitations. In Oto MA (ed): Practice and Progress in Cardiac Pacing and Electrophysiology. AA Dordrecht, The Netherlands, Kluwer Academic Publishers, 1996, pp. 47-61.
7. Rozanski JJ, Kleinfeld M. Alternans of the ST segment in Prinzmetal's angina. PACE 1982; 5: 359-365.
8. Nearing BD, Oesterle SN, Verrier RL. Quantification of ischaemia induced vulnerability by precordial T wave alternans analysis in dog and human. Cardiovasc Res 1994; 28: 1440-1449.
9. Rosenbaum DS, Jackson LE, Smith JM, et al. Electrical alternans and vulnerability to ventricular arrhythmia. N Engl J Med 1994; 330: 235-241.
10. Verrier RL, Nearing BD. Electrophysiologic basis for T wave alternans as an index of vulnerability to ventricular fibrillation. J Cardiovasc Electrophysiol 1994; 5: 445-461.
11. Konta T, Ikeda K, Yamaki M, et al. Significance of discordant ST alternans in ventricular fibrillation. Circulation 1990; 82: 2185-89.
12. Hashimoto H, Suzuki K, Miyake S, et al. Effects of calcium antagonists on the electrical alternans of the ST segment and on associated mechanical alternans during acute coronary occlusion in dogs. Circulation 1983; 68: 667-72.
13. Hirayama Y, Saitoh H, Atarashi H, et al. Electrical and mechanical alternans in canine myocardium in vivo dependence of intracellular calcium cycling. Circulation 1993; 88: 1363-66.
14. Mines GR. On functional analysis by the action of electrolytes. J Physiol 1913; 46: 188-235.
15. Bardaji A, Vidal F, Richard C. T wave alternans associated with amiodarone. Journal of Electrocardiol 1993; 26:155-57.
16. Okamoto S, Inden M, Konishi T, et al. ST segment alternans during percutaneous transluminal coronary angioplasty- A case report. Angiology 1991; 42: 30-34.

17. Adam DR, Smith JM, Akselrod S, et al. Fluctations in T-wave morphology and susceptibility to ventricular fibrillation. J Electrocardiol 1984; 17: 209-218.
18. Smith JM, Clancy EA, Valeri CR, et al. Electrical alternans and cardiac electrical instability. Circulation 1988; 77: 110-121.
19. Nearing B, Huangh A, Verrier RL. Dynamic tracking of cardiac vulnerability by complex demodulation of the T-wave. Science 1991;252: 437-440.
20. Zareba W, Moss AJ, leCessie S, et al. T wave alternans in long QT syndrome. J Am Coll Cardiol 1994; 23: 1541-1544.
21. Adachi K, Ohnishi Y, Shima T, et al. Determinant of microvolt level T-Wave Alternans in patients with dilated cardiomyopathy. J Am Coll Cardiol 1999;34:374 –80.
22. Murda'h MA, Nagayoshi H, Albrecht P, et al. T-wave alternans as a predictor of sudden death in hypertrophic cardiomyopathy (abstr).Circulation 1996; 94: 669.
23. Puletti M, Curione M, Righetti G, et al. Alternans of the ST segment and T-wave in acute myocardial infarction. J Electrocardiol 1980; 13: 297-300.
24. Joyal M, Feldman RL, Pepine CJ. ST-segment alternans during percutaneous transluminal coronary angioplasty. Am J Cardiol 1984; 54: 915-916.
25. Sutton PMI, Taggart P, Lab M, et al. Alternans of epicardial repolarization as a localized phenomenon in man. Eur Heart J 1991; 12: 70-78.
26. Verrier RL, Nearing BD, Gail BS, et al. T-wave alternans during ambulatory ischemia in patients with stable coronary disease. ANE 1996;1(2Pt. 1): 113-120.
27. Salerno JA, Previtali M, Panciroli C, et al. Ventricular arrhythmias during acute myocardial ischaemia. The role and significance of R-ST-T alternans and the prevention of ischaemic sudden death by medical treatment. Eur Heart J 1986;7: 63-75.
28. Kleinfeld MJ, Rozanski JJ. Alternans of the ST segment in Prinzmetal's angina. Circulation 1977; 55: 574-577.
29. Gilchrist IC. Prevalence and significance of ST-segment alternans during coronary angioplasty. Am J Cardiol 1991; 68: 1534-1535.
30. Sochanski M, Feldman T, Chua KG, et al. ST segment alternans during coronary angioplasty. Cathet Cardiovasc Diag 1992; 27: 45-48.
31. Batur MK, Oto A, Ider Z, et al. T-wave alternans in induced ischaemia in human. (Abstract) Eur Heart J 1998; 19:433.
32. Batur MK, Oto A, Ider Z, et al. Angiology, accepted for publication.
33. Armoundas AA, Rosenbaum DS, Ruskin JN, et al. Prognostic significance of electrical alternans versus signal averaged electrocardiography in predicting the outcome of electrophysiological testing and arrhythmia-free survival. Heart 1998;80:251-6.
34. Hohnloser SH, Klingenheben T, Li YG, et al. T wave alternans as a predictor of recurrent ventriculartachyarrhythmias in ICD recipients: prospective comparison with conventional risk markers. J Cardiovasc Electrophysiol 1998;9:1258-68.

4.
PULSE PROPAGATION IN EXCITABILITY CHANGING MEDIUM

Avinoam Rabinovitch, PhD[1], Ira Aviram[2], PhD, Menahem Friedman, PhD[3], Natalie Gulko[3], Eugene Crystal, MD[4], Ilya A. Fleidervish, MD[4], I. Eli Ovsyshcher, MD, PhD[4]

Physics Department, Ben Gurion University, Beer-Sheva 84105, Israel[1]; 35, Shderot Yeelim, Beer-Sheva 84730, Israel[2]; Mathematics Department, Ben Gurion University, Beer-Sheva 84105, Israel[3]; Cardiology & EP Lab., Soroka Medical Center, Ben Gurion University, Beer-Sheva 84105, Israel[4].

Introduction

The myocardium is a multicellular medium, whose cells respond in different ways to electrical excitations even in a healthy subject. In the atria, for example, the sinus node cells (e.g. ref. 1) are in a strong so called "limit cycle", periodic situation, the time constant of the relatively rapid cycle being of the order of 1 sec. Further away from the sinus node the limit cycle behavior becomes weaker, less rapid, and eventually converts into a so called "excitable"[2] situation whereby, in response to a driving excitation, an isolated impulse propagates through the medium. In scarred and injured tissues, drastic changes in the electrical response behavior of the afflicted cells might occur. The changes can be of two types: cells either become more 'limit cycle' - like, or more 'excitable' - like, depending on the type and location of the injury. The change in the electrical response behavior is evidently the result of changes in the membrane and surrounding tissues.
In this work we consider a 1D medium whose properties vary as a *function of position*. We first give a combined, simple definition for the concept of excitability for both the 'excitable' as well as the 'limit cycle' regions. The response to driving pulses in a variable excitability medium were discussed in detail in ref. 3, including a linearly continuous variation (of a type occurring in healthy tissues, as well as near a block, or an ectopic source), and a localized "scar" of lower or higher excitability. Here we present additional results concerning the presence of an excitability step in the way of a propagating train of pulses, showing under certain conditions, a prolonged transient gap in the train.

The model

The mathematical model used here (FHN) is described by a system of two coupled, non-linear dimension-less differential equations for the membrane 'action potential' $v(x,t)$, and the 'refractivity' $w(x,t)$:

From Ovsyshcher IE. *Cardiac Arrythmias and Device Therapy: Results and Perspectives for the New Century.* Armonk, NY: Futura Publishing Company, Inc., © 2000

$$\frac{\partial v}{\partial t} = \frac{\partial^2 v}{\partial x^2} + v(v-a)(1-v) - w + v_0(x)\delta(t)$$

$$\frac{\partial w}{\partial t} = b(v - dw)$$

(1)

The parameter a may take positive, as well as negative values, and is used here to define the excitability range (see below). The product bd gives the ratio between the fast {excitation), and the slow (recovery) time constants. We take $10^{-3} \leq b \leq 3 \times 10^{-2}$ and $d=3$. An initiating pulse (IP) of membrane potential $v_0(x)\delta(t)$, usually a narrow gaussian, is applied at a specific point in space, say $x=0$.

Consider first a, b, and d independent of position. Simulation runs showed that the smaller the value of a, the easier it was for the pulse to propagate. It is well known [3,4,5] that as a increases, the velocity decreases until, at some value of a_c characteristic of the pair b, d, the propagating pulse (PP) ceases to move and collapses, irrespective of the IP height. The velocity c shows at $a = a_c$ a jump from a finite value on the left, to zero on the right. We chose the propagation velocity c as the measure of the "ease" of propagation.

Figure 1 shows the velocity c as a function of a and b obtained from computer simulation runs. The open square on each curve of b=const marks the value $a = a_p$ separating two different regimes of pulse propagation: To the right $(a > a_p)$ we have the 'excitable' regime where the IP splits into two *isolated* PP's of *constant shape* moving symmetrically in opposite directions. To the left $(a < a_p)$ the (constant) values of the parameters a, b, d correspond to a limit cycle regime meaning that at the point $x = 0$, where the IP has been applied, new excitations will be generated at a *uniform* pace, thus creating "trains" of uniformly spaced PP's moving in opposite directions.

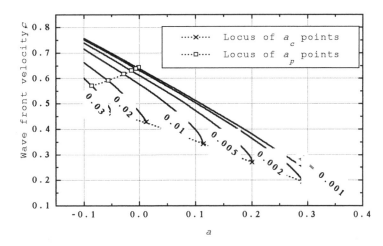

Figure 1. The wave front velocity c as function of a and b.

An important feature of a_p observed during simulations was that the curves $c(a)$ for each constant b are continuous through a_p, and most likely have a continuous derivative at this point. This feature allows using c as a good measure of 'excitability' for *all* types of propagation media.

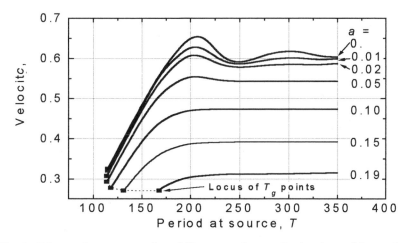

Fig 2. Dispersion curves for different values of a in the uniform domain, $b=0.005$. The locus of T_g points is the limit to the right of which there is a one to one correspondence between source pulses and those propagating through the medium.

Propagation of a train of pulses.

Investigations were carried out with a series of T-periodic IP's of the form $v_0(x)\sum_{j=1}^{\infty}\delta(t - jT)$, replacing the source term in Eq. (1). This series generates a pulse train propagating through the medium. Fig 2 represents a dispersion map summarizing simulation results for the steady state velocity as function of T, at values of a constant throughout the medium, i.e. uniform excitability. The velocity was measured far away from the source as well as from the train front. For large T the distance between successive pulses being large, they do not interact, and travel at a velocity exactly corresponding to that in Fig.1.For short interpulse periods however, the recovery tail of each traveling pulse becomes increasingly perturbed by the following one, and the velocity and distance between pulses drops rather sharply[6]. A threshold value $T=T_g(a)$ is reached for each a where the one to one correspondence between propagating and source pulses breaks down: some of them will collapse.

Next, the propagation of a train of pulses was considered through an inhomogeneous medium with a step-wise variation of excitability at a point x_s:

$$a(x) = \begin{cases} a_0, & x \le x_s \\ a_1, & x_s < x \end{cases} \qquad (2),$$

A source of T-periodic pulses is present at $x_0 \ll x_s$. If both $T > T_g(a_0)$, and $T > T_g(a_1)$, the train behaves in a perfectly expected manner. If however, $T_g(a_0) < T < T_g(a_1)$, and $a_1 > a_0$, then a rather interesting transient situation occurs described as follows: A train traveling through the region a_0 encounters the step and goes over it. All the leading pulses go through while shrinking and 'crowding' into each other, their density per unit length becoming higher and higher right after the crossing. At a certain stage, the latest pulse which crossed the step collapses. The preceding surviving pulse, say $\# j_1$, becomes the last of a finite pack detached from the rest of the oncoming train (phase 1), and keeps on traveling through the medium a_1. Starting with $j_1 + 1$, a finite number k of pulses collapse creating a wide gap (phase 2) in the train, until the pulse $j_2 = j_1 + k + 1$ manages to survive. This moment marks the beginning of phase 3, in which we witness a change of behavior, i.e. one of two successive pulses collapses, while the other goes through (1:2 regime). This verbal description is illustrated in Fig. 3 representing a snapshot of a train taken at $t=7570$, traveling through an inhomogeneous medium with $a_0 = 0.05$, $T_g(0.05) = 115$, $a_1 = 0.19$,

$T_g(0.19) = 168$, $x_s = 200$. The source is at $x_0 = -700$, sending pulses with $T = 165$. For this particular set of parameters we find: $j_1 = 16$, $k = 8$, $j_2 = 25$. After this, all even numbered pulses collapse, and $j = 34$ is just about to do so. Phase 3 eventually becomes stationary, and the train propagates through the a_1 medium at the asymptotic velocity $c = 0.315$.

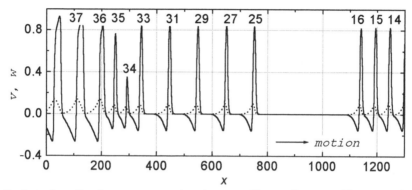

Fig 3. A train of pulses propagating in a medium of non-uniform excitability with a positive step variation in the value of a. See text for details.

The reason for pulse collapse is that it travels at a distance where the refractory tail of the preceding pulse has not decayed sufficiently, and the relatively large values of $w(x)$ in this region contribute negatively to $\partial v / \partial t$. Less well understood is phase 2 and the transition to phase 3. Figure 4 illustrates what happens in the region a_1 for several values of T. For each incoming pulse beyond j_1 the time elapsed between step crossing and its collapse was recorded and plotted as a function of the ordination number j of the pulse, showing a general decreasing trend. The line F marks the onset of phase 2. At some value j for each T we observe a bifurcation: in a pair of adjacent pulses the time elapsed for one continues to decrease, while for the other it increases. The ascending branches terminate after a few steps because the corresponding pulses j_2 cease to collapse (line P), marking the onset of phase 3. Line B is the approximate locus of bifurcation.

Conclusions

During normal operation, heart tissue propagates not a solitary pulse, but a wave train of nearly constant period. Localized inhomogeneities alter the train wave in various ways. We analyzed in this work a train wave crossing a sharp drop in the excitability parameter, and observed an interesting, prolonged transient including a temporary block, and a transition to a 1:2 regime.

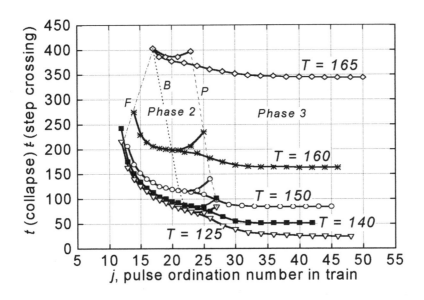

Figure 4. The time elapsed between crossing of the excitability step and collapse of pulses. See text for details.

References

1. Reiner VS, Antzelevitch C, : Phase Resetting and Annihilation in a Mathematical Model of the Sinus Node, Am. J. Physiol. 1985; 249: H1143-H1153.
2. Glass L, Mackey MC: From Clocks to Chaos, and references therein. Princeton University Press, 1988, pp.144-171.
3. Rabinovitch A, Aviram I, Gulko N, et. al.: A Model for Propagation of Action Potentials in Non-uniformly Excitable Media. J. Theor. Biol. 1999; 196:141-154.
4. Rinzel J, Ermentrout GB, Analysis of Neural Excitability and Oscillation. In Koch I, Segev (eds): Methods in Neuronal Modeling. Cambridge, Mass, MIT Press, 1989, pp. 135-169.
5. Cross MC, Hohenberg PC: Pattern Formation outside of Equilibrium. Rev. Mod. Phys. 1993; 65: 851-1112.
6. Elphick C, Meron E, Rinzel J, et. al., Impulse patterning and relaxational propagation in excitable media. J. Theor. Biol. 1990, 146:249-268.

5.
MODELLING OF DEFIBRILLATION THRESHOLDS

Marek Malik, PhD, MD, Karel FAA Smits, MSc, Fred Lindemans, PhD

St George's Hospital Medical School, London, England, Bakken Research Centre, Maastricht, The Netherlands

Introduction

Configurations of electrodes used with implantable defibrillators are difficult to optimise based purely on direct experiments. Frequent experimental repositioning of electrodes in human implants is neither practical nor ethical and animal studies have a limited validity because of the different geometries of animal thoraces. Because of these problems, several projects have been reported aimed at computer simulation of the electric field in the thorax and at modelling defibrillation thresholds of defibrillation systems involving both external and internal electrodes.[1-3] Unfortunately, most available models have rather high computational demands even when implemented on advanced workstations, which makes factorial analysis (the "Design of Experiments" approach) of electrode positions and combinations required for optimising defibrillation performance highly impractical or directly impossible.

Having this in mind, a computer model of the defibrillation field that is suitable for simulation of defibrillation thresholds has been developed with the particular aim of allowing a factorial analysis of different electrode configurations to be computed on affordable personal computers. In this text, we shortly describe the mathematical and computational background of the model and some key features of its computer implementation. As an example of the capabilities of the model, we also briefly report a simulation study that investigated the reduction of the defibrillation thresholds by adding subcutaneous coil electrodes to a right ventricular - active can defibrillator system.

Model

The model is based on the finite difference approach. This makes it possible to implement algorithms of step-wise computation that make the computation more flexible compared to the more usual finite element approach.

The shape and structure of the thorax including all relevant organs is described within a 3D rectangular network of the nodes of the model. The characteristics of each organ include homogeneous isotropic conductivity of the relevant nodes. In each experiment, electrodes are introduced as sets of nodes with predefined voltages. The goal of the model is to compute voltages of all other nodes. From the voltages and organ conductivity, the current densities throughout the structure of the model are derived and from these, simulated defibrillation thresholds are calculated based on the critical mass theory.[4] It is assumed that the current density must exceed a (tissue dependent) threshold J_{thr} in 90 percent of the myocardium. The electrode voltage required for $J_{90}=J_{thr}$ is the threshold voltage V_{90}-DFT, where J_{90} is the 90-th percentile of the current density distribution in the myocardium. The associ-

From Ovsyshcher IE. *Cardiac Arrythmias and Device Therapy: Results and Perspectives for the New Century.* Armonk, NY: Futura Publishing Company, Inc., © 2000

ated energy E_{90}-DFT is defined as the energy stored in a 120 μF capacitor at the V_{90}-DFT voltage.

The principles of the model are taken from basic Kirchhoff laws. In a 3D rectangular network, each node has 6 neighbours (with some exceptions on the borders) and the potential of the node is described by a linear formula incorporating the potentials of the neighbours. These linear formulae create a set of equations, which is solved by Gauss-Jordan elimination. In order to speed up this elimination process, the set of all nodes is divided into those in which the placement of electrodes is, in principle, not possible or illogical (e.g. nodes corresponding to the left ventricular cavity, tissue inside the lungs, etc.) and the others. The matrix of the complete linear equation system is rearranged in such a way that the equations corresponding to the nodes which cannot model electrode placement are separated first. After separating the equations of all the non-electrode nodes, an equivalent equation set is obtained which has the identical number of degrees of freedom and permits the same electrode combinations to be introduced. Individual experiments with the model may then be initiated from this pre-separated equation set rather than from the original equation system which greatly reduces the computational necessity of individual simulation experiments. It follows from the arithmetic complexity of the Gauss-Jordan elimination, that selecting 5% of the nodes as possible electrode places reduces the computational requirements of the equation separation phase of each experiment 8,000 times. The process of pre-separating the nodes which are not used as electrode positions is further repeated for individual batches of experiments that perform factorial analysis of different combinations of a small number of electrodes. The computational requirements of the model are further reduced in this way.

The programs of the model have been written in C++ language utilising object oriented programming. Programs are independent of the anatomy of the model and of its grid resolution. Because of the batch organisation, the model computation is organised in steps each having a separate executable phase. The individual phases communicate via binary files of interim results and are independent of the assumptions made by the previous phases. Hence, different anatomies of the thorax, isotropic or anisotropic organs, different grid resolutions, etc. can be introduced without the need of changing the computational core of the model. As the sequential separation of parts of the equation-set requires rather unusual algorithms to be employed, the programs do not utilise any commercial linear algebra library. Rather, all necessary routines were purpose built and the source text of all the programs of the model has in excess of 16,000 lines in C++.

The present implementation of the model has been tailored to the computational capacity of personal computers having 64 Mbytes of RAM. In this implementation, the anatomy of the model and of the organs has been designed artificially and incorporated into a network of $103 \times 69 \times 101$ nodes representing cubes with 3.5 mm edges. The modelled anatomy was checked visually in different cross sections and a reasonable correspondence between the model and true anatomical images was ensured. The conductivity of individual tissues has been based on previous laboratory measurements.[5-7]

The present implementation of the model exists in seven different versions. In addition to an anatomical image corresponding to the normal heart, three stages of left ventricular dilatation and three stages of left ventricular hypertrophy have been introduced. These range from mild dilatation and hypertrophy to anatomies modelling severe pathologies.

The model has been calibrated by comparing modelled impedance of realistic electrode configurations with data known from clinical measurements and experiments.

Experimental Series

Since the introduction of active can (AC) ICDs with biphasic defibrillation pulses, the average defibrillation thresholds have become sufficiently low to have a 10J safety margin with a 34J output device. Because of surgical simplicity, the configuration of choice is an AC ICD implanted in the left sub-pectoral area and combined with a single transvenous endocardial right ventricular (RV) electrode, eventually combined with a superior vena cava electrode. In few patients, however, the implant criteria for defibrillation efficacy are not met and the implantation of one or mode subcutaneous coil electrodes in the dorso-lateral thoracic area may resolve the problem by defibrillation threshold reduction. However, implantation of additional sub-cutaneous electrodes prolongs the implant procedure and requires additional surgical skills. It may also be of additional risk to the patient.

To study the expected reduction of the defibrillation thresholds by adding a subcutaneous coil to an RV-AC defibrillation system, the computer model has been used in an extensive series of experiments allowing factorial evaluation of different positions and different number of additional subcutaneous coil electrodes.

In this series, the projected surface area of the AC was 37 cm². The implant site was the sub-pectoral area of the left anterior chest wall. Subcutaneous electrodes of 25 cm were electrically connected to AC and positioned in the subcutaneous tissue in the dorso-lateral chest wall of the model. RV electrodes had a length of 5 cm and pointed from the base of the heart to the apex with a curvature approximately following the curvature of the septum and free lateral wall of the right ventricular cavity. Diameter of the modelled RV electrodes was approximately 3.5 mm and the diameter of the models of subcutaneous electrodes corresponded approximately to 2.5 mm (modelled by discontinuities in the 3.5 mm grid).

As in other studies with this model, the natural variation of anatomy and inter-patient variability of implant sites were modelled by adding additional factors to the factorial design of the investigations. Different combinations of 1 to 3 subcutaneous electrodes as well as systems without any subcutaneous electrodes were simulated with different positions of the RV electrode, active can placement and implant site of the subcutaneous electrode. The number of subcutaneous electrodes varied from 0 to 3 and individual electrodes were considered in three different vertical placements and at three different positions of the distal tip of the electrode (at 0, 5 and 10 cm from dorsal mid line). Twelve different positions of RV electrodes were considered ranging in both ventricular depth anterior/posterior position and longitudinal position. Finally, three left sub-pectoral positions of AC were introduced. All these combinations resulted in a set of 792 experiments that were simulated using all the different morphologies of the model.

Two sets of statistical analyses were performed: firstly, the number of subcutaneous electrodes was used as an independent variable while the other variables constituted experimental "noise", and secondly, the position of the distal tip of subcutaneous electrodes was used as the independent variable and the number of subcutaneous electrodes (1–3) was added to the experimental "noise".

For simplicity, only the results of the normal heart morphology model are shown here. The effects of adding subcutaneous (SQ) electrodes on defibrillation threshold (DFT, mean ± standard deviation), percentage of AC current and on impedance are shown in Table 1, corresponding effects of the distance of the tip of subcutaneous coil or multiple coils from dorsal mid line are shown in Table 2. (N indicates the number of experiments modelling experimental "noise".)

Table 1
Effects of adding subcutaneous electrodes

Configuration	N	DFT [J]	AC Current [%]	Impedance [Ω]
RV-AC	36	13.0 ± 4.6	100	50.4 ± 1.5
RV-AC+1SQ	324	6.7 ± 1.9	64.9 ± 2.5	43.0 ± 2.4
RV-AC+2SQ	324	5.5 ± 1.4	53.0 ± 2.9	40.5 ± 2.3
RV-AC+3SQ	108	5.0 ± 1.2	46.9 ± 3.1	39.2 ± 2.2

Table 2
Effects of the tip position of the subcutaneous coil/coils from dorsal mid line

Distance [cm]	N	DFT (J)	AC Current [%]	Impedance [Ω]
0	252	5.7 ± 1.5	56.4 ± 7.1	40.5 ± 2.6
5	252	5.8 ± 1.6	57.2 ± 7.3	41.4 ± 2.7
10	252	6.4 ± 1.9	58.0 ± 7.9	42.3 ± 2.8

It is obvious from these tables that the greatest improvement of defibrillation threshold is obtained by adding a single subcutaneous electrode. Not only the defibrillation threshold is reduced but, more importantly, the standard deviation of the threshold is also reduced (that is, RV electrode position is less critical). Addition of a second or third subcutaneous electrode yields only minor further improvement. Variations of implant depth (distance of the tip to dorsal mid line) and longitudinal position of subcutaneous electrode have only a minor effect on defibrillation threshold.

Conclusion

The major strengths of the present system for defibrillation threshold modelling is the computational flexibility that permits large series of experiments to be conducted and subjected to various statistical evaluations. This allows complete factorial analyses of the effects of different modifications of the electrode systems within a whole scale of possibilities. Using fast Pentium III powered personal computers, a single experiment with the model can be computed in less than 2 minutes which, together with the possibility of batch programming, allows a huge number of experiments to be completed in a practically acceptable time. The experimental series presented in this text is only one of many experiments that were already completed with this modelling system. The model was already implemented on a number of different personal computers and the total number of experiments computed so far exceeds 100,000. The model is useful mainly in the conceptual evaluation of the new designs of electrode systems since it permits every new idea to be initially tested without any substantial design and engineering work. Most of the experiments conducted so far were of this kind.

The main limitation of the present version of the model is the gross grid size and the restricted anatomy of electrode placements (for instance, coronary sinus electrodes are not incorporated in the present version). For these reasons, a new version of the model is presently being developed which uses a substantial part of the present computational core but slightly increases the precision of the grid and mainly the flexibility of electrode placement. The present version of the model also does not introduce the anisotropic conductivity of myocardium and skeleton muscles.

References

1. Sepulveda NG, Wikswo JP Jr, Echt DS. Finite element analysis of cardiac defibrillation current distributions. IEEE Trans Biomed Eng 1990: BME-37: 354-365.
2. Doin AM, Horacek BM, Rautaharju PM. Evaluation of cardiac defibrillation using a computer model of the thorax. Med Instrument 1978; 12: 53-54.
3. Fahy JB, Kim Y, Ananthaswamy A. Optimal electrode configuration for external cardiac pacing and defibrillation: an inhomogeneous study. IEEE Trans Biomed Eng. 1987; BME-34 : 743-748.
4. Zipes DP, Fischer J, King RM, et al. Termination of ventricular fibrillation in dogs by depolarising a critical amount of myocardium. Am J Cardiol 1975; 36: 37-44.
5. Geddes LA, Baker LE. The specific resistivity of biological material. Med Biol Eng Comp1967; 5: 271-293.
6. Van Oosterom A, De Boer RW, van Dam RTh. Intramural resistivity of cardiac tissue. Med Biol Eng Comput 1979: 17: 337-343.
7. Trautman ED, Newbower R.S. A practical analysis of electrical conductivity of blood. IEEE Trans Biomed Eng 1983; BME-30: 141-154.

6

SUBTHRESHOLD CONDITIONING STIMULI MODULATE REFRACTORINESS IN MURINE VENTRICULAR SLICES

Eugene Crystal, M.D., Ilya A. Fleidervish, M.D., Ph.D, Avinoam Rabinovitch, Ph.D., I. Eli Ovsyshcher, M.D., Ph.D..

Electrophysiology Laboratory and Arrhythmia Service, Cardiology Department, Soroka University Medical Center & Department of Physiology, Faculty of Health Sciences, Physics Department, Ben-Gurion University of the Negev, Beer Sheva, Israel

Introduction

During the last two decades, since implantable cardiac devices have become widely available, the role of electrical therapy in management of patients suffering from malignant ventricular arrhythmias is progressively increasing. Currently, the devices operate in two principal modes: pacing, to suppress the arrhythmia by overdrive stimulation (SS), and defibrillation. The possibility of use of low-energy subthreshold stimulation to manipulate the propagation and refractoriness for suppression of arrhythmia, although discussed in the experimental and clinical literature and found promising[1-5], has not yet been adequately explored.

The ability of SS to prevent a subsequent suprathreshold stimulus from depolarizing a ventricular myocardium was first described more than 70 years ago[6]. Since then, similar observations were made on whole animal heart models[5-8] and in human myocardium[1-3].

Here, we used an *in vitro* murine ventricular slice preparation to study the effects of SS on initiation and spread of excitation and on refractoriness.

Methods

Cardiac slices were obtained from 2-4 week old CD1 mice. Animals of either sex were deeply anesthetized with Nembutal (60 mg kg^{-1}), their chests were opened, and the hearts rapidly removed and placed in cold (6°C), oxygenated (95% O_2 – 5% CO_2) Ringer's solution. A vibratome (Pelco 1000) was used to obtain transversal slices (250-350 µm thick), in a plane parallel to the base of the heart (Fig. 1A), and the slices were placed in a holding chamber containing Ringer's solution at room temperature. They were transferred to an interface-type recording chamber after more than 1 hour of incubation.

From Ovsyshcher IE. *Cardiac Arrythmias and Device Therapy: Results and Perspectives for the New Century.* Armonk, NY: Futura Publishing Company, Inc., © 2000

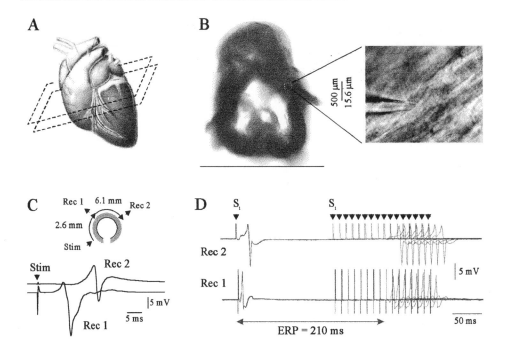

Fig. 1. Murine ventricular slice. **A.** Three to five 250-300 μm thick ventricular sections were cut from the murine heart in a plane parallel to the heart base. **B.** Live cardiac slice as seen under low-gain magnification. **C.** IR-DIC high-gain image of live cardiomyocytes under a thin layer of debris, about 50 μm below slice surface. **D.** Estimation of apparent propagation velocity by simultaneous recording of two electrograms at two different sites in the slice. The propagation velocity was calculated as the ratio of distance between recording electrodes 1 and 2 and times when the excitation wave reached these sites. *Inset:* the schematic drawing of the slice and location of stimulating and recording electrodes. Note that slice was cut in the paraseptal area to prevent propagation in a counter-clockwise direction. **E.** Determining of the effective refractory period. Under the same experimental conditions as in D, pairs of stimuli were delivered at decremental inter-stimulus intervals (S_1S_1) mode, to determine the longest S_1S_1, at which the second stimulus elicits a propagating excitation wave. The stimuli were of 100 μsec duration and had an amplitude 1.5 times higher than threshold. In these slices, ERP measured at two sites, was 210 msec.

Results

The experimental results were obtained using extracellular electrogram recordings in 37 ventricular slices from 11 mice. Being examined under low-gain magnification, slices usually had a "figure-8"-shape, with well recognizable free wall of left ventricle, ventricular septum and free right ventricular wall (Fig. 1B, left). With higher magnification infrared DIC video microscopy, live undamaged cardiomyocytes were clearly identified under the thin layer of debris on the surface of the slice (Fig. 1B, right). Rectangular 100 μs duration current pulses, delivered through a bipolar electrode, elicited action potentials that propagated throughout the slice with a velocity of 0.4-0.6 m/s (n= 6; Fig. 1C). The apparent refractory period as assessed using computer-driven double-pulse stimulation was in the range of 180-210 ms (n=37, Fig. 1D). The apparent propagation velocity and effective refractoriness were usually homogeneous throughout the slice, and remained stable for a period of more than 3 hours. Slices that showed heterogeneity and/or instability in refractoriness were discarded. Since the ventricular wall and septum of mice are extremely thin (about 500 µm, see Fig. 1), and slices were cut at thickness of not more than 350 µm, they represent virtually "two-dimensional" case, such that the electrical field between needles of stimulating electrode excites the myocardium in-depth, from subendocardial to subepicardial layers, and from the bottom to the top of the slice.

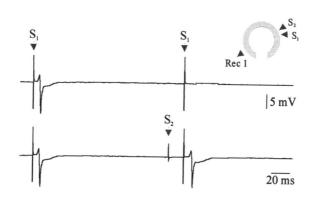

Fig. 2. Subthreshold stimulus shortens the refractory period (summation). Top, second stimulus S_1 does not elicit an excitation wave when delivered during the refractory period after the first S_1. Delivering of subthreshold stimulus, S_2, 20 ms prior to the second S_1 results in initiation of the excitation. *Inset:* the schematic drawing of the slice and location of stimulating and recording electrodes. Note the close location of two stimulation electrodes.

To examine how subthreshold stimulation affects ventricular refractoriness, the conditioning subthreshold stimuli were delivered through the separate bipolar electrode (S_2) at different times relative to the second of the pair of SS (S_1S_1). When the second S_1 of the pair fell during refractoriness, delivery of S_2 through the second stimulating electrode located at a distance less than 1 mm from the first one, at a time >20 ms prior to the second S_1, shortened the refractoriness, enabling the initiation of an excitation wave (Fig. 2). Under similar experimental conditions, when the second S_1 of the pair fell shortly after the end of refractoriness, delivery of S_2, 15-30 ms prior to the second S_1 frequently resulted in effective prolongation of the refractoriness, preventing the initiation of the excitation (Fig. 3).

Delivery of S_2 through the second stimulating electrode located at a distance of more than 1 mm from the first one, to prevent direct interference

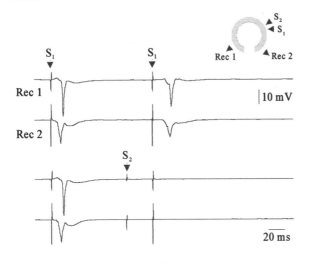

Fig. 3. Subthreshold stimulus inhibits generation of an excitation wave. Top, simultaneous recording from two different sites, Rec1 and Rec2 (see inset), shows that suprathreshold stimulus S_1 elicits excitation wave that propagates in both directions. The second stimulus S_1, applied right after the end of refractory period, elicits similar, but slower propagating wave. Bottom, subthreshold stimulus, S_2, delivered 30 msec before the second S_1, at a distance of about 1 mm from S_1 (see inset), prevents the wave generation. *Inset:* the relative location of stimulating electrodes, S_1 and S_2, and recording electrodes Rec1 and Rec2. Note that slice was cut in the paraseptal area to prevent consecutive excitation of sites Rec1 and Rec2 by the same excitation wave. Rec1 indicates propagation in a counter clock-wise direction, and Rec2, in a clockwise direction.

of the stimuli, apparently prolonged refractoriness in the area adjacent to the S_2, creating the inexcitable obstacle through which the excitation wave could not by-pass (Fig. 4). In this case, the subthreshold stimulus did not affect either initiation of a wave, or its propagation in the opposite direction.

Fig. 4. Inhibition of propagation of the excitation wave by subthreshold stimulus. Recording from a different slice, under conditions similar to those of Fig. 3. Top, suprathreshold stimulus S_1 elicits excitation wave that propagates in both directions. Bottom, when the subthreshold stimulus, S_2, is delivered at a distance of about 5 mm from S_1 (see inset), 20 msec before the delivery of second S_1, it blocked propagation towards Rec1 completely, while not affecting the propagation in a clockwise direction, towards Rec2. *Inset:* schematic location of the stimulating and recording electrodes. Note that S_2 electrode is located at a longer distance from S_1, than in Fig. 3.

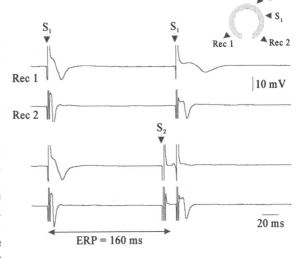

Discussion

The present study demonstrates that SS could affect initiation of excitation, and its propagation, by modifying the ventricular refractoriness. Earlier works in dog[7,8] and humane[1,2] ventricular tissue showed the ability of appropriately timed SS to prolong the refractory period for action potential generation. We found that, in murine ventricles, the SS could exert two opposite effects, either extending or shortening the tissue refractoriness, most likely depending on timing and location of the stimulus. The mechanisms underlying these effects are not completely clear. In our experiments, the subthreshold S_2 stimulus interfered with subsequent S_1 only when delivered during the relative refractory period, i.e. during rapid repolarization or immediately upon complete repolarization of cardiac tissue. In the case of close location of stimulating electrodes, this interference may be purely electrotonic. Thus, depolarization produced by S_2 may shift the membrane potential closer to the threshold, resulting in decrease in amount of current necessary to excite the tissue several milliseconds later. On the other hand, the same electrotonic depolarization could decrease the excitability by slowing down the time course of Na^+ channel reactivation. This might extend the refractory period, since action potential generation is critically dependent on availability of Na^+ channels. The second mechanism seems to prevail, since shortening of refractoriness by S_2 was only rarely observed.

When the stimuli were delivered at a distance, which prevented their direct electrotonic interaction, the appropriately timed SS produced a transmural area of prolonged refractoriness, that could only conduct an excitation in a decremental fashion (Fig. 4). Surprisingly, this inexcitable obstacle appeared to be long lasting and large enough to prevent even an electrotonic action potential propagation, like described by Anshelevitch and Moe[9,10].

SS has been shown to be able to terminate atrioventricular node reentrant tachycardia[4]. The atrioventricular propagation, however, even normally, is known to be fragile, with a tendency to become decremental. In human ventricles, precisely directed, ultra-rapid subthreshold stimulation was shown to be able to interrupt sustained ventricular tachycardia[3]. This can be related to interference of subthreshold stimuli with abnormal area of slow propagation[11], that also is fragile. The mechanism, however, might be similar to that described here: induction of prolonged refractoriness in an area of normal conduction.

Finally, in this preliminary report we demonstrated that SS could exert different effects. The one of possible clinical relevance is the potential ability of subthreshold stimulus to create the temporary inexcitable obstacle in a normal ventricular myocardium, that is large enough and lasts long enough to interrupt reentry, and to depress the focus of triggered activity. In the future, this could make the SS an additional mode for implantable cardiac devices.

References

1. Prystowsky EN, Zipes DP Inhibition in the human heart. Circulation 1983; 68: 707-713.

2. Windle JR, Miles WM, Zipes DP, et al. Subthreshold conditioning stimuli prolong human ventricular refractoriness. Am J Cardiol 1986; 57: 381-386.

3. Shenasa M, Cardinal R, Kus T, et al. Termination of sustained ventricular tachycardia by ultrarapid subthreshold stimulation in humans. Circulation 1988; 78: 1135-1143

4. Fromer M, Shenasa M Ultrarapid subthreshold stimulation for termination of atrioventricular node reentrant tachycardia. J Am Coll Cardiol 1992; 20:879-883.

5. Salama G, Kanai A, Efimov IR Subthreshold stimulation of Purkinje fibers interrupts ventricular tachycardia in intact hearts. Circ Res 1994; 74: 604-619.

6. Drury AN, Love WS The supposed lengthening of the absolute refractory period of frog's ventricular muscle by veratrine. Heart 1926; 68: 707-713.

7. Paya R, Chorro FJ, Sanchis J, et al. Changes in canine ventricular refractoriness induced by trains of subthreshold high-frequency stimuli. J Electrocardiol 1991; 24:63-69.

8. Skale BT, Kallok MJ, Prystowsky EN, et al. Inhibition of premature ventricular extrastimuli by subthreshold conditioning stimuli. J Am Coll Cardiol 1985; 6:133-140.

9. Antzelevitch C, Moe GK Electrotonically mediated delayed conduction and reentry in relation to "slow responses" in mammalian ventricular conducting tissue. Circ Res 1981; 49: 1129-1139.

10. Antzelevitch C, Moe GK Electrotonic inhibition and summation of impulse conduction in mammalian Purkinje fibers. Am J Physiol 1983; 245: H42-H53.

11. Podczeck A, Borggrefe M, Martinez-Rubio A et al. Termination of re-entrant ventricular tachycardia by subthreshold stimulus applied to the zone of slow conduction. Eur Heart J 1988; 9:1146-1150.

7.
ADENOSINE TRIPHOSPHATE IN CARDIAC ARRHYTHMIAS: FROM THERAPEUTIC TO BEDSIDE DIAGNOSTIC USE

Bernard Belhassen, MD

Electrophysiology Laboratory, Department of Cardiology, Tel-Aviv Sourasky Medical Center, Tel-Aviv University, Tel-Aviv, Israel

Introduction

More than 70 years ago, Drury and Szent-Gyorgyi[1] were the first to show that extracellular adenosine and related compounds exert pronounced electrophysiologic effects in the mammalian heart, including transient depressant effects on the sinus node and the atrioventricular (AV) node. In ensuing years, the effects of adenosine compounds were demonstrated in numerous animal preparations and in the human heart.[2] The earliest reports that we could find on the effects of adenosine triphosphate (ATP) in the acute management of paroxysmal supraventricular tachycardia (PSVT) are by Hungarian workers. In letters to the editor published in 1955, Somlo[3], Komor and Garas[4] reported on the termination of hundreds of episodes of PSVT using 10–70mg ATP injected intravenously as a rapid bolus. The effects of ATP on various types of tachycardia were subsequently studied in France by Motte[5], Puech[6], and their coworkers. These studies confirmed the high efficacy of ATP in the acute therapy of PSVT and showed that this drug could be used as a tool for diagnostic purpose. In 1983, we published[7] the first study of the electrophysiologic effects of ATP in AV nodal and AV reentrant tachycardias. Since the effect of ATP is mainly due to its degradation into its metabolite adenosine, similar clinical results with adenosine were reported beginning in 1983.[8] Both ATP and adenosine were shown to achieve a success rate of almost 100% for the conversion of PSVT, greater to that obtained with verapamil.[9] In most countries, adenosine compounds are presently the drugs of first choice used in the acute termination of PSVT and have supplanted verapamil for this indication.[10,11] Besides its utilisation in the acute management of PSVT, ATP has been shown to be very useful as a diagnostic tool in several clinical settings. The use of ATP as a diagnostic tool is mainly based on its marked transient depressant effects on the AV node.

Differential diagnosis of regular, narrow QRS supraventricular tachycardia

There are five main possible diagnosis of regular, narrow QRS supraventricular tachycardia: a) AV nodal reentry tachycardia (AVNRT);

From Ovsyshcher IE. *Cardiac Arrythmias and Device Therapy: Results and Perspectives for the New Century.* Armonk, NY: Futura Publishing Company, Inc., © 2000

b) AV reentrant tachycardia (AVRT) involving a retrogradely conducting accessory pathway; c) atrial tachycardia; d) atrial flutter; e) sinus tachycardia. The mechanism of the first two tachycardias involve the AV node in the reentry circuit and therefore both are abruptly terminated by ATP. In most instances, these tachycardias terminate due to conduction block in the antegrade slow pathway and the AV node in patients with the common slow/fast form of AVNRT and AVRT, respectively. Atrial flutter and most cases of atrial tachycardia are insensitive to ATP and therefore only transient slowing of the ventricular rate is observed upon occurrence of AV nodal block following ATP administration, allowing a clear demonstration of the atrial activity. Some cases of atrial tachycardia are adenosine sensitive and, as such, are terminated by ATP. Sinus tachycardia is transiently slowed by ATP. Taking in account that the great majority (85-90%) of PSVT are due to either AVNRT or AVRT, one can assume that a sudden termination of a PSVT during ATP administration strongly suggests that the mechanism of PSVT is related to any of these two mechanisms.

Differential diagnosis of regular, wide QRS tachycardia
There are four main diagnosis of regular, wide QRS tachycardia: a) ventricular tachycardia (VT); b) SVT with preexisting or rate-dependent intraventricular aberration; c) antidromic AVRT involving an accessory pathway in the antegrade direction and the AV node in the retrograde direction; d) atrial flutter/tachycardia with antegrade conduction over an accessory pathway. ATP is ineffective in the acute management of the vast majority of VT, especially those occurring in patients with organic heart disease. The only types of VT that can be terminated by ATP are those with a right or left bundle branch block pattern occurring in patients with no demonstrable heart disease. The mechanism of these adenosine-sensitive VT is attributed to cyclic-AMP dependent triggered activity.[12] As emphasized in the previous chapter, SVT with intraventricular aberration is either transiently slowed or terminated by ATP, depending on the actual mechanism of the tachycardia. Antidromic AVRT is terminated by ATP since its mechanism involves the AV node in the reentry circuit. Finally, atrial tachyarrhythmias with antegrade conduction over an accessory pathway are almost never terminated by ATP; in contrast, the administration of ATP in such cases may have severe deleterious consequences owing to adenosine-induced shortening of the atrial and accessory pathway refractoriness. This can result in either transformation of an atrial tachycardia into atrial fibrillation and/or significant acceleration of the ventricular rate, which can both lead to potentially lethal arrhythmias.[13] In clinical practice where the differential

diagnosis is between VT and SVT with aberration, termination of a wide QRS tachycardia with ATP suggests AVNRT or AVRT while a lack of effect of ATP rather supports a diagnosis of VT.

Diagnosis of preexcitation in patients with minor or latent forms

While the diagnosis of ventricular preexcitation is obvious during sinus rhythm in the great majority of patients with the Wolff-Parkinson-White (WPW) syndrome based on the association of short PR interval, delta wave and wide QRS complex, some patients may exhibit minor degrees of preexcitation ("minor preexcitation") or no preexcitation despite the presence of antegrade conduction over the accessory pathway ("latent preexcitation").[14] These types of preexcitation result from the presence of one or several of the following conditions: 1. Distal location of the accessory pathway (for example left lateral accessory pathways) 2. Slow conduction properties of the accessory pathway (for example in case of right-sided atriofascicular accessory pathways); 3. Enhanced AV nodal conduction; 4. Intraatrial conduction disturbances. All these situations result in shorter conduction time from the sinus node to the ventricles over the normal AV nodal route as compared to that over the accessory pathway. In such patients, the administration of ATP, by creating a marked AV nodal delay, allows to maximize transiently the degree of preexcitation, and thereby an accurate ECG accessory pathway location.[14-16]

Assessment of the effects of ajmaline test on "minor preexcitation"

Another diagnostic use of ATP in patients with "minor" forms of preexcitation is in the assessment of the effects of ajmaline test. The latter is useful for the noninvasive evaluation of the refractory period of the accessory pathway in patients with the WPW syndrome since it has been shown to abolish preexcitation in most patients with a refractory period of the pathway greater than 250 msec.[17,18] The effects of ajmaline on preexcitation are easily appreciated in patients with overt WPW but not in patients with minor or latent forms. The potent AV nodal depressant effects of ATP unmask these forms of preexcitation and allow the assessment of the results of ajmaline test.[19]

Revelation of accessory pathway conduction in patients with intermittent WPW syndrome.

In patients with intermittent preexcitation, antegrade conduction over the accessory pathway may disappear for undetermined, long periods of time despite the use of isoproterenol. In such instances, adenosine[20] and ATP (unpublished data) may elicit the manifestation of the preexcitation, albeit transiently. The mechanism underlying this phenomenon seems to be related to the shortening of the action potential duration of the accessory pathway secondary to adenosine administration.

Noninvasive diagnosis of dual AV nodal physiology

AVNRT is the most frequently encountered type of regular, PSVT in clinical practice. In patients with the common form of AVNRT, the circus movement involves a slow pathway in the antegrade direction and a fast pathway in the retrograde direction. In about 85% of these patients, the evidence of antegrade dual AV nodal physiology is given by electrophysiologic testing. Since the antegrade refractory period of the fast pathway is usually greater than that of the slow pathway, we postulated that ATP could have a differential effect on these two pathways when injected during *sinus rhythm* and thereby may be useful in the noninvasive diagnosis of dual AV node physiology. In a pilot study involving 41 patients, we found that   76% of patients with inducible sustained slow / fast AVNRT exhibited ECG signs suggesting dual AV node physiology following ATP administration during sinus rhythm.[21] An almost similar incidence (75%) was found in a larger group of patients (n=96)   In whom a simplified protocol of administration of ATP was tested.[22]

Noninvasive assessment of the results of radiofrequency ablation of the slow pathway

We also found that ATP test could be used in the noninvasive assessment of the results of radiofrequency ablation.[23] Dual AV node physiology by ATP test disappeared in 27 (96%) of 28 patients who underwent slow pathway abolition and in 18 (60%) of 30 patients who underwent slow pathway modification. In the 12 patients who showed persistent dual AV node physiology by ATP test after slow pathway modification, the number of beats conducted over the slow pathway was significantly reduced (2.5 ± 2.2 vs 6.3 ± 3.3, p<0.002). In 10 (83%) of these 12 patients, the number of beats conducted over the slow pathway decreased by ≥ 2 beats.

Noninvasive diagnosis of concealed accessory pathway

Since ATP exerts a transient depressant effect on AV nodal conduction, we postulated that in patients with concealed accessory pathways, such conduction delay caused by the administration of ATP during *sinus rhythm* could allow the occurrence of AV reentrant orthodromic echo beats (AVRE) or AVRT. Therefore we evaluated the value of the intravenous administration of   ATP during sinus rhythm in the noninvasive diagnosis of the presence of a concealed accessory pathway and associated dual AV node physiology in 33 patients with inducible sustained AVRT and in 27 control patients.[24] We found AVRE or AVRT in 24 (73%) study patients and in none of the control group. We also found that ECG signs suggestive of dual AV node physiology were observed after ATP administration in 7 (21%) study patients and in none of the control group.

Noninvasive diagnosis of the mechanism of tachycardia in patients with palpitations or SVT of undetermined mechanism

Based on our previous findings on the use of ATP in the diagnosis of dual AV node physiology and concealed accessory pathway, we evaluated in 66 patients, the predictive accuracy of a simple bedside ATP test for identifying patients with palpitations or supraventricular arrhythmias of unclear mechanism who actually have AVNRT or AVRT and would benefit from invasive electrophysiologic evaluation.[25] The results of the ATP test were correlated with the results of a subsequent electrophysiologic study. A positive ATP test predicted the presence of AVNRT or AVRT with a positive predictive value of 92% (sensitivity=70%) but a negative predictive value of 21% (specificity=57%). Moreover, signs of dual AV node physiology by ATP test predicted the induction of AVNRT with a predictive positive value of 89%. Therefore, our bedside ATP test identifies patients with palpitations who are likely to have AVNRT or AVRT (and therefore may benefit from electrophysiologic evaluation) with a high positive predictive value.

Conclusion

First used as a major agent in our therapeutic arsenal for terminating PSVT, ATP has gained importance as a bedside, diagnostic tool in a variety of clinical settings, especially in the noninvasive diagnosis of dual AV node physiology and concealed accessory pathway. Further studies are required to assess the potential use of ATP test in the noninvasive identification of other types of tachyarrhythmias, such as atrial fibrillation, taking in account the well known fibrillatory effects of adenosine compounds at the atrial level.[26]

Acknowledgments

I express my deep gratitude to Gilbert Motte, MD (Clamart, France), Amir Pelleg, PhD (Hahneman University, Philadelphia, USA), Sami Viskin, MD, Aron Glick, MD and Roman Fish, MD (Tel-Aviv Medical Center, Israel), Michael Glikson, MD and Michael Eldar, MD (Sheba

Medical Center, Israel), for their invaluable help and support in the performance of the studies which form the basis of this review.

References

1. Drury A, Szent-Gyorgyi A: The physiological activity of adenine compounds with especial reference to their action upon mammalian heart. J Physiol (Lond) 1929;68:213-237.

2. Belhassen B, Pelleg A: Electrophysiologic effects of adenosine triphosphate and adenosine on the mammalian heart: clinical and experimental aspects. J Am Coll Cardiol 1984;4:414-424.

3. Somlo E: Adenosine triphosphate in paroxysmal tachycardia. Lancet 1955; 268: 1125 (letter).

4. Komor K, Garas Z: Adenosine triphosphate in paroxysmal tachycardia. Lancet 1955; 269:93-94 (letter).

5. Motté G, Waynberger M, Lebars A, et al.:L'adénosine triphosphorique dans les tachycardies paroxystiques. Intérêt diagnostique et thérapeutique. Nouv Presse Med 1972;1:3057-3061

6. Puech P, Grolleau R, Sat M: L'adénosine-5-triphosphorique (Striadyne) dans les arythmies cardiaques. Nouv Presse Med (Paris) 1972;1:606.

7. Belhassen B, Pelleg A, Shoshani D, et al.: Electrophysiologic effects of adenosine- 5'-triphosphate on atrioventricular reentrant tachycardia. Circulation 1983;68:827-833.

8. DiMarco J, Sellers T, Berne R, et al.: Adenosine: electrophysiologic effects and therapeutic use for terminating paroxysmal supraventricular tachycardia. Circulation 1983;68:1254-1263.

9. Belhassen B, Glick A, Laniado S: Comparative clinical and electrophysiologic effects of adenosine triphosphate and verapamil on paroxysmal reciprocating junctional tachycardia. Circulation 1988;77:795-805.

10. Belhassen B, Pelleg A: Acute management of paroxysmal supraventricular tachycardia: verapamil, adenosine triphosphate or adenosine? Am J Cardiol 1984;54:225-227.

11. Viskin S, Belhassen B: Acute management of paroxysmal atrioventricular junctional reentrant tachycardia: pharmacologic strategies. Am Heart J 1990; 120:180-188.

12. Lerman B, Stein K, Markowitz S: Adenosine-sensitive ventricular tachycardia: a conceptual approach. J Cardiovasc Electrophysiol 1996;7:559-569.

13. Rankin A, Rae A, Houston A: Acceleration of ventricular response to atrial flutter after intravenous adenosine. Br Heart J 1993;69:263-265.

14. Grolleau R, Slama R: Les faisceaux de Kent inapparents. In: Le groupe de rythmologie de la société française de cardiologie (ed): Les troubles du rythme cardiaque. Nanterre, éditions Corbière, 1978, pp.187-197.

15. Valeix B, Faugère G, Chabrillat Y, et al.: Intérêt et limites de la Striadyne injectable dans la détection des faisceaux de Kent inapparents en conduction antérograde. L'information cardiologique (Paris) 1979;2:363-369.

16. Garrat C, Antoniou A, Griffith M, et al.: Use of intravenous adenosine in sinus rhythm as a diagnostic test for latent preexcitation. Am J Cardiol 1990;65:868-873.

17. Wellens H, Bär F, Gorgels A, et al.: Use of ajmaline in patients with the Wolff- Parkinson-White syndrome to disclose short refractory period of the accessory pathway. Am J Cardiol 1980;54:130-135.

18. Eshchar Y, Belhassen B, Laniado S: Comparison of exercise and ajmaline tests with electrocardiographic study in the Wolff-Parkinson-White syndrome. Am J Cardiol 1986;57:782-786.

19. Belhassen B, Shoshani D, Laniado S: Unmasking of ventricular preexcitation by adenosine triphosphate: its usefulness in the assessment of ajmaline test. Am Heart J 1989;118: 634-636.

20. Morgan-Hughes N, Griffith M, McComb J: Intravenous adenosine can reveal accessory pathways not revealed by routine electrophysiologic testing. PACE 1993;16:2059-2063

21. Belhassen B, Fish R, Glikson M, et al.: Noninvasive diagnosis of dual AV node physiology in patients with AV nodal reentrant tachycardia by administration of adenosine-5'-triphosphate during sinus rhythm. Circulation 1998;98:47-53.

22. Fish R, Belhassen B, Eldar M, et al.: Non invasive diagnosis of dual AV node pathways by intravenous adenosine triphosphate : prospective evaluation of a simplified protocol. PACE 1999;22:836 (abstract)

23. Belhassen B, Fish R, Eldar M, et al.: Assessment of the results of radiofrequency ablation of the slow pathway with administration of adenosine triphosphate during sinus rhythm. PACE 1999 ;22:796 (abstract)

24. Belhassen B, Fish R, Viskin S, et al.: Adenosine -5'-triphosphate test for the non invasive diagnosis of concealed accessory pathway. (submitted for publication)

25. Viskin S, Fish R, Glick A, et al.: ATP test : A bedside diagnostic tool for identifying patients with palpitations who are likely to benefit from electrophysiologic evaluation. Eur Heart J 1999;20:583 (abstract)

26. Tebbenjohanns J, Schumacher B, Pfeiffer D, et al.: Dose and rate-dependent effects of adenosine on atrial action potential duration in humans. J Interv Card Electrophysiol 1997;1:39-40.

8.

LONG QT SYNDROME: PHENOTYPE-GENOTYPE CONSIDERATIONS

Arthur J. Moss, M.D., Wojciech Zareba, M.D., Ph.D., and Jennifer L. Robinson, M.S.

Cardiology Unit, Department of Medicine, University of Rochester Medical Center, Rochester, New York, USA

Introduction

The hereditary Long QT Syndrome (LQTS) is a familial disorder with prolonged ventricular repolarization on the electrocardiogram and a propensity to recurrent syncope, polymorphous ventricular tachycardia of the torsades de pointes type, and sudden arrhythmic death.[1,2] Six genetic loci have been identified involving 5 mutant genes with over 150 different mutations. The 5 mutant LQTS genes include KVLQT1 (LQT1)[3], HERG (LQT2)[4], SCN5A (LQT3)[5], KCNE1 [minK] (LQT5)[6], and KCNE2 [MiRPI] (LQT6)[7]. KVLQT1, HERG, KCNE1, and KCNE2 encode potassium channel subunits. Four KVLQT1 subunits coassemble with the KCNE1 protein to form I_{Ks} channels that are involved in the slowly activating delayed rectifier potassium current.[8] Four HERG subunits coassemble with the KCNE2 protein to form I_{Kr} channels that are involved in the rapidly activating delayed rectifier potassium current.[7] Mutant components of these channels result in a reduction of I_{Ks} and I_{Kr} currents by a dominant-negative loss-of-function. SCN5A encodes the cardiac sodium channel that is involved in the sodium current I_{Na}, with mutations of this encoded protein associated with a gain-of-function.[9] Reduced function of the repolarizing potassium channels or gain-of-function of the sodium channel prolong the cardiac action potential with resultant QT prolongation and a tendency to ventricular arrhythmias. The classical Romano-Ward syndrome with QT prolongation and normal hearing is due to single dominant mutations of any of the identified 5 ionic LQTS genes. Double-dominant (recessive) mutations involving KVLQT1-KCNE1 result in the Jervell Lange-Nielsen syndrome, a severe form of LQTS with deafness. Double-dominant mutations of HERG-KCNE2 result in a severe phenotype in infancy, but with normal hearing.

The identification of the 5 mutant genes at loci LQT1, LQT2, LQT3, LQT5, and LQT6 was largely derived from patients enrolled in the International Long QT Syndrome Registry. During the past 20 years, 865 families with LQTS have been enrolled in the Registry. This study

From Ovsyshcher IE. *Cardiac Arrythmias and Device Therapy: Results and Perspectives for the New Century.* Armonk, NY: Futura Publishing Company, Inc., © 2000

expands on the phenotype characteristics of the carriers of mutant KVLQT1, HERG, and SCN5A genes that were previously reported.[10-12]

Methods

The study population was drawn from the individuals enrolled in the International Long QT Syndrome Registry, with 246 subjects from 38 families identified as having a mutant LQTS gene.   Clinical and electrocardiographic data were obtained at the time of enrollment into the Registry.   The measured QT interval was corrected for heart rate (QTc) using the Bazett formula.   Cardiac events occurring before age 41 years included syncope, aborted cardiac arrest, and death.   Statistical analysis utilized routine univariate techniques, as appropriate.   The Kaplan-Meier life-table method was used to evaluate the cumulative probability of a first cardiac event, with results compared between groups by the log-rank test. The Cox survivorship method was utilized to evaluate the significance and independence of the genotype as a predictor of cardiac events.

Results

1. Deafness – five percent of the probands in the Registry have the Jervell and Lange-Nielsen syndrome with congenital deafness, marked QT prolongation, and severe clinical manifestations with a high frequency of recurrent syncope, overt T-wave alternans, and a high lethality.   To date, all reported cases have involved homozygous or mixed heterozygous mutations of KVLQT1 and/or KCNE1 genes, with marked reduction in I_{Ks} current.   The parents, each with only a single copy of the gene mutation, generally have a mild form of LQTS, and in one family reported from the Registry both parents had normal or borderline QTc intervals in the range of 0.43 to 0.44 sec.[13]

2. Gender and age-related issues – among LQTS gene carriers, no sex preference was observed, with similar cardiac event rates in males and females.   However, among LQT1 carriers, males were significantly younger than females at first cardiac event (9 vs. 13 years; p<0.05), and the cumulative age-related probability of first event by age 15 years was higher in males than females (69% vs. 32%; p<0.05).

2. ECG morphology – five quantitative electrocardiographic repolarization parameters, i.e., four Bazett-corrected time intervals (QTonset$_c$, QTpeak$_c$, QTc, and Tduration$_c$ in msec) and the absolute height of the T wave (Tamplitude in mV) were measured in 76 LQTS-affected individuals (Table 1).   Each of the three LQTS genotypes were associated with somewhat distinctive electrocardiographic repolarization features. Among affected individuals, the QTonset$_c$ was unusually prolonged in those with

LQT3 mutations involving the SCN5A gene; Tamplitude was generally quite small in those with LQT2 (HERG/KCNE2) mutations; and Tduration$_c$ was particularly long in those with LQT1 (KVLQT1/KCNE1) mutations.

Table 1. Repolarization Parameters in Lead II in Subjects with LQT1, LQT2, and LQT3 Gene Mutations

Variables	LQT1 (n=40)	LQT2 (n=17)	LQT3 (n=19)	P-value*
QTonset$_c$ msec	243±76	290±56	**341±42**	<0.001
QTpeak$_c$ msec	415±43	392±44	433±40	0.04
QTc msec	502±43	480±50	529±44	0.01
Tduration$_c$ msec	**262±64**	191±51	187±33	<0.001
Tamplitude mV	0.37±0.17	**0.13±0.07**	0.36±0.14	<0.001

Values are mean ±sd. P-values for differences among the three gene-loci groups. Bold values indicate most distinctive differences. Modified from Circulation 1995;92:2929-2934,[10] with permission.

4. <u>Clinical course</u> – the cardiac event rate differed by genotype. The LQT1 and LQT2 groups had significantly higher frequencies and cumula-

Table 2. Cardiac Events in Subjects with LQT1, LQT2, and LQT3 Gene Mutations

Cardiac Events	LQT1 (n=112)	LQT2 (n=72)	LQT3 (n=62)	P-value*
≥1 cardiac event-%	62	46	18	<0.001
≥2 cardiac events-%	37	36	5	<0.001
Mean age 1st event-yr	9	12	16	<0.05
Cum. probability of cardiac event by age 40-%	70	56	20	<0.001
Aborted arrest -%	7	6	3	ns
Death-%	2	0	3	ns

P-values for differences among the three gene-loci groups. Modified from N Engl J Med 1998;339;960-965,[11] with permission.

tive probabilities of cardiac events than the LQT3 subjects (Fig. 1). By the age of 15 years, 53% of the LQT1 subjects, 29% of the LQT2 subjects, and 6 percent of the LQT3 subjects had a first cardiac event. Multiple cardiac events were more frequent in the LQT1 and LQT2 groups than in LQT3. Cox regression analysis confirmed that after adjustment for

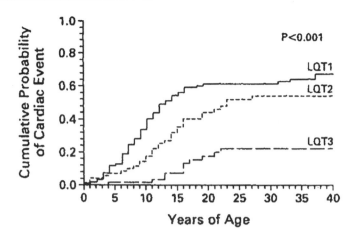

Figure 1. Cumulative probability of cardiac events by genotype.
From N Engl J Med 1998;338:960-965,[11] with permission.

baseline QTc, subjects with LQT1 and LQT2 mutations were 3 to 5 times more likely to experience a cardiac event by age 40 than the LQT3 subjects. A longer QTc was associated with an increased risk of cardiac events (hazard ratio 1.06 per 10-msec increase in QTc; P=0.003), and this association was independent of genotype. Although the cumulative probability of death through age 40 was similar in the three groups, death as a function of the frequency of cardiac events, i.e., lethality, was quite different in the three genotypes. Twenty-three percent of all cardiac events were fatal in LQT3, whereas only 4% of events were fatal in LQT1 and LQT2 subjects (P<0.001).

5. Beta-blocker effectiveness – the effectiveness of beta-blockers was evaluated during matched periods of time before and after initiation of this therapy. In a subset of 139 genotyped patients, beta-blocker therapy had minimal effects on QTc in all three genotypes. Following initiation of beta blockers, there was a significant (P<0.001) reduction in the number of cardiac events and the cardiac event rate (events/patient/year) in LQT1 and LQT2 subjects when compared to the pre-beta-blocker period, but not in LQT3 subjects.

6. Arousal and non-arousal related events – the precipitating factors associated with cardiac events were evaluated in 78 genotyped subjects with classifiable first cardiac events (Table 3). A significant association was observed between genotype and susceptibility to arousal/non-arousal-related cardiac events. The majority of patients with LQT1 and LQT2

Table 3. First Arousal and Non-arousal-related Cardiac Events in Subjects with LQT1, LQT2, and LQT3 Gene Mutations.

Genotype	Arousal (n=60)	Non-arousal (n=18)
LQT1	85%	15%
LQT2	67%	33%
LQT3	33%	67%

The distribution of arousal and non-arousal frequencies by genotype is significantly different from chance at P=0.008.

genotypes experienced a first cardiac event associated with arousal, while a majority of those with LQT3 genotype experienced their first cardiac event without arousal. Among 25 genotyped subjects who had cardiac events precipitated by loud noise or swimming activity, all 19 subjects with swimming-related episodes occurred in those with LQT1 whereas 5 of 6 subjects with auditory-related events occurred in subjects with LQT2 mutation (P<0.001).

Discussion

This study from the International Long QT Syndrome Registry involving only a limited number of genotyped LQTS subjects reveals that there are gender, age-related, ECG T-wave pattern, clinical course, beta-blocker efficacy, and arousal-related differences among subjects with the three major genotypes.

These different phenotypic manifestations relate in one way or another to the ionic current disturbances associated with the LQT1, LQT2, and LQT3 mutations. The different time- and voltage dependence of I_{Ks}, I_{Kr}, and I_{Na} involved in LQTS may explain the variable phenotype. Exercise and acute arousal-related events occur most frequently in mutations affecting I_{Ks}, and this current predominates in conditions with augmented sympathetic activity. Reduced I_{Ks} current due to LQT1 or LQT5 mutations would be associated with reduced action potential shortening during sympathetic hyperactivity, thus explaining the frequent occurrence of events during exercise and acute non-auditory arousal. Subjects with I_{Kr} mutations (HERG) experience cardiac events triggered by loud auditory stimuli, but this is not the case with subjects having mutations involving I_{Ks} (KVLQT1/KCNE1). Subjects heterozygous for KVLQT1/ KCNE1 mutations have normal hearing, but the startle response to loud noises may be attenuated due to subclinical hearing deficiency.

Subjects with LQT3 (SCN5A) mutations seem to experience a majority of their cardiac events during relative inactivity and not with acute arousal. It may be that the presence of normal potassium currents (I_{Ks} and I_{Kr}) in LQT3 patients is associated with appropriate action potential shortening during exercise and associated hyperadrenergic states.

There are a lot of gaps in our understanding of the phenotype-genotype relationships associated with LQTS. It is estimated that only about 50 percent of the subjects with LQTS have identifiable mutations involving the currently known five LQTS genes (LQT1, LQT2, LQT3, LQT5, LQT6), so additional genetic mutations will surely be identified. In addition, among the five LQTS genes, there are already over 150 different nonsense, missense, frameshift, deletion, and splice-site mutations that have been identified. These mutations produce a variety of alterations in the membrane-spanning channel proteins, with involvement of pore regions, as well as intracellular, extracellular, and transmembrane segments. These different types and positions of the mutations may well explain the variable expression and disease severity among different mutations involving a specific LQTS gene. In addition, the associated genetic environment may contribute to modifier effects that can result in variable penetrance of the disease.

Conclusion

LQTS is a paradigm for investigating the phenotype-genotype associations of an autosomal genetic disorder with both dominant and recessive forms of inheritance. The LQTS genotype has a major influence on the clinical manifestations of this disorder, but a complex interplay of mutation type and location as well as modifying genetic and environmental factors contribute to the clinical diversity of this genetic cardiac syndrome. An understanding of the genetically altered ion currents mechanisms in LQTS may permit the development of pharmacologically tailored, gene-specific therapy.

References

1. Moss AJ, Schwartz PJ, Crampton RS, et al. The long QT syndrome: a prospective international study. Circulation 1985;71:17-21.
2. Moss AJ, Schwartz PJ, Crampton RS, et al. The long QT syndrome: prospective longitudinal study of 328 families. Circulation 1991;84:1136-1144.
3. Wang Q, Curran ME, Splawski I, et al. Positional cloning of a novel potassium channel gene - KVLQT1 mutations cause cardiac arrhythmias. Nat Genet 1996;12:17-23.

4. Curran ME, Splawski I, Timothy KW, et al. A molecular basis for cardiac arrhythmia: HERG mutations cause long QT syndrome. Cell 1995;80:795-803.

5. Wang Q, Shen J, Splawski I, et al. SCN5A mutations associated with an inherited cardiac arrhythmia, long QT syndrome. Cell 1995;80:805-811.

6. Splawski I, Tristani-Firouzi M, Lehmann MH, et al. Mutations in the hminK gene cause long QT syndrome and suppress I_{Ks}. Nat Genet 1997;17:338-340.

7. Abbott GW, Sesti F, Splawski I, et al. MiRP1 forms Ikr potassium channels with HERG and is associated with cardiac arrhythmia. Cell 1999;97:175-187.

8. Sanguinetti MC, Curran ME, Zou A, et al. Coassembly of KVLQT1 and minK (IsK) proteins to form cardiac Iks potassium channel. Nature 1996;384:80-83.

9. Bennett PB, Yazawa K, Makita N, et al. Molecular mechanism for an inherited cardiac arrhythmia. Nature 1995;376:683-685.

10. Moss AJ, Zareba W, Benhorin J, et al. Electrocardiographic T-wave patterns in genetically distinct forms of the hereditary long-QT syndrome. Circulation 1995;92:2929-2934.

11. Zareba W, Moss AJ, Schwartz PJ, et al. Influence of the genotype on the clinical course of the long-QT syndrome. N Engl J Med 1998;339:960-965.

12. Moss AJ, Zareba W, Hall WJ, et al. Effectiveness and limitations of beta-blocker therapy in congenital long QT syndrome. Circulation (in press).

13. Chen Q, Zhang D, Gingell RL, et al. Homozygous deletion in KVLQT1 associated with Jervell and Lange-Nielsen Syndrome. Circulation 1999;99:1344-1347.

QT SYNDROME:
ELECTROPHYSIOLOGICAL AND CLINICAL ASPECTS

Melvin M. Scheinman, M.D.

Cardiac Electrophysiology Service, Cardiology Division, University of California, San Francisco, San Francisco, CA

The congenital long QT syndrome was first recognized by Jervell and Lange-Nielsen in 1954. They described a Norwegian family[1] in whom 4 of 6 children had prolonged QT interval, congenital sensorineural hearing loss, recurrent syncope and sudden death in 3. In 1963, Romano[2] and in 1964, Ward[3] described a similar syndrome but without deafness. Over the past four decades since the initial clinical description, the molecular basis for this disorder has been unraveled and yielded an incredible link between genetic abnormalities producing specific ion channel abnormalities with plausible explanations for the lethal arrhythmias suffered by these patients. In this essay, we shall review the burgeoning literature of known pathogenetic mechanisms, clinical expression of the disorder as well as current therapy.

Ion Channel Function

The ionic currents responsible for various phases of the action potential has been well delineated. The resting potential Ik_1 is due to outward K^+ current, rapid depolarization (phase 0) is due to rapid ingress of Na^+ ions, phase 2 is caused by continued activation of L type Ca^{++} current while restoration of the action potential to baseline is due to activation of the delayed K^+ rectifier currents Ik_r and Ik_s. The Ik_s current has slower activation kinetics and its current becomes dominant with increase of the heart rate. Prolongation of the QT interval may be caused by any combination of ionic mechanisms leading to enhanced flow of inward positive ions or impaired ejection of positive ions from the cell. The known genetic abnormalities are summarized in Table 1.

It is immediately obvious that LQT_1, LQT_2, LQT_4 and JLN are due to abnormalities in K^+ ion function. Of the patients in whom specific genetic abnormalities have been identified, Ik_s (LQT_1) appears to be the most common while JLN forms are quite rare. The

From Ovsyshcher IE. *Cardiac Arrythmias and Device Therapy: Results and Perspectives for the New Century.* Armonk, NY: Futura Publishing Company, Inc., © 2000

reason for the latter is that affected individuals must inherit an abnormal gene from each parent. So, while each parent has the Romano-Ward syndrome, affected children are homozygous for KVLQT1 or KCNE1 genes. The deafness is due to the fact that Ik_S is crucial from proper endolymphatic middle ear function. It should be emphasized that KCNE1 (Mink) is a protein subunit which, when combined with KVLQT1, makes up the Ik_S channel.

Recent studies have shown links between genetic abnormalities, abnormal ionic currents and the genesis of polymorphic ventricular tachycardia. These studies have used agents which impair specific ionic function and thus tend to mimic various types of long QT syndrome. For example, Dofetilide is a pure Ik_r block which might mimic the LQT2 genetic disorder. Anthoplerin A (AP-A) block Na^+ inactivation and hence would expect to mimic LQT3 dynamics[5].

Pathogenesis of the Long QT Interval, T Wave Alternans and Polymorphous Ventricular Tachycardia

From the above, it is evident that genetic abnormalities that interfere with K^+ conductance (i.e.; LQT1, LQT2, LQT5 or JLN) will result in prolongation of the QT interval owing to impaired egress of K^+ ions hence prolonging action potential duration. On the other hand, abnormalities involving inactivation of Na^+ current would also prolong the QT interval because of continuous leakage of Na^+ ion into the cell. Alternation of the T waves has been recognized as a potential precursor to development of malignant arrhythmias. Recent elegant studies by Shimizu[6], using a perfused wedge preparation has clarified the mechanism of this finding. Perfusion of the preparation with ATX (which enhances the Na^+ current) resulted in marked prolongation of the QT interval, primarily by prolonging the action potential duration from mid-myocardial cells. With rapid pacing, action potential duration from mid-myocardial and epicardial cells alternated resulting in striking T wave alternans. Similar findings were described by El-Sherif[5] and Pastore et al[7] using an optical mapping system.

It was found that rapid pacing produced conduction block in the mid-myocardial cells and initiated ventricular fibrillation. Further understanding of the genesis of polymorphic ventricular tachycardia comes from the elegant work of El-Sherif et al[5]. They studied mongrel puppies with hearts exposed, who were instrumented with 256 to 384 plunge electrodes. In this preparation, application of Anthopleurin-A resulted in pacing induced T wave alternans followed by functional block between Epi and mid-myocardial cells and the induction of polymorphic ventricular tachycardia. The initiating impulse always arose from the endocardial surface (? Purkinje cells), tended to rotate around the more refractory M cells and then usually spontaneously terminated, similar to that observed in patients.

Clinical Manifestations
Diagnosis

The diagnosis rests largely on measurement of the QT interval from a 12 lead ECG. Lead II is usually used in an effort to avoid the confounding effects of normal low amplitude U waves best seen in the pericardial leads. The diagnosis can be made with relative certainty if the corrected QT (QTc) is ≥0.48 seconds in females and 0.47 seconds in males[8]. On the other hand, the diagnosis is unlikely in the face of QTc≤0.41 seconds in males or ≤0.43 seconds in females. Of importance is the finding (LQT1 patients) that 10% of affected individuals will have a normal QTc and 30% will have borderline values. Because the baseline QTc may not be definitive, other features should be explored, including notching of the T wave or prominent U wave. In addition, a history of exercise, emotionally triggered or startle induced syncope is commonly observed for those with LQT1 while those with LQT2 or LQT3 may have symptoms at rest or during sleep. Screening of family members is important for both establishing the diagnosis and for finding affected individuals.

Exercise stress testing may be of value, particularly for LQT1 patients since exercise may result in a less than expected decrease in the QT interval. The QT interval on a 24 hour Holter may be helpful, but it must be appreciated that the QT interval will be longer on the Holter compared to the standard ECG. Some suggests that QTc>0.50 seconds is abnormal in a Holter recording[8]. A standard invasive electrophysiologic study is of no value but measurement of monophasic action potential during infusion of epinephrine may be helpful in difficult cases. Genetic testing still remains a research tool and is only of help if a positive result is found. It should be appreciated that only 50% of affected patients will have a specific genetic abnormality found.

Electrocardiographic Manifestations

Ventricular bigeminy or any short-long short sequence preceding torsades was initially emphasized as being characteristic of acquired torsades. It has recently been emphasized that the sequence is often found for patients with the congenital long QT syndrome[9]. The pause sets up prolongation of the QT for the beat which terminates the pause, which in turn is thought to encourage initiation of early afterdepolarizations which produce ectopic ventricular complexes. These complexes occurring in a milieu of marked inhomogeneity is thought to generate episodes of torsade de pointes. T wave alternans is infrequently observed in patients with the congenital long QT syndrome but has been found to occur predominately in patients with marked prolongation of the QT interval and was associated with higher risk for cardiac events compared to those without this finding[10]. The actual pattern of torsade may vary widely. It may be manifest by alternate changes in QRS amplitude (cardiac ballet) or by obvious changes in QRS resulting in a pattern in which the apex of the QRS rotates around baseline. In patients where torsade has been recorded in the course of recording a 12 lead ECG shows that a wide variety of patterns are observed in the different leads. It is, therefore, clear that recognition of the pattern of polymorphic ventricular tachycardia is the important issue rather than any specific pattern.

Demographics and Natural History

It is estimated that one in 10,000 persons is a gene carrier and the disease causes 3,000 to 4,000 sudden deaths/year[11]. Symptoms usually appear in preteen or teenage years. Sudden death occurs in 10 to 30% of symptomatic patients. It is estimated that untreated patients have a very high mortality approaching 10%/year. Treatment with beta blockers appear to reduce mortality to less than 2%/year. The importance of prompt correct diagnosis is highlighted by the fact that 30 to 40% of the deaths occur as the first event[11].

Treatment

The mainstay for therapy of the long QT syndrome is use of beta blockers. The international long QT registry has clearly documented the efficacy of beta blocker therapy[12]. The rationale behind beta blocker therapy rests on several factors, including block of Ca^{++} ingress into the cell or failure to achieve high heart rates that may trigger lethal arrhythmias[5]. Beta blocker would appear to be especially beneficial for patients with LQT1 since these are the patients who show the least change in QT with increase in heart rate. Beta blockers would appear to be less effective for patients with LQT3 since the QT shows rapid decline with exercise[13]. There is no evidence that one beta blocker is superior to another. However, most experience has been accumulated with use of long-acting propranolol or Nadolol therapy. For patients who cannot take non-selective beta blockers, use of selective agents are indicated. If beta blockers cannot be tolerated, then trials of calcium channel blockers are appropriate since the importance of cellular Ca^{++} ingress in the initiation of torsade is well appreciated in experimental settings. There is only very limited experience in use of calcium channel blockers as chronic therapy in humans.

For patients who fail beta blocker therapy, a host of other treatments have been suggested. The first suggested was use of left cervical sympathectomy which was subsequently expanded to include removal of the left cervico-thoracic chain of ganglion. This approach rested on observations in animals of QT prolongation with either stimulation of the left cervico-sympathetic chain or by excision of the right cervical sympathetics. Left cervico-thoracic sympathectomy has been associated with a decrease in symptoms but the incidence of sudden cardiac death is still approximately 8%. Our personal experience has shown that this operation is associated with a high recurrence rate.

We first reported use of chronic pacemaker therapy for treatment of patients with the long QT syndrome in 19[15]. In our initial experience, we found that use of chronic pacing and beta blockers (combined therapy) was associated with excellent results in compliant patients. The rationale behind this therapy rested on the avoidance of pauses which often triggered episodes of torsade de pointes. In addition, we found that cardiac pacing was the only modality that resulted in chronic normalization of the QT interval for most patients with the long QT syndrome. We also appreciated that dual chambered pacing was more appropriate for these young/active individuals, both for obtaining optimal hemodynamics as well as avoidance of periods of atrioventricular block (for those with atrial based pacing systems) during vagal dominance. Use of pacemaker therapy was arranged to achieve a normal or near-normal QT interval at the lowest achievable paced rate. For adults, the paced rate was usually in the 80 to 90 range. Higher paced rates were required in children. We found that recurrence of symptoms was quite common for those who experienced pacemaker failure[15]. Our most recent studies include observations for 37 patients treated over a mean of almost 7 years[16]. We found that the failure rate in terms of recurrence of syncope and/or sudden cardiac death was approximately 20%. The high failure rate occurred even in patients totally compliant with drug therapy and with normal pacemaker function. This experience has led us to suggest that all symptomatic patients be treated with beta blockers and dual chamber pacemaker with defibrillator backup. It should be emphasized that triple therapy (as described) is required to avoid exposure of the patients to repeated shocks. In our experience, only one patient had defibrillator "storm" with 17 shocks in four hours. Similar results have been described in reports of ICDs inserted in children with the long QT syndrome[17].

Since the disease is so lethal and since sudden death may appear with minimal or no symptoms, it is our practice to initiate beta blocker therapy for asymptomatic affected family members. We also occasioned use of the pacemaker-defibrillator for all patients with syncope (not clearly associated with other causes) or sudden cardiac death.

Future Therapeutic Options
Based on the recent molecular/genetics studies, a number of very potentially promising therapies have been proposed. It should be emphasized that all such treatments are still experimental and associated with very limited follow-up. For example, K^+ loading with oral K^+ and K^+ retaining diuretics[18] or flecainide[19] for

treatment of patients with HERG genotype. Verapamil[20] or K^+ channel openers (i.e., Pinacidyl) may potentially benefit all patients with abnormal K^+ channel function[21-23]. For patients with SCNSA genotype, a Na^+ channel blocker (Mexiletine) has been shown to normalize the QT interval[24]. It should be emphasized that these suggested therapies are totally investigational and it is not known whether they will replace existing treatments.

General Recommendations

It is well to remember that episodes of torsades may be initiated by any of a number of drugs that prolong the QT interval. The patients and family should be provided with a list of drugs to avoid. These drugs include class IA and III antiarrhythmic agents, various psychotropic drugs (i.e., Thorazine, tricyclic antidepressants), antihistamines (Terfanidine, Histaminal), antibiotics (Macrolide), Antifungal agents (Ketoconazole), etc. The patient and family should be advised to check with their physician before initiating any new drug. Avoidance of electrolyte depletion, use of beverages containing K^+ during hot weather should be encouraged. We previously curtailed participation in competitive sports but in our patients with defibrillators, we have become more lenient. Competitive sports are very much part of the growing up process and restriction in this area may prove to be quite onerous for younger patients. Our own policy is evolving towards allowing even competitive athletics in patients treated with triple therapy.

Summary

Remarkable strides have been made in both understanding the fundamental abnormalities as it relates to disease pathogenesis. This disease is the first arrhythmia traced to a genetic abnormality which is responsible for a specific ion channel malfunction which is responsible for lethal arrhythmias. We await with great anticipation the further unraveling of this exciting adventure, especially as it relates to gene specific therapy for our patients.

References

1.   Jervell A, Lange-Nielsen F: Congenital deaf-mutism, functional heart disease with prolongation of the Q-T interval, and sudden death. Am Heart J 1957;54:59-68.

2.   Romano C, Gemme G, Pongiglione R: Aritmie cardiache rare dell'eta' pediatrica. II. Accessi sincopali perfibrillazione ventricolare parossistica. Clin Pediatr (Bologna) 1963;45:656-683.

3.   Ward OC. A new familial cardiac syndrome in children. J Irish Med Assoc 1964;54:103-106.

4.   Ackerman MJ: The long QT syndrome: ion channel diseases of the heart. Mayo Clinic Proceedings,1998,73(30:250-269.

5.   El-Sherif N, Chinushi M, Caref EB, et al: Electrophysiological mechanism of the characteristic electrocardiographic morphology of torsade de pointes tachyarrhythmias in the long QT syndrome. Detailed analysis of ventricular tridimensional activation patterns. Circulation 1997;96:4392-4399.

6.   Shimizu W, Antzelevitch C: Cellular and ionic basis for T-wave alternans in the long QT syndrome. Circulation, in press, 1999.

7.   Pastore JM, Girouard SD, Laruita KR, et al: Mechanism linking T-wave alternans to the genesis of cardiac fibrillation. Circulation 1999;99:1385-1394.

8.   Vincent GM, Timothy K, Leppert M, et al: The spectrum of symptoms and QT interval in carriers of the gene for the long QT syndrome. N Eng J Med 1992;;327:846-852.

9.   Molnar J, Zhang F, Weiss J et al: Diurnal pattern of QTc interval: How long is prolonged? Possible relation to circadian triggers of cardiovascular events. J Am Cool Cordial 1996;27:76-83.

10.   Moss JA: Long QT syndrome. In Podrid PJ, Kowey PR (eds): Cardiac Arrhythmias. Mechanisms, Diagnosis, and Management. Baltimore, MD, Williams and Wilkins, 1995, pp 1110-1120.

11.   Vincent GM: The molecular basis of the long QT syndrome: Genes causing fainting and sudden death. Ann Rev Med 1998;49:263-274.

12.   Vincent GM, Fox J, Zhang L, et al: Beta-blockers markedly reduce risk and syncope in KVLQT1 long QT patients. Circulation 1996;94(Suppl. 1):I-204.

13.   Schwartz PJ, Priori SG, Locati EH, et al: Long QT syndrome patients with mutations of the SCN5A and HERG genes have differential responses to Na+ channel blockade and to increases in heart rate. Implications for gene-specific therapy. Circulation 1995;92:3381-3386.

14.   Weitkamp L, Vincent M, Garson A, et al: The long QT syndrome: prospective longitudinal study of 328 families. Circulation 1991;84:1136-44.

15.   Eldar M, Griffin JC, Abbott JA, et al: Permanent cardiac pacing in patients with the long QT syndrome. J Am Coll Cardiol 1987;10:600-607.

16.   Dorostkar P, Eldar M, Belhassen B, et al: Long-term follow-up of patients with the long QT syndrome treated with beta blockers and chronic pacing. Circulation, in press, 1999.

17.   Groh WJ, Silka MJ, Oliver RP, et al: Use of implantable cardioverter-defibrillators in the congenital long QT syndrome. Am J Cardiol 1996;78:703-706.

18.   Compton SJ, Lux RL, Ramsey MR, et al: Genetically defined therapy of inherited long QT syndrome. Correction of abnormal repolarization by potassium. Circulation 1996;94:1018-1022.

19.   Hallman K, Carlsson L: Prevention of class III-induced proarrhythmias by flecainide in an animal model of the acquired long QT syndrome. Pharmacol Toxicol 1995;77:250-254.

20.   Shimizu W, Ohe T, Kurita T, et al: Effects of verapamil and propranolol on early after depolarizations and ventricular arrhythmias induced by epinephrine in congenital long QT syndrome. J Am Cool Cordial 1995;26:1299-309.

21.   Chinch M, Aiwa Y, H, et al: suppresses a hump on the monophasic action potential and torsade de pointes in a patient with idiopathic long QT syndrome. Jpn Heart J 1995;36:477-481.

22.   Vincent GM, Fox J, Zhang L, et al: Effects of a potassium channel   opener in KVLQT1 long QT gene carriers. J Am Coll Cardiol 1997;29:183A.

23.   Sato T, Hata Y, Yamamoto M, et al: Early after depolarizations abolished by potassium channel opener in a patient with idiopathic long QT syndrome. J Cardiovasc Electrophysiol 1995;6:279-282.

24.   Priori SG, Napolitano C, Cantu F, et al: Differential response to Na^+ channel blockade, beta-adrenergic stimulation, and rapid pacing in a cellular model mimicking the SCN5A and HERG defects present in the long QT syndrome. Circ Res 1996;78:1009-1005.

Table 1.
Romano-Ward Syndrome (autosomal dominant, normal hearing)[4]

Designation	Chromosome	Gene	Channel
LQT1	11p15.5	KVLQT1	I_{Ks}
LQT2	7q35-36	HERG	I_{Kr}
LQT3	3p21-24	SCN5A	I_{Na}
LQT4	4q25-27	--	--
LQT5	21q22.1-22.2	KCNE1 (Mink)	I_{Ks}
LQT6	--	--	--

Jervell and Lang-Nielsen

JLN1	11p15.5	KVLQT1	I_{Ks}
JLN2	2q22.1-22.2	KCNE1 (Mink)	I_{Ks}

LQTS with syndactyl ? gene

10.
LEFT ATRIAL "ISTHMUS" CONCEPT: PITFALLS IN LATERAL ACCESSORY PATHWAY ABLATION

David Luria, M.D., Jan Nemec, M.D., Paul A. Friedman, M.D.
Mayo Clinic, Rochester, MN, USA.

Introduction

A narrow "isthmus" of conduction between anatomical obstacles is a known part of many right atrial (RA) arrhythmia circuits[1]; however, recent observations have suggested the presence of a left atrial isthmus as well. In one series of four patients, local delay in coronary sinus (CS) activation was observed during left lateral accessory pathway (AP) ablation[2]. It was proposed that a narrow isthmus of tissue between left inferior pulmonary vein and mitral anulus, altered during radiofrequency (RF) energy delivery, was responsible for these findings. Further recent observations have confirmed the presence of a left atrial isthmus, and shed light on the important electrophysiologic phenomena, which may mislead the electrophysiologist in the absence of an understanding of the isthmus concept. The purpose of this report is to present these observations, and to illustrate the clinical implications of the left atrial isthmus for patients undergoing left lateral AP ablation.

Electrophysiologic Observations

Three patients were referred to the EP study due to paroxysmal supraventricular tachycardia. Two had manifest ventricular preexcitation on 12-lead ECG, consistent with the presence of a left lateral AP. During right ventricular (RV) pacing, retrograde pathway conduction with earliest activation in the lateral (one case) and posterolateral (two cases) left atrium was evident. Orthodromic tachycardia (ORT) with eccentric atrial activation was easily inducible in all cases.

RF energy delivery during RV pacing (two patients) or ORT (one patient) led to prolongation of the local ventriculoatrial (VA) interval (68.3±34 msec) at the mid/distal CS and reversal of the atrial activation sequence. **(Fig1,2).** ORT remained easily inducible in all patients. Tachycardia morphology, cycle length (CL) and His VA intervals remained unchanged, but the atrial activation changed from an eccentric to a concentric pattern in two patients in the absence of a second accessory pathway, and without repositioning of the CS catheter. **(Fig 3,4).** In the third patient, the ORT CL and the His VA interval increased along with mid/proximal CS VA interval prolongation, but the distal CS VA interval remained constant. **(Fig 5).**

From Ovsyshcher IE. *Cardiac Arrythmias and Device Therapy: Results and Perspectives for the New Century.* Armonk, NY: Futura Publishing Company, Inc., © 2000

Fig 1   **Fig 2**

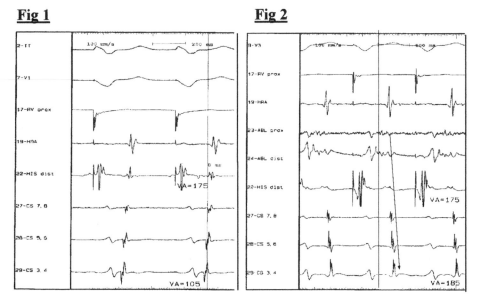

Patient 1. RV pacing before (fig1) and after (fig2) RF energy application.
Note prolongation of the local VA interval (CS recording) with a constant His VA
conduction time. Eccentric atrial activation is lost after the ablation. Earliest atrial
activation, however, remains at the site of the ABL catheter, just distal to CS 3,4.
CS 7,8 is proximal, CS 3,4 is distal.

Fig 3   **Fig 4**

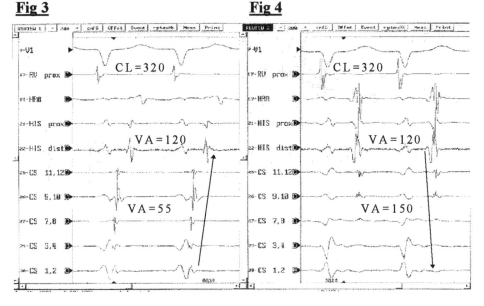

Patient 2. Electrograms at the beginning (fig 3) and at the end (fig 4) of the RF energy
application. ORT persists with constant CL and His VA interval. Note the local VA
prolongation at the mid/proximal CS with reversal of atrial activation sequence.
CS 11,12 is proximal; CS 1,2 is distal.

Fig 5.

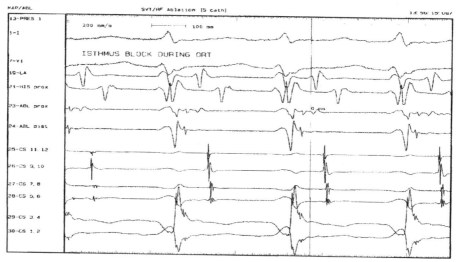

Patient 3. Reversal of mid/proximal CS activation sequence (CS 5-8/9-12) with significant VA delay after RF energy delivery.

In all cases, successful eradication of AP conduction resulted after RF ablation in a slightly more lateral/distal location than the initial lesion site.

"Isthmus" concept.

Several potential mechanisms may invoked to account for the observed EP phenomena. First, accessory pathway damage due to RF ablation may lead to local VA prolongation. However, the lack of change in tachycardia cycle length and the constant local VA interval at a distal left atrial site during RV pacing and/or ORT, exclude this possibility. Retrograde AV nodal conduction with fusion can lead to change in atrial sequence during ventricular pacing, but not during ORT. Alternatively, a second (paraseptal) AP or a Y-shaped AP with two atrial insertion sites could account for ongoing ORT with apparent concentric retrograde conduction subsequent to ablation. However, the fact that the tachycardia cycle length was unaltered, the fact that the local VA interval was unchanged, and most importantly, the successful elimination of all AP conduction at a site in close proximity to the first energy delivery exclude these alternative hypotheses. However, the concept of a narrow low left atrial isthmus of conduction, which is damaged by the first energy delivery concisely accounts for the observed phenomena. **(Fig 6).** Pacing distal to the ablation site with a multipolar catheter positioned across the left atrial "isthmus" confirmed this hypothesis in one patient. Clear evidence of local conduction block was observed. **(Fig 7).**

Fig 6

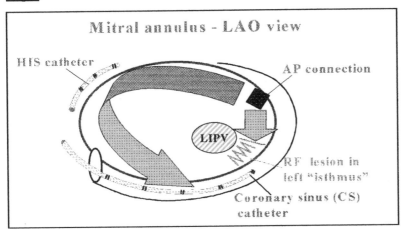

The "left atrial isthmus" concept. The presence of conduction block between the left inferior pulmonary vein (LIPV) and the mitral annulus after the first RF lesion results in a concentric atrial activation sequence (arrow) during RV pacing or ORT despite the persistence of the left lateral accessory pathway.

Fig 7

LA isthmus block.
CS 1,2 is distal, CS 11,12 is proximal.
Pacing from low lateral left atrium after isthmus block development.
CS 1,2, positioned distal (lateral) to the ablation site. Conduction proceeds from CS 1,2 to CS 5,6, where it is halted by LA isthmus block (note double potentials on CS 5,6).
A counterclockwise wavefront excites the proximal CS poles from near the septum (CS 11,12) laterally until the isthmus block is encountered again at CS 5,6, inscribing the second of electrogram of the double potentials.

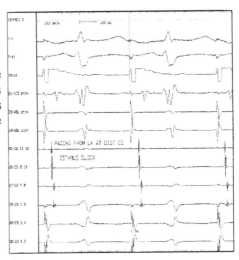

Anatomical considerations.

Anatomical obstacles have been shown to have a major role in right atrial conduction patterns and arrhythmogenesis[1]. Giving the fluoroscopically demonstrated location of the left atrial isthmus in low lateral atrium, the mitral annulus and the left inferior pulmonary vein seems to be the most fitting borders of this narrow conduction zone. **(Fig 8).** Further investigations should demonstrate if narrow and vulnerable isthmus in this area is a universal structure or specific for patients with a lateral AP.

Fig 8

Anatomy of the left atrial isthmus. Human atria in a patient who died of non cardiac causes. Dissection is performed along AV grove, with the CS open. The atria are viewed from the cardiac apex, analogous to an LAO projection. Ablation catheter is positioned through foramen ovale to he left atrial isthmus area.

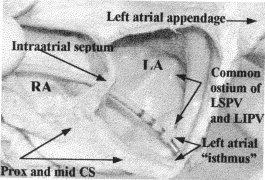

Clinical importance.

Awareness of the left atrial isthmus can prevent misinterpretation of the atrial activation sequence change during RF ablation as AP damage or a second AP conduction. The loss of eccentric conduction during RF ablation with persistent tachycardia would often suggest the presence of an additional, septal accessory pathway. However, in the presence of an isthmus block, *lateral* movement of ablation catheter led to successful AP eradication in our patients **(fig 9).**

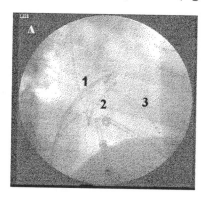
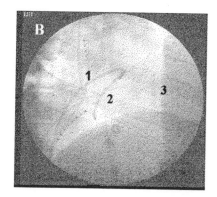

Fig 9. Two fluoroscopic images (RAO projection) demonstrating catheter positions during isthmus block (A) and successful AP ablation (B). Note small lateral (distal) movement of ablation catheter (1) from A to B position. (2)-CS catheter, (3)-RV catheter

References

1. Olgin JE, Kalman JM, Fitzpatrick AP, et al. Role of right atrial endocardial structures as barriers to conduction during human type I atrial flutter. Circulation 1995;92:1839-1848.
2. Etheridge SP, Compton SJ, Klein RC: A left side isthmus? Conduction block following single RF lesion in human left atria. Circulation 1998; 17 (suppl):A2972

11.
HOW DOES SPONTANEOUS VENTRICULAR TACHYCARDIA INITIATE: ANALYSIS OF STORED INTRACARDIAC ELECTROGRAMS

Maria Trusz-Gluza, MD, Wlodzimierz Kargul, MD,
Tadeusz Zajac, MD, Artur Filipecki, MD,
Ewa Konarska-Kuszewska, MD, Maciej Pruski, MD,
Zbigniew Michalak, MD, Krzysztof Szydlo, MD

I Department of Cardiology, Silesian University School of Medicine,
Katowice, Poland

Introduction

Historically, the mechanisms of initiation of malignant ventricular arrhythmias were usually studied by Holter or other surface electrocardiographic (ECG) monitoring or programmed ventricular stimulation. The analysis of Holter ECG registration in patients experiencing sudden cardiac death showed that frequently episodes are initiated by ventricular tachycardia degenerating to ventricular fibrillation[1,2]. In recent years dynamic development of implantable defibrillator-cardioverter (ICD) has allowed effective treatment of malignant arrhythmias[3]. The newest generation of ICD's has among its therapeutic and diagnostic options the capability to store the intracardiac electrograms from episodes of arrhythmia - this enables investigation of ventricular tachycardia or fibrillation (VT/VF) initiation mechanism. There are few publications on this subject[4-8].

The purpose of the study was to analyze the mode of initiation of ventricular tachyarrhythmia from the intracardiac electrogram registered during arrhythmic episode. Heart rate before the episode, type of initiating dysrrhythmia and type of provoked arrhythmia were assessed.

Material and methods

The study population consisted of 23 patients with implanted ICD with the possibility to store intracardiac electrogram with at least one episode of VT/VF treated by ICD. The patients were 16 to 68 years old with a mean age of 48. Sixteen of them were males (details - table I). The implanted ICD's were Biotronik Phylax 06, XM and MycroPhylax.

The episodes qualified to analysis fulfilled the following criteria:
1. The registration of the onset of ventricular tachyarrhythmia was preceded by at least 5 depolarisations of the baseline rhythm
2. The graphic analysis of RR intervals was available.

From Ovsyshcher IE. *Cardiac Arrythmias and Device Therapy: Results and Perspectives for the New Century.* Armonk, NY: Futura Publishing Company, Inc., © 2000

Table I. Characteristics of the study population

Underlying disease:	
- Ischaemic heart disease	13
- Post myocardial infarction	11
- Hypertrophic cardiomyopathy	2
- Dilative cardiomyopathy	2
- Arrhythmogenic right ventricular dysplasia	2
- Left ventricular ejection fraction <40%	10
- Arrhythmia recorded before ICD implantation:	
- Ventricular tachycardia/Ventricular fibrillation	11
- Ventricular tachycardia	8
- Ventricular fibrillation	4

The parameters assessed included:
- Type of baseline rhythm and cycle lengths preceding VT,
- Prematurity index (IP) - ratio of the coupling interval of depolarization inducing VT/VF to the preceding baseline rhythm cycle length,
- VT cycle length,
- Intra-patient reproducibility of mechanism of arrythmia initiation if at least 6 episodes in one patient were registered.

Results
The entry criteria were fulfilled in 172 episodes - from 1 to 23 per patient, mean 7.4/patient. The half of the episodes were terminated by antiarrhythmic pacing and the other 50% by electric shock. The baseline rhythm before VT/VF in 24% of the episodes showed moderate bradycardia (<60 bpm), in 23% it was between 81 and 100 bpm and in 27% of the episodes arrhythmia was preceded by sinus tachycardia.
During 63 episodes (37%) the baseline rhythm was regular, in 54 events (31%) frequent premature depolarisations were observed and in 9 episodes sequences of nonsustained VT. Only 3 episodes were initiated during atrial fibrillation and only one during antibradycardia pacing.

Table II. Analysis of the episodes initiated by "short-long-short" sequence and the others

	All episodes	„short-long-short" sequence		
		(+)	(-)	p.
	(n = 172)	(n = 52)	(n = 120)	
Preceding rhythm cycle length (ms)	796 〉 220	954 〉 232	728 〉 176	<0,001
Prematurity index	0,64 〉 0,2	0,48 〉 0,1	0,71 〉 0,2	<0,001
VT/VF cycle (ms)	326 〉 76	279 〉 52	347 〉 76	<0,001

In 52 (30%) episodes VT was preceded by a short-long-short sequence in 8 (35%) patients. Early premature beat (IP≤0.4) was found in 12 (7%) episodes in 3 patients whereas late premature beats (IP≥0.75) initiated 56 (33%) events in 11 patients. More detailed characteristics of the events are shown in table II. Episodes initiated by a short-long-short sequence had smaller IP (0.48 vs. 0.71) and shorter VT cycle length (279 ms vs. 347 ms). Slow monomorphic VT was most frequently preceded by late-coupled premature beats (IP=0.74) as opposed to the fast, usually polymorphic tachycardia (IP=0.53) - table III.

Table III. Impact of VT/VF initiation mechanism on tachycardia cycle

	VT/VF cycle		
	> 350 ms n = 74	277 - 349 ms n = 31	< 277 ms n = 67
Preceding rhythm cycle length (ms)	786 〉 195	743 〉 211	832 〉 246
Prematurity index	0,74 〉 0,15	0,66 〉 0,14	0,53 〉 0,13

Prematurity index: p<0,05 1 vs 2,   p<0,001 1 vs 3, 2 vs 3

To analyze the reproducibility of tachycardia initiation in a single patient the mean and standard deviation of IP and VT cycle were determined. Table IV shows that in the majority of patients mechanism of VT/VF initiation was stable. In 5 patients VT/VF was always induced after short-long-short sequence, in 2 other patients some episodes were also initiated by late premature beats.

Discussion

The third generation ICD not only improved the treatment of spontaneous ventricular tachyarrhythmias, but also contributed to a better understanding of arrhythmia mechanisms. The intracardiac electrogram analysis enables analysis of rhythm immediately preceding VT, initiation mechanism and last but not least effectiveness of delivered therapy[5-8]. The analyzed tachycardia episodes in our patients in 50% events were preceded by moderate tachycardia (>80 bpm) whereas only 24% were initiated during rhythm below 60 bpm. This finding suggests important contribution of adrenergic stimulation in arrhythmogenesis - similar to the data of Myerfeldt[7]. However, Roelke[6] observed more often (5-20%) the incidence of supraventricular tachyarrhythmias, especially atrial fibrillation preceding VT/VF - found only in 3 events in our population.

The intracardiac electrograms showed that initiation by R/T premature beats is very rare in patients with chronic paroxysmal ventricular arrhythmias[7]. It was also observed in our study. However, it should be stressed, that intracardiac electrogram is specially filtered to minimize T wave amplitude and improves specificity of arrhythmia detection but makes QT calculation impossible. In our series only 7% of episodes were initiated by premature beats with IP ≤ 0.4. More often VT/VF was induced by late premature beats (similarly to other investigators) or short-long-short sequence, which was recorded in 30% of events. Others estimated this sequence to be responsible for 14-25% of arrhythmic episodes[6-10]. The short-long-short sequence is known to initiate torsade de pointes[1,2] but it seems to precede other types of VT as well. In our group it was responsible for faster VT's. Since in 11 patients we registered at least 6 episodes of VT/VF we tried to assess the intrapatient reproducibility of initiating arrhythmia mechanism. Our results demonstrated that the onset was rather constant[7]. In 5 patients all episodes were initiated by a short-long-short sequence, so in some of them the elevation of antibradycardia pacing frequency smoothed heart rate variability and in further follow up prevented recurrence of arrhythmia. The presented analysis of intracardiac electrograms has some limitations[5,7,12]. In ICDs implanted in our patients local signal is recorded from a bipolar lead, thus it is difficult to differentiate ventricular from supraventricular arrhythmias as well as monomorphic from polymorphic tachycardia.

Conclusions

In patients with implanted ICD ventricular tachyarrhythmias are usually initiated by rather late premature beats and are characterized by high intrapatient reproducibility. The short-long-short sequence is a little bit less frequent but also plays an important role. Fast ventricular tachycardias are more frequently initiated by premature depolarisations with shorter coupling interval or by short-long-short sequence.

References

1. Bayes de Luna A, Guindo J, Vinolas X, et al.: Sudden cardiac death. In Moss AJ, Stern S (ed): Noninvasive Electrocardiology. London, Saunders, 1995, pp.73-91.

2. Olshausen KV, Witt T, Pop T et al.: Sudden cardiac death while wearing a Holter monitor. Am. J. Cardiol. 1991; 61:381-385.

3. Mirowski M, Reid PR, Mower MM et al.: Termination of malignant ventricular tachyarrhythmias with an implanted automatic defibrillator in human beings. N. Engl. J. Med. 1980; 303:322-324.

4. Callans DJ, Hook BG, Marchlinski FE: Use of bipolar recordings from patch - patch and rate sensing leads to distinguish ventricular tachycardia from supraventricular rhythms in patients with implantable cardioverter defibrillators. PACE 1991; 14:1917-1922.

5. Marchlinski FE, Gottlieb CD, Sarter B et al.: ICD data storage: value in arrhythmia management. PACE 1993: 16:527-534.

6. Roelke M, Garan H, McGovern BA, Ruskin JN: Analysis of the initiation of spontaneous monomorphic ventricular tachycardia by stored intracardiac electrograms. JACC 1994; 23:117-122.

7. Meyerfeldt U, Schirdewan A, Wiedemann M., et al.: The mode of onset of ventricular tachycardia. A patient - specific phenomenon. Eur. Heart J. 1997; 18:1956-1965.

8. Grubman EM, Pavri BB, Shipman T, et al.: Cardiac death and stored electrograms in patients with third - generation implantable cardioverter-defibrillators. JACC 1998; 32:1056-1063.

9. Auricchio A, Hartung W, Geller C, Klein H: Clinical relevance of stored electrograms for implantable cardioverter-defibrillators (ICD) troubleshooting and understanding of mechanisms for ventricular tachyarrhythmias. Am J. Cardiol. 1996:78 (suppl. 5A):33-41.

10. Zaim S, Zaim B, Rottman J, et al.: Characterization of spontaneous recurrent ventricular arrhythmias detected by electrogram-storing defibrillators in sudden cardiac death survivors with no inducible ventricular arrhythmias at baseline electrophysiologic testing. Am. Heart J. 1996; 132:274-279.

11. Marchlinski FE, Callans DJ, Gottlieb CD, et al.: Benefits and lessons from stored electrogram information in implantable defibrillators. J.Cardiovasc Electrophysiol. 1995; 6:832-851.

Part II.

Atrial Fibrillation, Common Aspects

CONTROL OF ATRIAL FIBRILLATION: A THEORETICAL PERSPECTIVE

Leon Glass[†], PhD, Marc Courtemanche[‡], PhD

[†]Department of Physiology,
McGill University, Montréal, QC, Canada H3G 1Y6

[‡]Institut de cardiologie de Montréal et Département de physiologie,
Université de Montréal, Montréal, QC, Canada H1T 1C8

Introduction

Atrial fibrillation (AF) is a common arrhythmia that presents various treatment options. Pharmacologic therapy[1, 2, 3] is used to maintain sinus rhythm, to control the ventricular response, or to convert AF to sinus rhythm. Ablation[4, 5] has been used to modify the atrioventricular node to control the ventricular response, to destroy ectopic foci that initiate and maintain AF, or to modify the geometry of the atria so that they no longer provide a substrate for AF. Cardioversion shocks[6] are applied through surface or intrathoracic electrodes to convert AF to sinus rhythm. Implanted dual chamber pacemakers[7] are also an effective therapy for AF and may help to maintain sinus rhythm and control the ventricular response. The many different strategies in current clinical use and the high level of research underway by drug companies, device manufacturers, and basic scientists attest to the medical and economic importance of AF, and to fact that there is a need to improve on currently available treatments for AF.

The development and analysis of mathematical models of AF appears to have played a minimal role in the development of current therapies. This relative lack of theory is curious in view of the important role that theoretical models have played in the development of current conceptual models of AF. Early experimental work[8] led to theoretical models of AF[9, 10] proposing that AF was sustained by multiple wavelets propagating through atria with heterogeneous electrical properties. Although insights from these models have shaped current understanding of AF[11], the models have not yet led to mathematically based analyses of new methods to control AF.

In this paper we describe several strategies to potentially control AF that involve detailed theoretical analyses of underlying dynamics. In Section 2, we summarize the current three main conceptual models of AF. In Section 3, we discuss control and ablation of ectopic foci. Then in Section 4, we summarize recent uses of nonlinear dynamics to control rhythms using electrical stimulation in model systems, and the initial attempts to extend these techniques to control AF. In Section 5, we discuss how realistic theoretical models of ionic currents might help to selectively design drugs to control AF.

From Ovsyshcher IE. *Cardiac Arrythmias and Device Therapy: Results and Perspectives for the New Century.* Armonk, NY: Futura Publishing Company, Inc., © 2000

2. Mechanisms of AF

AF can be associated with many different underlying mechanisms. The most appropriate therapy or method of control would depend on the particular mechanism. At the moment, three main mechanisms for AF have been proposed. Nattel et al.[12] provide an extensive historical survey and should be consulted for additional references.

Some AF is associated with an accelerated *ectopic focus* that acts as source of excitation[4, 5]. If the ectopic focus is sufficiently rapid, the atrial tissue cannot follow the excitation in a 1:1 fashion. This leads to wavebreaks at regions of slower conduction or longer refractory period. The resulting reentrant waves would be expected to circulate in the atria in a complex fashion leading to AF. Theoretical analyses in model systems have shown how rapid focal excitation can lead to the establishment of fibrillatory activity[13]. It is not necessary that the ectopic focus be continually active. Depending on the atrial substrate, a short burst or even a single ectopic beat arising from an ectopic focus might be adequate to initiate AF that is sustained by reentrant circulation[14].

AF could also be associated with a *mother reentrant wave* that acts as source of waves that break up as they propagate through the atria, a view propounded by Lewis (for an early discussion see Garrey[8]). For example the mother wave could be a typical flutter wave in the right atrium. As with AF due to an ectopic focus, once the AF is initiated, it might be sustained even if the flutter wave terminates. During electrophysiological study, AF associated with a mother wave would most likely show strong monomorphic periodic activity from some endocardial sites, and irregular disorganized activity at other sites.

Finally, AF might be associated with *multiple circulating wavelets*[8, 10]. This rhythm could be preceded by a more regular rhythm originating from an ectopic focus or a mother reentrant wave. Evidence suggests that for AF to be stably maintained, it is necessary for there to always be multiple circulating wavelets[11]. Thus, strategies that would reduce the number of circulating wavelets, might lead to termination of AF.

Even in a single patient, there might be different mechanisms present at different times. For example, some patients display flutter-fibrillation rhythms so it would be likely that during the fibrillation phase there is a mother wave present at least some of the time.

3. Control and ablation of ectopic foci

Premature atrial contractions (PACs) often initiate AF[14]. Therapies that suppress premature atrial contraction might therefore be useful to maintain sinus rhythm. However, in order to design therapies to suppress PACs it would be useful to understand their mechanisms and dynamics. Though we are not aware of careful analyses of the dynamics of PACs, there have been numerous studies of the dynamics of premature ventricular contractions (PVCs). There are many different ways to characterize PACs and PVCs including: measuring the coupling interval from the preceding beat to the premature beat, determining the frequency dependence of the premature beat on the underlying rhythm, determining the number of normal beats between the premature beats. The situation can lead to unexpected subtleties. For example, in ventricular parasystole, there is an ectopic focus that has its own fixed rhythm that competes with the intrinsic rhythm set by the sinus node, leading to a set of complex different rhythms depending on the relative frequencies of the sinus and parasystolic focus, as well as the refractory period of the ventricles. In such rhythms the time interval between PVCs depends on the phase in the sinus cycle of the preceding PVC[15]. However, not all PVCs are associated with a parasystolic focus, and PVCs can also be generated by other mechanisms such as reentrant excitation, and early and late afterdepolarizations. For the case of PACs, we anticipate a similar range of potential mechanisms. Strategies to suppress PACs would best be launched following an analysis of mechanism of PAC formation in particular patients or classes of patients. For example, from theoretical and experimental models of the effects of periodic stimulation on autonomous pacemakers, we expect that for PACs caused by an ectopic focus, it should be possible to suppress the PACs by overdrive pacing from a locus near the ectopic focus at a rate faster ($70 - 90\%$) than the ectopic frequency[16]. However such a strategy might not work for other mechanisms of PAC formation. It would be important to identify the mechanism of PACs in particular patients or particular classes of patients.

In recent years ablation has been used to successfully treat AF due to rapidly firing ectopic foci in the pulmonary veins[4, 5]. In such a situation, or in situations in which ectopic foci might be in other locations, a major issue is to locate the ectopic focus. Recent work describes a new method to locate ectopic foci by first measuring carefully the timing of excitation at three or more sites. Based on the timing differences between the arrival of excitations at the different locations, it is possible to define a triangulation algorithm that targets the ectopic focus[17]. Though the method works in idealized models, the effects of heterogeneity and complex geometry may lead to problems in clinical settings. However, if a putative location for an ectopic focus has been determined, then by resetting the focus using stimuli delivered throughout the pacemaker cycle it is possible to estimate the distance of the stimulator from the ectopic source, and to confirm when the stimulus is in the near vicinity of the source.

4. Control and Ablation of Reentrant Circuits

The basic theory for circulation of reentrant excitation in a fixed ring was first developed by Wiener and Rosenblueth[9]. Assume that the excitation travels in a fixed path of length L with a velocity v, and that θ is the refractory time. Then the period of circulation is L/v, the wavelength is $v\theta$, and a stable wave can circulate only if $L > v\theta$. However, this analysis is extremely crude since both the refractory period and the velocity decrease for waves that closely follow in the wake of a preceding excitation[10]. These additional factors lead to the possibility of instabilities in the dynamics of reentrant waves. If the parameters for propagation are fixed, then reentry in a smaller ring may lead to complex fluctuations in circulation time in which circulation times alternate in complex fashion[18]. Because such fluctuations in conduction time may precede the occurrence of local block and hence be arrhythmogenic, it may be of interest to develop methods to control them.

Advances in mathematical analyses of nonlinear systems have led to suggestion of new strategies of control that may be useful. Though the implementation may be subtle, the basic idea is simple. Though some rhythms may be complex, the systems that generate these rhythms often may allow simpler periodic motions, but these may be unstable. However, by selectively applying stimuli it is possible to stabilize the more complex rhythm.

In cardiac alternans there is a beat to beat alternation of timing or morphology of cardiac complexes. In an in vitro model of AV reentrant tachycardia consisting of the rabbit atrioventricular node and an artificial accessory pathway in which the atria are stimulated at a fixed delay after ventricular activation, alternans in the conduction time from the atria to the ventricles is observed for certain short values of the fixed delay in the artificial accessory pathway[19]. However, using a computer algorithm to subtly modify the delay, leads to a regularization of the rhythm at a value approximately equal to the mean value of conduction time during the alternans[20].

Nonlinear control techniques have also been applied to control more complex cardiac rhythms. The initial study applied stimuli to an in vitro preparation of interventricular rabbit septum that had been treated with ouabain and epinephrine to induce complex rhythms[21]. Application of the nonlinear control led to a regularization of the rhythm, but the interpretation of the mechanism underlying the regularization has been questioned[22]. Very recently, a similar algorithm has been tested clinically during AF in patients. Intracardiac electrical activity is first recorded, and an algorithm scans to the data to detect an unstable periodic orbit. Another algorithm is then used to deliver stimuli to target the dynamics to that unstable orbit. This procedure resulted in local control of atrial frequency, but not global control. The local control was superior to what could be achieved with fixed pacing or pacing using a demand pacemaker algorithm[23].

Finally, if there is a combination of flutter and AF in a single patient, then during the flutter phase, a properly timed stimulus should be capable of stopping the reentrant rhythm[8, 24]. Computer analysis might be used to identify the time segments during which there is flutter rather than AF. Alternatively, in patients with flutter-AF ablation might successfully interrupt the flutter circuit and thus reduce the incidence of AF. A recent clinical trial suggests that such a procedure may be useful in some patients with AF[25].

The above results point the way to the many different directions that can be used to control AF based on the notion of controlling or eliminating reentrant excitation using either stimulation or ablation. Nonlinear control methods could help to design new classes of pacemakers in which the timing of each stimulus is based on ongoing computations of activation. Data analysis of recordings during AF might help to identify different classes of patients thereby optimizing therapy. At the moment, the computer and pacemaker technology appear to be adequate, but we do not yet understand how to maximally design algorithms to take advantage of the computer technology.

5. Pharmacological Approaches

Antiarrhythmic drug therapy is widely prescribed for patients with AF[1, 2]. However, since antiarrhythmic agents are frequently proarrhythmic in at least some subclasses of patients[1], there are serious concerns about the long range efficacy of antiarrhythmic agents to control AF. There is clearly a need to better understand the global effects of pharmacological agents used to treat AF in order to develop improved therapeutic approaches. We are working towards developing realistic ionic models of the atrial action potential with a long term view of assessing the effects of pharmacological agents on the stability of atrial fibrillation based on theoretical mechanisms of reentrant arrhythmias.

Based on the discussion of the dynamics of reentry in Section 4, we know that factors that increase the refractory period and conduction velocity tend to destabilize reentrant excitation[26]. Because the refractory period is most often proportional to action potential duration (APD), interventions that prolong APD and speed up conduction tend to prevent sustained reentry[26]. This is thought to be the mechanism of action of drugs that decrease the likelihood of AF by prolonging APD[27]. However, many of these drugs also prolong ventricular APD, increasing the likelihood of ventricular arrhythmias through other mechanisms in certain patients[28, 29]. Thus, to better develop methods to control AF, it would be helpful to have theoretical models of atrial and ventricular tissue so that the effects of interventions can be compared in both atrial and ventricular models.

With the increased availability of electrophysiological data from human atrial samples, realistic models of the human atrial action potential (AP) have recently been developed[30, 31]. These models successfully reproduce and explain the major features of human atrial APs. The models also allow for direct manipulation of ionic channel conductances in order to mimic the action of putative, highly-specific drugs. Recent work using one such model has attempted to reproduce the electrophysiological changes associated with AF at the cellular level in order to compare the behavior of normal cells and cells that experienced AF[32]. Experiments have shown a variety of changes in atrial cells exposed to

AF, including, importantly, a decreased APD. This AF-induced remodeling of atrial cells could contribute to the observation that prolonged exposure to AF tends to stabilize the arrhythmia[33].

Since activation of potassium currents shortens the action potential, drugs that block potassium currents would prolong APD and potentially reverse AF-induced remodeling, thereby reducing the likelihood of sustaining AF. Model testing of various targets for AF drug therapy revealed that normal and AF-altered myocytes respond similarly to potassium channel blockade[32]. Since most atrial potassium channels are also present in the ventricles, prolongation of normal APD could be pro-arrhythmic. One exception, however, was observed in the response to inhibition of the ultrarapid delayed rectifier current (I_{Kur}). Applying a 90% reduction in I_{Kur} channel conductance to the model resulted in no net change in APD in normal myocytes, but resulted in a significant increase in APD of AF-altered myocytes. I_{Kur} being absent in human ventricular myocytes, the modeling results point to I_{Kur} as a promising target for the development of a non-arrhythmogenic, AF- and atrial-specific drug for the treatment of AF.

The above analysis is necessarily incomplete. Although having an accurate model of a single atrial cell indicates potential drug targets, most antiarrhythmic drugs have effects on multiple channels. Moreover, atrial tissue is heterogeneous, and there is some evidence that heterogeneity is increased under conditions of atrial fibrillation. Therefore, an accurate assessment of the effects of drug therapy using mathematical models necessarily requires models that incorporate the anatomical aspects underlying propagation in both normal and diseased tissue. Initial attempts at incorporating geometrical factors into propagation in the atria have used highly over-simplified models[34]. There is a need for more realistic models that account for both the anatomy as well as the physiology of atrial conduction in normal and diseased tissue.

6. Conclusions

AF is a serious disorder that can arise in a wide variety of different settings, and may be associated with a wide range of different mechanisms. Theoretical analysis offers the prospects of new methods for improving the control of AF: (i) computer analysis of dynamics during AF may offer insight into the mechanisms of the arrhythmia in the individual patient, thereby enabling selection of an optimal therapy; (ii) new methods for identifying and locating ectopic foci are being developed that rely on intracardiac recording of activity coupled with pacemaker protocols; (iii) a new generation of pacemakers should be able to deliver pulses based on processing of the immediatedly preceding rhythm in order to control AF or to convert AF to sinus rhythm; (iv) computer models for the propagation of the action potential in the atria should give insights into targets for drug therapy that would be useful in converting or controlling AF. Further, such models should be useful for optimally designing ablation procedures.

References

[1] Coplen SE, Antman EM, Berlin JA, et al.: Efficacy and safety of quinidine therapy for maintenance of sinus rhythm after cardioversion: A meta-analysis of randomized control trials. Circulation 1990;82:1106-1116.

[2] Ruffy R. Atrial fibrillation. In: Zipes DP, Jalife J (eds): Cardiac Electrophysiology, Philadelphia, WB Saunders, 1995, pp. 682-690.

[3] Olgin JE, Viskin S: Management of intermittent atrial fibrillation: drugs to maintain sinus rhythm. J Cardiovasc Electrophysiol 1999;10:433-441.

[4] Haissaguerre M, Marcus FI, Fischer B, et al.: Radiofrequency catheter ablation in unusual mechanisms of atrial fibrillation: Report of three cases. J Cardiovasc Electrophysiol 1994;5:743-751.

[5] Guerra PG, Lesh MD: The role of nonpharmacologic therapies for the treatment of AF. J Cardiovasc Electrophysiol 1999;10:450-460.

[6] Miller JM, Jayachandran JV, Coppes et al.: Optimal management of the patient with chronic atrial fibrillation: whom to convert? J Cardiovasc Electrophysiol 1999;10:442-449.

[7] Pollak A, Falk RH: Pacemaker therapy in patients with atrial fibrillation. Am Heart J 1993;125:824-830.

[8] Garrey WE: Auricular fibrillation. Physiol Rev 1924;4:215-250.

[9] Wiener N, Rosenblueth A: The mathematical formulation of the problem of conduction of impulses in a network of connected excitable elements, specifically in cardiac muscle. Arch Inst Cardiol Mex 1946;16:205-265.

[10] Moe GK, Rheinboldt WC, Abildskov JA: A computer model of atrial fibrillation. Am Heart J 1964;67:200-220.

[11] Allessie MA, Rensma PL, Brugada J, et al.: Pathophysiology of atrial fibrillation. In Zipes DP, Jalife J (eds): Cardiac Electrophysiology. Philadelphia, WB Saunders, 1990, pp. 548-559.

[12] Nattel S, Li D, Yue L: Basic mechanisms of atrial fibrillation: ery new insights into very old ideas. Ann Rev Physiol 2000;62:51-77.

[13] Cao JM, Qu Z, Kim YH et al.: Spatiotemporal heterogeneity in the induction of ventricular fibrillation by rapid pacing: importance of cardiac restitution properties. Circ Res 1999;84:1318-1331.

[14] Bennett MA, Pentecost BL. The pattern of onset and spontaneous cessation of atrial fibrillation in man. Circulation 1970;41:981-988.

[15] Courtemanche M, Glass L, Bélair J et al.: A circle map in a human heart. Physica 1989;40D:299-310.

[16] Zeng WZ, Courtemanche M, Sehn L, et al.: Theoretical computation of phase-locking in embryonic atrial heart cell aggregates. J Theor Biol 1990;145:225-244.

[17] K. Hall, L. Glass: Locating ectopic foci. J Cardiovasc Electrophysiol 1999;10:387-398.

[18] Courtemanche M, Glass L, Keener JP. Instabilities of a propagating pulse in a ring of excitable media. Phys Rev Lett 1993;70:2182-2185.

[19] Amellal F, Hall K, Glass L, et al.: Alternation of atrioventricular nodal conduction time during atrioventricular reentrant tachycardia: Are dual pathways necessary? J Cardiovas Electrophysiol 1996;7:943-951.

[20] Hall K, Christini DJ, Tremblay M, et al.: Dynamic control of cardiac alternans. Phys Rev Lett 1997;78:4518-4521.

[21] Garfinkel A, Spano ML, Ditto WL, et al.: Controlling cardiac chaos. Science 1992;257:1230-1235.

[22] Glass L, Zeng W. Bifurcations in flat-topped maps and the control of cardiac chaos. Int J Bif Chaos 1994;4:1061-1067.

[23] Langberg JJ, Bolmann A, McTeague K, et al.: Control of human atrial fibrillation. Int J Bif Chaos 1999; In Press.

[24] Nomura T, Glass L: Entrainment and termination of reentrant wave propagation in a periodically stimulated ring of excitable media. Phys Rev E 1996;53:6353-6360.

[25] Nabar A, Rodriguez LM, Timmermans C, et al.: Effect of right atrial isthmus ablation on the occurrence of atrial fibrillation. observations in four patient groups having type I atrial flutter with or without associated atrial fibrillation. Circulation 1999;99:1441-1445.

[26] Rensma PL, Allessie MA, Lammers WJEP, et al.: Length of excitation wave and susceptibility to reentrant atrial arrhythmias in normal conscious dogs. Circ Res 1988;62:395-410

[27] Wang Z, Pelletier LC, Talajic M, et al.: Effects of flecainide and quinidine on human atrial action potentials: role of rate-dependence and comparison with guinea pig, rabbit, and dog tissues. Circulation 1990;82:274-283

[28] Jackman WM, Clark M, Friday KJ, et al.: Ventricular tachyarrhythmias in the long QT syndromes. Med Clin North Am 1984;68:1079-1109

[29] Roden DM, Thompson KA, Hoffman BF, et al.: Clinical feature and basic mechanisms of quinidine-induced arrhythmias. J Am Coll Cardiol 1986;8:73A-78A

[30] Courtemanche M, Ramirez RJ, Nattel S. Ionic mechanisms underlying human atrial action potential properties: insights from a mathematical model. Am J Physiol 1998;275: H301-H321.

[31] Nygren A, Fiset C, Firek L, et al.: Mathematical model of an adult human atrial cell: the role of K^+ currents in repolarization. Circ Res 1998;82:63:81.

[32] Courtemanche M, Ramirez RJ, Nattel S: Ionic targets for drug-therapy and AF-induced electrical remodeling: insights from a mathematical model. Cardiovasc Res 42 (1999): 477-489.

[33] Wijffels MCEF, Kirchhof CJHJ, Dorland R, et al.: Atrial fibrillation begets atrial fibrillation: a study in awake chronically instrumented goats. Circulation 1995;92:1954-1968.

[34] Gray RA, Jalife J: Ventricular fibrillation and atrial fibrillation are two different beasts. Chaos 1998;8:65-78.

13.
SLOW DEVELOPMENT OF ATRIAL FIBRILLATION IN A TRANSVENOUSLY PACED SHEEP MODEL

Rik Willems, M.D., Hugo Ector, M.D., Ph.D., Hein Heidbüchel, M.D., Ph.D.

Department of Cardiology, University of Leuven, Leuven, Belgium

Introduction

Rapid atrial pacing induces electrophysiologic changes leading to the development of atrial fibrillation (AF) in goat[1] and dog models[2-4]. The keystone of this "electrical remodeling" is attributed to shortening and maladaptation to rate of the atrial effective refractory period (AERP). These findings introduced the concept of AF as a self-perpetuating arrhythmia: "AF begets AF"[1]. In these animal models there is a discrepancy between the slow development of AF and the time-course of the electrophysiological changes. Therefore we developed a transvenous paced sheep model of AF to study the development of electrical and hemodynamic changes and their correlation with the development of AF.

Methods

We instrumented 25 ewes with pacemakers to activate the atria at high rates. Fourteen sheep were instrumented with a pacing device capable of continuously stimulating the atria at rates > 300 bpm (6 modified pacemakers (Marathon, Intermedics®); 5 regular dual chamber pacemakers (Thera D(R), Medtronic®) with both the atrial and ventricular lead in the right atrial appendix; 3 neurostimulators (Itrel, Medtronic®)). Eleven sheep were instrumented with pacemakers (Thera D(R), Medtronic®) modified to deliver bursts of high rate atrial pacing on detection of sinus rhythm (SR). Below a ventricular rate of 120 bpm an algorithm assessing A-V synchrony was activated. SR was defined as 1/1 AV-synchrony during 4 consecutive heart cycles. On the detection of SR the pacemaker delivered a 2.5 sec burst of 42 Hz. All animals were followed for 30 weeks. Five animals died during follow-up. At regular intervals we deactivated the rapid atrial pacing and assessed the underlying rhythm. AF was considered to be

Table: Effect of rapid atrial pacing on electrical and hemodynamical parameters

parameters	baseline	1 week	3 weeks	9 weeks
n	13	13	12	5
AERP (ms)	177 ±18	124 ±19 *	120 ±12 *	111 ±9 *
PR (ms)	148 ±18	170 ±19 *	180 ±20 *†	179 ±19 *†
WeCL (ms)	259 ±25	296 ±39 *	300 ±37 *	289 ±44
CSNRT (ms)	273 ±153	358 ±151 *	480 ±174 *	596 ±184 *†
RAP (mmHg)	3.8 ±1.6	7.3 ±3.2 *	10.1 ±3.0 *†	11.6 ±2.8 *†
RVP$_{diast}$ (mmHg)	1.8 ±1.7	4.0 ±2.5 *	6.3 ±3.0 *†	6.5 ±2.5 *†

* p < 0.05 vs. baseline; † p < 0.05 vs. 1 week of rapid atrial pacing.

From Ovsyshcher IE. *Cardiac Arrythmias and Device Therapy: Results and Perspectives for the New Century.* Armonk, NY: Futura Publishing Company, Inc., © 2000

sustained if it lasted > 1 hour. In 13 animals (6 continuously paced, 7 burst-paced) an invasive electrophysiologic study was performed at baseline and at 1, 3, 6, 9 and 12 weeks of rapid atrial pacing. The AERP at a pacing cycle length (CL) of 500 ms, the sinus node recovery time (CSNRT = SNRT – basic CL), the Wenckebach CL (WeCL) and the PR-interval at a pacing CL of 500 were determined. The right atrial pressure (RAP) and right ventricular diastolic pressure (RVP_{diast}) were measured in SR and during apnea. In 8 sheep (4 in each group) at baseline, after 6 and 12 weeks of pacing an atrial angiography was performed. The distance between the tip of the atrial lead and the vena cava superior was measured. The animals were sedated with xylazine (0.2 mg/kg) and ketamine (10 mg/kg). Anesthesia was induced with halothane 5% using facemask. The sheep were intubated and ventilated with a mixture of 100% O2 and 0.5% halothane. The values reported are mean ± S.E.M.. For the analysis of the cumulative incidence of AF Kaplan-Meier survival curves with log-rank statistics were used. In the assessment of the evolution within one group we used a paired t-test. A.N.O.V.A. for repeated measurements was used for between group analyses. A two-sided p-value < 0.05 was considered statistically significant.

Results

There was a slow increase in the cumulative incidence of AF: 55% of the paced sheep had developed sustained AF after 15 weeks of pacing and 84% after 30 weeks (time-constant = 12 ±3 weeks). Chronic AF developed in 68% of the animals after 13 ±8 weeks. In contrast, AERP shortened much faster (time-constant = 3 ±1 days). After one week of pacing, it fell from 177 ±18 ms to 124 ±19 ms (p < 0.05).

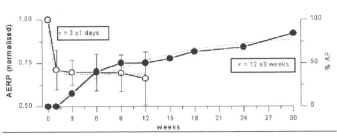

Fig. 1: Cumulative incidence of sustained AF (●), increasing slowly during rapid pacing. The dotted line shows the mono-exponential curve fitting of the "sustained" curve. It had a time-constant (τ) of 12 ±3 weeks. In contrast, the AERP (○) decayed much more rapidly with a time-constant of 3 ±1 days.

There was no further significant shortening of the AERP over time (Fig. 1). The changes in the other electrophysiologic parameters showed a somewhat slower time course and were accompanied by a increase in right atrial and ventricular pressure (Table). Continuous rapid atrial pacing was more effective in inducing AF. Sustained AF developed after 15 and 30 weeks in respectively 82% and 100% of continuously paced sheep vs. only 22% and 56% of burst-paced sheep (Kaplan-Meier log-rank analysis p < 0.05). In contrast, there was no difference between both groups concerning the rapid shortening of the AERP (Fig. 2).

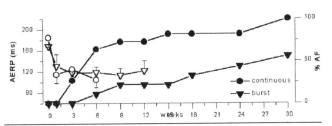

Fig. 2: Cumulative incidence of sustained AF in the continuously paced (●) vs. the burst-paced (▼) group. Continuous rapid atrial pacing was significantly more effective in inducing AF (Kaplan-Meier log-rank p < 0.05) Evolution of the AERP in the 2 pacing groups (○ continuous, △ burst atrial pacing). Analysis of variance showed no difference between the 2 pacing protocols.

There were however differences in the effects on other parameters. There was a statistical significant more pronounced effect on the PR-interval and WeCL and a trend toward the development of higher atrial pressure in the continuously paced group (p = 0.077). There was a significant enlargement of the right atrium, due to rapid atrial pacing. The distance between the tip of the atrial lead and the vena cava superior increased from 21 ±3 mm to 27 ±6 mm after 12 weeks of pacing. The effect on the atrial dimension was significantly more pronounced in the continuously paced group.

Discussion

Our results confirm that rapid atrial pacing leads to a fast shortening of AERP, already maximal after 1 week of pacing. There is however an obvious discrepancy between this fast AERP shortening and the much slower development of AF. Continuous atrial pacing was more effective in inducing AF then burst atrial pacing, contrasting with their equal effects on the AERP. This implies that other factors play a role in the development of sustained AF. Studies using rapid atrial pacing in dogs identified a slower decrease of conduction velocity and impairment of sinus node function as possible cofactors[3,4]. These findings are consistent with the lengthening of PR-interval, and with the increase in CSNRT in our sheep model. In addition we found an involvement of the AV node in atrial remodeling. These slower electrophysiologic changes on atrial conduction and nodal function corresponded better with the time course of development of AF and were more pronounced during continuous pacing. In humans AF is often the result of diseases that cause increased atrial pressure, like valvular disease, hypertrophic cardiomyopathy and hypertension[5]. Atrial stretch has been shown to facilitate by itself the induction of AF[6]. In dog models iatrogenic valvular regurgitation leads to atrial enlargement and increased susceptibility to long-lasting atrial arrhythmias[7]. Concomitantly significant histological and ultrastructural changes (hypertrophy and increased connective tissue), but no significant abnormalities of cellular electrophysiology could be demonstrated[7]. Also the persistence of AF after reverse electrical remodeling (i.e. AERP normalization), as has been shown by others[8], may indicate the importance of other changes than AERP-shortening in the development of AF. Before AF became sustained in our model we demonstrated conduction slowing and binodal dysfunction paralleled by an increase in right atrial pressure and atrial enlargement, more pronounced in the continuously paced group. These changes take more than 6 weeks to develop and may parallel the structural changes that were described in AF. Structural changes in atrial myocytes, resembling those seen in hibernating myocardium have been reported in animal models of AF[2] and took 8 to 16 weeks to develop[9].

Clinical Implications

Epidemiological series showed that only 25-33% of patients with paroxysmal AF developed permanent AF[10]. The difference in induction of AF in our 2 pacing groups also indicates that sporadic paroxysms of AF by itself may not be sufficient to initiate the spiral of "AF begets AF". In our model continuous rapid atrial activation led to atrial enlargement and the development of AF, while intermittent rapid rates were less arrhythmogenic and were not associated with an increase in atrial dimensions. This is concordant with recent echocardiographic findings that showed that chronic AF (as opposed to intermittent) was an independent predictor of left atrial size[11]. Our data suggest a causative relationship between atrial dilatation and the development of AF. Therefore, a limitation of the paroxysms of AF and a control of atrial size might be a justified therapeutic goal in the treatment of AF, without a rigorous restoration of SR being obligatory.

Conclusion

We have shown in a purely transvenously instrumented sheep model of rapid atrial pacing that fast shortening of the AERP contrasts with slow development of AF. Moreover, continuous rapid atrial pacing was more effective then burst atrial pacing in inducing AF, without a difference in effect on the AERP. We have identified slower co-factors in the inducibility of AF, being not only electrophysiologic changes (slowing of conduction, sinus- and AV-nodal dysfunction), but also a rise in atrial pressure and atrial enlargement. These changes were more pronounced in the continuously paced group. These findings may indicate that structural changes, possibly induced by the elevated pressure, are mandatory co-factors for the development of AF.

Acknowledgments

Rik Willems is a Research Assistant of the Fund for Scientific Research - Flanders. This study was supported in part by a research grant from Astra Pharmaceuticals Belgium and by Research Project nr. G.0264.98 and mandate Clinical Investigator F 6/15 DB D 8948 of the Fund for Scientific Research – Flanders.

References

1. Wijffels MC, Kirchhof CJ, Dorland R, Allessie MA: Atrial fibrillation begets atrial fibrillation. A study in awake chronically instrumented goats. Circulation 1995;92:1954-68.

2. Morillo CA, Klein GJ, Jones DL, Guiraudon CM: Chronic rapid atrial pacing. Structural, functional, and electrophysiological characteristics of a new model of sustained atrial fibrillation. Circulation 1995;91:1588-95.

3. Elvan A, Wylie K, Zipes DP: Pacing-induced chronic atrial fibrillation impairs sinus node function in dogs. Electrophysiological remodeling. Circulation 1996;94:2953-60.

4. Gaspo R, Bosch RF, Talajic M, Nattel S: Functional mechanisms underlying tachycardia-induced sustained atrial fibrillation in a chronic dog model. Circulation 1997;96:4027-35.

5. Kannel WB, Abbott RD, Savage DD, McNamara PM: Epidemiologic features of chronic atrial fibrillation: the Framingham study. NEJM 1982;306:1018-22.

6. Ravelli F, Allessie M: Effects of atrial dilatation on refractory period and vulnerability to atrial fibrillation in the isolated Langendorff-perfused rabbit heart. Circulation 1997;96:1686-95.

7. Boyden PA, Hoffman BF: The effects on atrial electrophysiology and structure of surgically induced right atrial enlargement in dogs. Circ Res 1981;49:1319-31

8. McRury ID, Mitchell MA, Haines MD: Natural history of chronic atrial fibrillation in canines: fibrillation despite reverse electrical remodeling. PACE 1997;20:1155.

9. Ausma J, Lenders MH, Mast F, et al: Time course of structural changes due to atrial fibrillation in the goat. Circulation 1998;98:I683.

10. Godfredsen J: Atrial fibrillation: course and prognosis - a follow-up study of 1212 cases. In: Kulbertus HE, Olsson SB, Schlepper M, ed. Atrial Fibrillation. AB Hässle, Mölndal (1982) 134-145.

11. Dittrich HC, Pearce LA, Asinger RW, et al: Left atrial diameter in nonvalvular atrial fibrillation: An echocardiographic study. Stroke Prevention in Atrial Fibrillation Investigators. Am Heart J 1999;137:494-9.

14

CATHETER MAPPING OF ATRIAL FIBRILLATION IN PATIENTS WITH SPONTANEOUS ATRIAL FIBRILLATION

Sanjeev Saksena, MD, FACC, FESC, Atul Prakash, MD, MRCP, Ryszard B. Krol, MD, PhD, Steven Kim, George Philip, MS

Arrhythmia & Pacemaker Service, Eastern Heart Institute, Passaic; Electrophysiology Research Foundation, Millburn; & Robert Wood Johnson School of Medicine, New Brunswick, New Jersey, U.S.A.

Introduction

Recent efforts at evaluating atrial fibrillation [AF] have provided new insights into the mechanisms of initiation of the arrhythmia. Among these have been the observations that a focal origin exists in a subgroup of patients with recurrent AF, and that periods of organized wavefront activity may exist in experimental AF.[1,2] In these studies, electrogram recordings have been restricted to a few locations, and either temporal analysis or frequency analysis of single electrograms. In experimental studies high density regional recordings and in intraoperative procedures, multiple right and left atrial regions have been examined.[3,4] However, simultaneous mapping of initiation, perpetuation and termination of AF in man has been unavailable. The absence of a simultaneous global atrial view can limit interpretation of the onset arrhythmia and its interaction with atrial substrate(s) for evolution of AF. Behavior of other atrial regions also cannot be understood in the absence of this information. We have recently described a method for simultaneous biatrial regional catheter mapping of AF in patients with spontaneous AF.[5,6] Further innovations in simultaneous mapping include the use of non-contact balloon electrodes hitherto used in monomorphic tachycardias.[7] We have recently combined these two methods for improved resolution. In this report, we describe our insights from regional catheter mapping and our early experience with combination contact and non-contact mapping.

Atrial Fibrillation Initiation

Initial studies were performed in induced AF. The earliest activation site of the first AF beat was generally in the vicinity of the triggering extrastimulus and the onset arrhythmia showed a single or two activation sequences in over 90% and three wavefronts in the remainder. These wavefronts are usually reproducible. These sites of early activation are distinct from regions of atrial conduction delay. Significant conduction delay emerged at the mid-interatrial septum, His bundle region, coronary

From Ovsyshcher IE. *Cardiac Arrythmias and Device Therapy: Results and Perspectives for the New Century.* Armonk, NY: Futura Publishing Company, Inc., © 2000

sinus ostium and distal coronary sinus recording sites with atrial premature beats. This progressive conduction delay usually becomes apparent usually at coupling intervals of <300 ms. At AF onset, the beat-to-beat activation sequence showed a single repetitive wavefront in significant proportion of patients; it showed variability ≥1 right or left atrial region during every episode of induced AF in over one-half of all patients; and both stable and changing activation sequences at different inductions were also observed in some patients. Upon AF initiation, there is relative organization of intracardiac atrial activation at the onset of induced AF despite surface electrocardiographic findings consistent with typical coarse or fine AF. Evidence suggesting reentry as the basis of the initial arrhythmia could be gleaned from the inverse relationship between the coupling interval of the extrastimulus and first AF cycle. Figure 1 shows the onset and organization of induced AF in a patient undergoing biatrial regional catheter mapping.

Mapping of Spontaneous Atrial Fibrillation

Spontaneous AF event mapping from onset to perpetuation and event termination, has been impeded in part by a lack of a global mapping technique for both atria. In addition, the occurrence of such events during electrophysiologic study is sparse in most experiences. It is impeded by administration of anesthetic or sedative drugs, the resting patient and the low event rate. Yet this examination of an AF event from initiation to termination provides critical insights as to mechanisms and management techniques that may be appropriate. Investigators have attempted to enhance yield by seeking patients with very frequent AF, provocative measures such as drug administration (isoproterenol, adenosine, etc.) or after cardioversion of spontaneous or induced sustained AF. We have found this latter technique to be of particular value. If spontaneous event rates are low, induced AF is elicited by programmed stimulation using a standardized protocol.[8] After mapping of this arrhythmia, internal or external cardioversion may be followed by early recurrences of spontaneous AF. In our experience, these episodes have similar origin to those that occur distant from any cardioversion attempt in most patients. In over 125 AF patients mapped, spontaneous AF onset, and evolution has been successfully mapped in approximately 20%.[9]

Early experience with spontaneous AF mapping is influenced by the patient population under study. Jais and coworkers demonstrate frequent origin of the triggering atrial premature contraction in the pulmonary veins in patients with paroxysmal AF.[10] However, multiple pulmonary vein origin and in a minority, other atrial sites were noted. Figure 1 shows our experience in patients with heart disease. We have noted diverse regions of origin of triggering atrial premature contractions, with left atrial sites predominating in patients without serious heart disease.

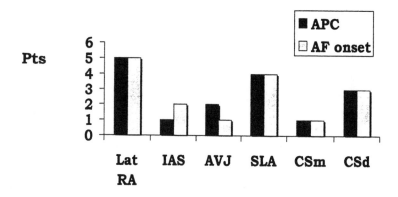

Figure 1. Location of triggering spontaneous atrial premature contraction and onset arrhythmia in patients with spontaneous AF as determined by biatrial regional catheter mapping. Abbreviations: APC = atrial premature contraction; AVJ = atrioventricular junction; CSd = distal coronary sinus; CSm = mid coronary sinus; IAS - interatrial septum; Lat RA = lateral right atrium; SLA = superior left atrium.

The onset arrhythmia for spontaneous AF is also organized and arises in the vicinity of the triggering beat as shown in Figure 2. This rapidly evolves into two or more wavefronts by the time 20 to 30 AF cycles have occurred. In this evolution, right atrial F-F cycle lengths often increase and concomitant acceleration of superior left atrial F-F cycles is noted. Emergence of delayed and fibrillatory conduction occurs at this time but this is usually absent at the onset of AF, particularly at the earliest regions of initiation of AF.[11] Spontaneous termination of AF is characterized by disappearance of such fibrillatory conduction, coalescence of activation wavefronts into one or two dominant wavefronts.[12] There may or may not be abrupt slowing at the moment of AF termination.

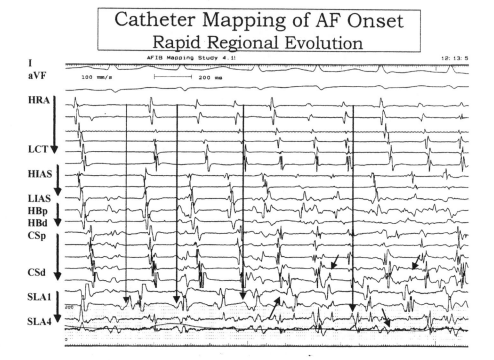

Figure 2. Onset and evolution of AF in a patient undergoing biatrial catheter mapping. Arrows represent intermediate locations between labeled recordings. Abbreviations: CSd = distal coronary sinus; CSp = proximal coronary sinus; HBd = distal His bundle; HBe = proximal His bundle; HIAS = high interatrial septum; HRA = high lateral right atrium; LCT = low lateral right atrium; LIAS = low interatrial septum; SLA1 = superior left atrium lateral; SLA4 = superior left atrium medial.

New Directions

More recently we have applied non-contact balloon mapping to examine the onset and perpetuation of AF with higher resolution in the right atrium. These studies are in progress and should help elucidate regional mechanisms. Preliminary data suggest that the onset arrhythmia is indeed in the vicinity of the triggering atrial premature contraction as indicated by contact mapping.

Conclusions

Catheter mapping of AF is now in evolution. Rapid progress is likely in the immediate future with new tools and techniques for this purpose.

References

1. Haissaguerre M, Jais P, Shah DC, et al: Spontaneous initiation of atrial fibrillation by ectopic beats originating in the pulmonary veins. N Eng J Med 1998;339:659-666.

2. Jalife J, Berenfeld O, Skanes A, et al: Mechanisms of atrial fibrillation: Mother rotor or multiple daughter wavelets or both. J Cardiovas Electrophysiol 1998;9:S2-S12.

3. Konings KTS, Kirchhof CJHJ, Smeets JRLM, et al: High density mapping of electrically induced atrial fibrillation in humans. Circulation 1994;89:1665-1680.

4. Cox JL, Canavan TE, Schuessler RB, et al: The surgical treatment of atrial fibrillation. II. Intraoperative electrophysiologic mapping and description of the electrophysiologic basis of atrial flutter and atrial fibrillation. J Thorac Cardiovasc Surg 1991;101:406-426.

5. Saksena S, Giorgberidze I, Mehra R, et al: Electrophysiology and endocardial mapping of induced atrial fibrillation in patients with spontaneous atrial fibrillation. Am J Cardiol 1999;83:187-193.

6. Saksena S, Prakash A, Krol RB, et al: Regional endocardial mapping of spontaneous and induced atrial fibrillation in patients with heart disease and refractory atrial fibrillation. Am J Cardiol 1999;84:880-889.

7. Schilling RJ, Peters NS, Davies DW: Simultaneous endocardial mapping in the human left ventricle using a non-contact catheter: comparison of contact and reconstructed electrograms during sinus rhythm. Circulation 1998;98:887-898.

8. Krol RB, Saksena S, Prakash A, et al: Prospective clinical evaluation of a programmed atrial stimulation protocol for induction of sustained atrial fibrillation and flutter. J Intervent Cardiac Electrophysiol 1999;3:19-25.

9. Prakash A, Saksena S, Krol R, et al: Simultaneous biatrial catheter mapping of the onset and perpetuation of spontaneous atrial fibrillation in man. PACE 1999;22(I):817.

10. Jais P, Haissaguerre M, Shah DC, et al: A focal source of atrial fibrillation treated by discrete radiofrequency ablation. Circulation 1997;95:572-576.

11. Saksena S, Prakash A, Krol RB, et al: Spontaneous and induced atrial fibrillation onset correlates with trigger location rather than sites of atrial conduction delay. Circulation 1999;100(I):I-653.

12. Krol RB, Prakash A, Saksena S, et al: Mapping of termination of spontaneous atrial fibrillation in humans. PACE 1999;22(II):A61.

15.
QUALITY OF LIFE IN ATRIAL FIBRILLATION

Berndt Lüderitz, MD, Susanne Herwig, MD, Werner Jung, MD

Department of Medicine - Cardiology,
University of Bonn, Bonn, Germany

Introduction
The efficacy of the therapy of atrial fibrillation has been primarily based on objective criteria such as mortality and morbidity. In addition to these objective criteria, interest has increased in recent years in the measurement of quality of life in relation to health care. Quality of life is now the new "catch phrase" in medicine. Like happiness, it is one of those terms that we all understand but for which adequate definitions do not exist. It is generally agreed that quality of life should be measured as an integral component of most trials, particularly where treatments are given with an intention to palliate or reduce symptoms (1). The term quality of life suggests an abstract and philosophical approach, but in reality most approaches used in medical contexts do not attempt to include more general notions such as life satisfaction or standard of living, and rather tend to concentrate on aspects of personal experience that might be related to health and health care (2). The incorporation of quality of life measurements in clinical studies is fortunately receiving a higher priority and often provides information that would be unobtainable by other means. It is important to distinguish the different applications of quality of life measure because instruments that have proven useful when applied in one context may be less appropriate elsewhere. A good research tool may be impractical for clinical uses. Generally, more attention has been given to the use of quality of life instruments in clinical trials than to an examination of their value in routine clinical care, medical audit, or resource allocation (1-4).

Definition of Quality of Life
Unfortunately, many trials dealing with aspects of quality of life do not assess the construct properly, or they assess only a single or limited aspect of what is really a multidimensional construct. Moreover, multidimensional endpoints such as quality of life present particular problems of design, analysis and interpretation (2). Although the concept of quality of life is inherently subjective and definitions vary, it can be assessed on the basis of health profiles including four components (5, 6, 7): physical condition, psychological well-being, social activities, and everyday activity. All four

From Ovsyshcher IE. *Cardiac Arrythmias and Device Therapy: Results and Perspectives for the New Century.* Armonk, NY: Futura Publishing Company, Inc., © 2000

dimensions can be subdivided into various aspects. For instance, physical function includes mobility and self-care, whereas the emotional dimension includes aspects such as anxiety and depression. The social dimension includes aspects such as intimacy, social support, and family contact. Each of these items can be measured in a quantitative way, hence the selection of appropriate instruments allows an extensive description of quality of life. Many instruments consist of a large number of questions in order to consider as many subscales and dimensions as possible. However, the evaluation of each question individually is not useful; it is necessary to assess quality of life scores for specific dimensions. The scores of each scale in a given instrument are summarized and expressed in a total quality of life score (6, 7, 8, 9).

Atrial fibrillation

Atrial fibrillation is a frequent and costly health care problem representing the most common arrhythmia resulting in hospital admission. Symptoms of atrial fibrillation may be caused by many factors (Table 1).

Table 1	Consequences of Atrial Fibrillation on Ventricular Function and Structure
	- Reduction of ejection fraction - Diastolic dysfunction - Elevation of filling pressure - Increase of end-systolic volume - Increase of end-diastolic volume - Reduction of cardiac output - Elevation of pulmonary artery pressure - Elevation of systemic vascular resistance - Reduction of contractile reserve - Increase in plasma levels of atrial natriuretic peptide, epinephrine, norepinephrine, aldosterone - Loss of myocytes with reactive cellular hypertrophy

The high prevalence of atrial fibrillation (2 to 4% in people over the age of 65 years) and its clinical complications, the poor efficacy of medical therapy for preventing recurrences, and dissatisfaction with alternative modes of therapy stimulated also the interest in an implantable atrial defibrillator. Two thirds of patients with atrial fibrillation report that symptoms such as fatigue, presyncope, palpitations, and dizziness significantly disrupt their lives (10) (Figure 1).

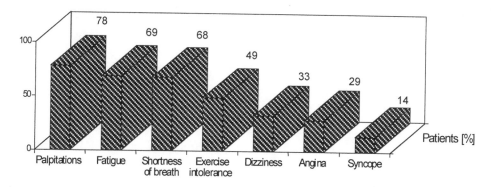

Figure 1.
Quality of life in atrial fibrillation (AF). Symptoms of 147 patients during AF (8).

Constructing Scales of Measurement

The measurement of quality of life should address each objective and subjective component that is important to members of the patient population and susceptible to being affected, positively or negatively, by interventions. In order to compare quality of life with other patient groups it is strongly recommended to use standardized instruments. Many new instruments reflect the multidimensionality of quality of life. There are several factors influencing the selection of appropriate instruments to assess quality of life (3). The first and most important issue when selecting an instrument is how well it will perform in the required situation. This can be assessed from the instruments psychometric properties. Validity and reliability are necessary for all contexts. Reliability means that all instruments must produce the same results on repeated use under the same conditions. This can be examined by test-retest reliability, although practically it may be difficult to distinguish measurement error from real changes in quality of life (2). Reliability is often assessed by examining internal reliability - the degree of agreement of items addressing equivalent concepts. Inter-rater reliability also needs to be established for interview based assessments. The validity of quality of life measures is more difficult to assess because instruments are measuring an inherently subjective phenomenon. An informal but essential approach is to examine face validity by evaluating whether instruments seem to cover the full range of relevant topics. This process may be enhanced by including people with a wide range of backgrounds in the assessment process. In addition, in depth descriptive surveys of the relevant patient group should be consulted as these provide invaluable evidence of the range of patients' experiences. Once validity has been shown for one purpose it cannot be assumed for all possible populations or applications. Measures of quality of life that can distinguish between patients at a point in time are not necessarily as sensitive to changes (responsiveness) in patients over time when repeated. Responsiveness is a measure of the association between the change in the observed score and the change in the true value of the construct. Responsiveness is a crucial requirement for most applications, especially in clinical trials. The absence of a standard against which to assess the measurement properties of a quality of life instrument is a particular problem when examining instruments sensitive to change. Although a measure may be responsive to changes in the true value of the construct, graduations in the metric of the observed score may not be adequate to reflect these changes. Sensitivity refers to the ability of the measurement to reflect true changes or differences in the true quality of life value. Problems such as an inadequate range or delineation of the response can mask important and therapeutically meaningful changes in quality of life. One of the most important areas for further development is in making quantitative change scores for quality of life more clinically meaningful. To ensure that the quality of life measure used is the most appropriate, the health problem and likely range of impacts of the treatment being investigated need to be carefully considered. Established instruments cannot be assumed to be most appropriate. One approach to improving the appropriateness of quality of life measures is to use instruments that let patients select the dimensions of most concern. Quality of life measures that are to be used routinely should be brief and simple. Brevity may mean, however, that potentially important information about patients' experiences is missed and the validity and responsiveness of shorter instruments need to be studied (2). Thus, the basic requirement of quality of life assessments are: multidimensional construct, reliability, validity, sensitivity, responsiveness, appropriateness to question or use and practical utility.

Summary
The efficacy of antiarrhythmic therapy in patients with atrial fibrillation has been based primarily on objective criteria, such as mortality and morbidity. However, therapies have also come to be evaluated on the basis of quality-of-life issues, as interest in measuring quality of life as it relates to

healthcare has piqued during recent years. Since 1948, when the World Health Organization defined health as being not only the absence of disease and infirmity but also the presence of physical, mental, and social well-being, quality-of-life parameters have become steadily more important in healthcare practice and research. Some authors have defined quality of life as an individuals' overall satisfaction with life and his general sense of well-being. Most definitions include several such broad domains as physical function, emotional state, social interaction, and somatic sensation. In some definitions two additional domains are included: personal productivity and intimacy. Personal productivity is the ability to contribute to society (eg, work or pursuit of a hobby), and intimacy includes sexual functioning as well as the ability to be intimately involved with other individuals. In an ongoing prospective study we are applying two different types of instruments questionnaires and standardized and validated instruments. The questionnaires were designed specifically to cover the following dimensions: social demographic data including age, education, occupation level, driving behavior, return to work and sexual activity. In addition, several standardized instruments are being completed by the patients at preselected times. Realizing that as quality of life is a multidimensional construct, our description of quality of life should take into account many different factors.

References

1. Slevin ML. Quality of life: philosophical question or clinical reality? Brit Med J 1992;305:466-469

2. Fitzpatrick R, Fletcher A, Gore S, et al. Quality of life measures in health care. I: Applications and issues in assessment: Brit Med J 1992;305:1074-1077

3. Fletcher A, Gore S, Jones D, et al. Quality of life in health care. II: Design, analysis, and interpretation: Brit Med J 1992;305:1145-1148

4. Spiegelhalter DJ, Gore SM, Fitzpatrick R, et al. Quality of life measures in health care. III: Resource allocation. Brit Med J 1992;305:1205-1209

5. Lüderitz B, Herwig S, Jung W. Quality of life in patients with atrial fibrillation. G Ital Cardiol 1998;28:586-589

6. Olschewski M, Schumacher M. "Lebensqualität" als Kriterium in der Therapieforschung. Intensivmed 1993;30:522-527

7. Schumacher M, Olschewski M, Schulgen G. Assessment of quality of life in clinical trials. Stat Med 1991;10:1915-1930

8.   Jung W, Lüderitz B. Quality of life in patients with atrial fibrillation. J Cardiovasc Electrophysiol 1998;9:S177-S186 (Suppl)

9.   Bubien RS, Knotts-Dolson SM, Plumb VJ, Kay GN. Effect of radiofrequency catheter ablation on health-related quality of life and activities of daily living in patients with recurrent arrhythmias. Circulation 1996;94:1585-1591.

10.   Hamer ME, Blumenthal JA, McCarthy EA, Phillips BG, Pritchett ELC. Quality-of-life assessment in patients with paroxysmal atrial fibrillation or paroxysmal supraventricular tachycardia. Am J Cardiol 1994; 74:826-829

Part III.

Atrial Fibrillation, Treatment

16.
COMBINED ANTIARRHYTHMIC THERAPY FOR THE PREVENTION OF PAROXYSMAL ATRIAL FIBRILLATION

Boris Strasberg, M.D. , Jairo Kusniec, M.D., Ronit Zabarsky, M.D.

Cardiology Department, Rabin Medical Center, Beilinson Campus, Sackler School of Medicine, Tel Aviv University, Petach Tikva/Tel Aviv.

Introduction

Even though new and promising techniques for the cure of atrial fibrillation are being evaluated, antiarrhythmic drug therapy still remains one of the main pillars in the prevention of atrial fibrillation. Despite the wide variety of drugs available, the long-term efficacy of these drugs has been quite disappointing[1].

Prospective or comparative studies of antiarrhythmic agents in the prevention of atrial fibrillation have studied only single agents at a time.[2] Drugs that slow AV nodal conduction (such as digoxin, beta blockers and calcium channel blockers) have been used only as adjuvants to slow ventricular response in case of recurrence of atrial fibrillation. No studies have been reported on the use of a combination of antiarrhythmic regimens. In this report we present our initial experience with the use of a combined antiarrhythmic regimen (class IC and III antiarrhythmic drugs according to the Vaughn-Williams classification) in the prevention of atrial fibrillation.

Material and Methods

Patients with paroxysmal atrial fibrillation who failed at least two attempts of prophylactic antiarrhythmic therapy using separately a type IC and type III antiarrhythmic drug, were recruited for this study.

Type IC agents used were propafenone (450mg to 600mg/day) or flecainide (100mg to 200mg/day). Type III agents used were sotalol (120mg to 320mg/day) or amiodarone (100mg to 200mg/day).

The combination used and the final dose of each combination drug was not controlled and was left up to the treating physician.

Patients were closely followed during the first week for the occurrence of side effects especially ECG changes (QT and QRS changes) and later on for the recurrence of atrial fibrillation. Patients with bundle branch block or significant left ventricular dysfunction were excluded.

From Ovsyshcher IE. *Cardiac Arrythmias and Device Therapy: Results and Perspectives for the New Century.* Armonk, NY: Futura Publishing Company, Inc., © 2000

Results

Eighteen patients were included, 10 women and 8 men, with ages ranging from 45 to 78 years, mean 62 years. Twelve patients had organic heart disease; hypertensive heart disease in 6; ischemic in 2, rheumatic in 4; six patients had lone atrial fibrillation.

Left ventricular function (estimated by echocardiography) was normal in all except 4 patients who had mild left ventricular dysfunction. Left atrial diameter ranged from 38 to 55mm, mean 46mm.

Twelve patients received sotalol, in combination with propafenone in 7 and in combination with flecainide in 5.

Six patients received amiodarone; in combination with propafenone in 4 and in combination with flecainide in 2.

Clinical follow-up has lasted between 4 to 20 months, mean 10 months.

Recurrences of atrial fibrillation were detected in 11 patients (61%), however amelioration of symptoms and reduction of duration of atrial fibrillation attacks permitted the continuation of the drug combination in 6 of these patients. In no case was the drug combination stopped due to side effects related to the combination.

Discussion

The tendency for recurrence of atrial fibrillation is high[1]. Treatment with antiarrhythmic drugs has decreased its recurrence but it is still far from satisfactory. All investigation up to date, studying the efficacy of antiarrhythmic drugs for the prevention of atrial fibrillation have used single agents at a time.[2] Drugs that slow conduction through the AV node (such as digoxin, beta blockers and calcium channel blockers) have been used as adjuvants to therapy but not investigated (in combination) for the prevention of atrial fibrillation. Drugs used for the prevention of atrial fibrillation are antiarrhythmic drugs of class IA and C, and type III. The combination of these drugs has been seldom reported in the literature and only in the treatment of ventricular arrhythmias. No such study has been reported for the prevention of atrial fibrillation.

In this preliminary study we tested the efficacy of the combination of antiarrhythmic drugs of class IC and III in the prevention of recurrence of atrial fibrillation. We chose not to include type IA agents because of their higher incidence of side effects and possible "QT interval complications" when given with class III antiarrhythmics. Considering that our patient population had already failed each drug individually and usually previously a type IA agent (higher risk group for recurrence of atrial fibrillation) we found that 39% of these patients responded to the drug combination. Obviously a longer observation period and a larger number of patients will determine the true usefulness of drug combination for the prevention of atrial fibrillation.

Is there a theoretical advantage for using a combination of antiarrhythmic agents? The most accepted explanation for established atrial fibrillation is the theory of reentry with multiple wavelets having a short excitable gap.[3] Reduction in the number of wavelets may terminate atrial fibrillation[4]. Increasing the wavelength for reentry can be accomplished only by prolongation of refractoriness.[5] Class III antiarrhythmic drugs prolong action potential duration and refractoriness primarily by blocking the outward potassium currents that control repolarization. Class IC antiarrhythmic drugs prolong refractoriness by blockade of sodium channels. They produce a rate-dependent increase in refractoriness. This rate accommodation of refractoriness increases the wavelength for reentry and decreases the number of circulating wavelets in the atrium. Thus, theoretically, drug combination acting through different electrophysiological channels and mechanisms may prove beneficial in the prevention of atrial fibrillation.

References

1. Levy S, Breithardt G, Campbell RWF, et al. Atrial fibrillation: current knowledge and recommendations for management. Eur Heart J 1998; 19:1294-1320
2. Costeas C, Kassotis J, Blitzer M, et al. Rhythm management in atrial fibrillation – with a primary emphasis on pharmacological therapy. PACE 1998; 21;742-752
3. Allessie MA, Konings K, Kirchhof CJHJ, et al. Electrophysiologic mechanisms of perpetuation of atrial fibrillation. Am J Cardiol 1996; 77;10A-23A
4. Wang J, Bourne GW, Wang Z, et al. Comparative mechanisms of antiarrhythmic drug action in experimental atrial fibrillation. Circulation 1993 ; 88:1030-1044
5. Grant AO. Mechanisms of atrial fibrillation and action of drugs used in its management. Am J Cardiol 1998; 82:43N-49N

17.
THE ABLATION OF ATRIAL FIBRILLATION

Boaz Avitall MD, PhD, Arvydas Urbonas MD,
Scott C. Millard BSE

The University of Illinois at Chicago, Chicago IL, USA.

Ablation of Focal paroxysmal Atrial fibrillation

It is now well established that in a subset of patients with paroxysmal Atrial Fibrillation (AF), one or several foci which initiate premature atrial activity (PACs), or recurrent runs of atrial tachycardia (AT) results in the initiation of paroxysmal AF[1]. The most intriguing aspect of this arrhythmia is that the foci were often identified to be within the pulmonary veins (PV), specifically the superior left and right PV. It is hypothesized that bursts of AT, or even PACs, may lead to atrial electrical remodeling, which in turn leads to persistent, chronic AF[1]. The clinical experience with the ablation of paroxysmal AF points to a triggering foci that initiates the runs of AT. Additional support to the hypothesis that focal activity may be the cause of chronic AF is provided by a recent publication[2]. In this report, linear lesions (LL) in the LA were directed at the regions of maximal electrical fractionated (Fx) activity which resulted in termination of the AF and unmasking of focal AT originating from PV ostium, trabeculated portions of the atrium, and LA appendage in humans. However, it is likely that the AT is a result of non-contiguous and/or transmural LL.

Paroxysmal AF ablation is now becoming a common procedure in clinical cardiac electrophysiology. The PVs have become an important site for lesion location, leading clinicians to direct the atrial mapping exclusively to the PV[3]. The trigger points of AF were found in the LSPV (12 patients), RSPV (8 patients), and both superior PVs (19 patients). From the trigger points found in the PVs (total 61 points), 18 were (30%) in the ostium of PVs and 43 inside the PVs (9 to 40 mm into the vein). After 6±3 applications of radiofrequency (RF) energy, 57 of 61 triggers were completely eliminated, and the other 4 triggers were partially eliminated. During a follow-up period of 8±2 months, 37 patients (88%) were free of symptomatic AF without any antiarrhythmic drugs. Further support of initiation and inhibition of AF induction after PV isolation has been reported in an acute AF induction protocol. Whereas pre PV isolation AF could be induced in 8 sheep, none could be induced following surgical isolation of the PVs [4].

It is now established that AT utilizes anatomical barriers such as the tricuspid ring, coronary sinus orifice, the isthmus, SVC and the IVC for the reentry circuit of type I atria flutter[5]. Although it is possible that automatic foci, unique to the PVs, is the cause of the reported clinical paroxysmal AF,

From Ovsyshcher IE. *Cardiac Arrythmias and Device Therapy: Results and Perspectives for the New Century.* Armonk, NY: Futura Publishing Company, Inc., © 2000

the structural anatomy of the PV insertion into the LA strongly supports the argument that the LA tissues spiraling deep into the PV may provide the substrate for atrial reentry arrhythmia[6,7]. If AT is persistent, it will cause atrial electrical remodeling and the initiation of AF.

Studies of AF ablation technologies and methodology:

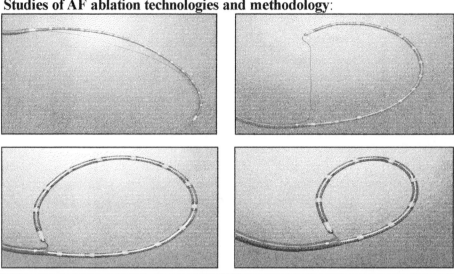

Figure 1. The catheter system: 8F with fourteen 12-mm long coil electrodes. A soft, braided pull-wire attached to the distal tip of the catheter can be retracted to deflect the catheter into loops of various sizes

In a recent publication we summarized the outcome of our evaluation[8,9] of a loop catheter (shown in Fig. 1) with 24 4-mm ring electrodes that can create loops in the atria. The electrodes can be used to record electrical activity and deliver RF power for ablation. In 33 dogs, 82 LL were generated principally in four left and right atrial positions as shown in Fig. 2. The lesions were generated using 3 power titration protocols: fixed levels, manual titration guided by local electrogram activity, and temperature-control. Bipolar activity was recorded from the 24 electrodes before, during, and after lesion generation. Data was gathered regarding lesion contiguity, transmurality, and dimensions, the changes in local electrical activity amplitude, the incidence rate of rapid impedance rises and desiccation or char formation, and rhythm outcomes. Catheter deployment requires <60 seconds. LL (12-16 cm in length and 6±2 mm wide) can be generated in 24-48 minutes without moving the catheter. Effective lesion formation can be predicted by a marked decrease in the amplitude of bipolar recordings (67±34%). Splitting or fragmentation of the electrogram and increasing pacing threshold (3.1±3.3 mV to 7.1±3.8 mV, $p<0.01$) are indicative of effective lesion formation. Impedance rises and char formation occurred at 91±12 °C. Linear lesion creation did not result in the initiation of AF; however, AT was recorded after the final lesion in 3/12 hearts. When using temperature-control, no char was noted in the LA; however, 8% of the RA burns had char. Based on these results we have concluded that the adjustable loop catheter which forces the atria to conform around the catheter is capable of producing linear, contiguous lesions up to 16 cm long with minimal effort and radiation exposure. Pacing thresholds, electrogram amplitude and character are markers of effective lesion formation. Although AF could not be induced after the ablation, sustained AT could be induced in 25% of the hearts[10]. To increase the efficiency of the ablation, a loop catheter was designed with 14x12 mm long coil electrodes 2 mm apart (Fig. 1) and equipped with two thermistors, which were positioned at the edges of each coil. The power is regulated to the maximal temperature measured between the two thermistors[10].

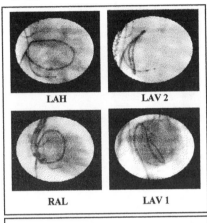

Figure 2. Loop catheter deployed in LA and RA positions. Standard HRA and CS catheters and a transesophageal echo probe are visible in some panels.

We reported this catheter system to be effective and efficient when compared to the 24X4 mm ring type electrodes[11]. Although temperature monitoring has been shown to be essential for the prevention of over-heating and char formation[12,13], we used local electrogram amplitude reduction as a marker for transmural lesion creation with the 12 mm long coil electrodes[14]. In this study, the R wave reduction of greater than 50% was a marker of transmural lesion formation.

Linear lesion efficacy and outcomes: In multiple reports we have addressed the issue of LL' efficacy and outcome. We reported that the creation of incomplete LL promotes the initiation of AT[15]. Although skipped lesions do not result in the induction of AF in the normal dog, these lesions placed in the RA resulted in the induction of an incessant type of non-overdrivable AT. Furthermore, in dogs with chronic AF induced with rapid pacing, LL in both atria resulted in 83% conversion of the AF. However in 33% of the dogs overdrivable AT was induced with burst pacing[16,17]. These results imply that lesion creation for the ablation of AF must be kept to a minimum and that the lesions have to be contiguous and transmural, terminating at a non-conductive barrier. While noncontiguous and nontransmural lesions have been shown to promote AT, the ablation of AF does not require contiguous and transmural lesions[18]. In the identification of the atrial tissues that promote AF in the rapid pacing dog model, we hypothesized that LL placed at regions of maximal Fx activity will cause generalized changes in the rate and character of the AF. These lesions would eventually lead to the termination of AF, and imply localized dominance of these regions. In dogs with chronic AF induced by the rapid pacing, atrial mapping and linear contiguous lesions were placed in the regions of maximal Fx activity. The heterogeneity of localized electrical activity was divided into 5 types: 1) NSR or AT, 2) High voltage (HV) AF no base line Fx activity, 3) Low voltage (LV) AF no Fx activity, 4) HV Fx activity, or 5) LV Fx activity. In these dogs, LA lesions connecting the PV and the mitral valve were associated with sudden termination of local electrical activity of Types 5 to 1 and were regionalized to the PV. In the

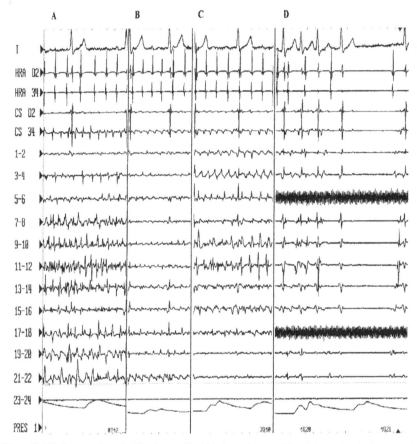

Figure 3. This is a recording of a 24-pole recording/ablation catheter positioned above the mitral valve and under the PVs.
- **A.** The electrical activity is continuous and Fx, especially in electrodes 7-14, which is under the left superior PV, HRA and CS organized
- **B.** After completion of the LA sub-PV lesion, the amplitude of the electrical activity decreased.
- **C.** The catheter was then placed in a vertical position bisecting the roof of the atria and showing highly fractionated activity in electrodes 13-18
- **D.** The Afib fractionated activity decreased and converted to discrete electrogram activity followed by NSR during RF delivery to electrodes 17.

remaining dog, a lesion anterior to the sub PV changed the local electrical activity from Type 5 to 3. Based on this study we can conclude that regionalized LL targeted at Fx localized recorded activity cause global changes in AF electrical activity, which lead to the termination of AF (example of AF termination during LA linear lesion shown in Fig. 3). This finding implies localized dominance in driving the AF (usually type 5) for these regions. Thus, the identification of highly Fx local activity provides a mappable target for regionalized ablation, the majority of which is under the PVs[19]. The Fx activity that was recorded in the dog model was found to be similar to the activity that in humans with AF whose local atrial electrical activity was mapped prior to mitral valve replacement and the creation of the MAZE operation for the treatment of chronic AF [20,21].

Chronic outcome of AF ablation in the rapid pacing dog model. A study of 29 dogs was conducted whereby spontaneous AF was established 6 months prior to ablation and further monitoring continued 6 months after the ablation. In 7/29 (24%) the AF was converted to NSR with lesions which were only placed in the left (6/7) or (1/7) right atria. In 4/7, the rhythm was converted to AT and in 2/7 only one lesion was needed to convert the AF. In 26/29 dogs the AF was converted to NSR or to overdrivable AT.

Only 3 dogs could not be converted with LL in both atria (7%). The number of lesions that were placed until AF rhythm conversion to either NSR or AT was 5±2 lesions. In 15/21 (73%) dogs LA LL resulted in AF conversion to atria tachycardia and only 6/21 (27%) RA lesion resulted in the conversion of the AF to AT. The conversion rate to either NSR or AT was similar with the use of 4-mm rings (92%) and 12-mm coil electrodes (87%). However, acutely, the 12-mm coil electrode multi-electrode loop catheter design is more likely to convert the AF to AT (60%) vs. 4-mm ring (42%), and similar differences were noted with the non-conversion. Only 5 dogs post 4-mm ring loop catheter ablations were followed for 6 months, and all (100%) were in NSR at the terminal study. Of the 10 dogs post 12-mm coil loop catheter ablation 7/10 (70%) were in NSR: one in overdrivable AT (10%), one in sustained AT (10%) and one in AF (10%). The 6 month combined chronic rhythm outcome was 80% in NSR, and 7% (one dog) in each of the other rhythm states.

The linear lesion location and conversion: Of the 26 dogs that were converted from AF, 12 had LA vertical and sub-PV lesions (connecting the mitral valve ring to the dome of the atria in the anterior posterior position), and 5 only had LA horizontal type lesions (encircling the PVs above the mitral ring). Nine had RA lesions that resulted in conversions: one RA isthmus, and 8 RA loop connecting the tricuspid valve anteriorly to the RA appendage, SVC, and SVC to IVC[22].

AF prevention: More recently we investigated whether linear atrial lesions provide protection from AF in two sets of dogs. One group (7 dogs, 35±3 kg) previously had chronic AF due to rapid atrial pacing, but was converted to NSR after the creation of LL. This group is referred to as "AF" dogs. The other group (5 dogs, 30±4 kg) included "Normal" dogs in NSR in which LL have been created. Rapid-pacing pacemakers were implanted in 7 mongrel dogs. Rapid atrial pacing was maintained for 56±9 days. Spontaneous sustained AF was recorded after 21±8 days. The dogs maintained spontaneous AF for 178±64 days. Creation of LL was performed in both groups of dogs using a loop catheter with 14X12-mm coil electrodes capable of creating expanding loops. RF power was titrated with automatic temperature control to attain an average target temperature of 70° C for 60 seconds. In the 7 AF dogs NSR was attained after 5±2 lesions were placed in LA and 2±1 in RA. In 5 Normal dogs LL were placed in the LA (3±1) and RA (2±1) using the loop catheter. Post ablation rhythm status was monitored weekly. After 6 months of recovery, arrhythmia inducibility was tested with burst pacing (10 times at 50 msec cycle length for 5 sec).

In the AF group: after the termination of burst pacing, 2 dogs remained in NSR, 4 dogs exhibited AT, and 1 dog had nonsustained AF.

In the Normal dogs: a run of nonsustained AT was induced in 1 dog. RA rapid pacing at 400 B/M was initiated in both groups for 33 ±7 days. Rhythm was evaluated daily during rapid pacing and 2 weeks after the pacemaker was turned off. After 5±1 weeks of repacing rapidly, AF and AT were induced in all the dogs. Within 3 days of cessation of pacing, none of the Normal dogs were in AF and 2 of the AF group remained in AF. Within 2 weeks, all of the Normal dogs returned to NSR and 1 dog from the AF group remained in AF. Based on the result from this study it was concluded that rapid pacing induced sustained AF in all paced dogs within 1 month of rapid pacing without the LL. The LL were highly effective in ablating the AF in this model. During the 6 months of post LL recovery, no AF was recorded in both groups. In the AF group, after burst pacing for 5 seconds (10 times) NSR returned immediately in 2/7, and in 4/7 AT was induced, and only 1/7 had sustained AF. In the AF dogs, after 4 weeks of rapid re-pacing only 2/7 had sustained AF following linear lesion placement. LL in the LA and RA prevented the re-initiation of sustained AF in all of the NSR dogs. Only one NSR dog had non-sustained AT. LL did not prevent induction of AF in both sets of dogs as a result of rapid pacing but resulted in SHORT LIVED (1-2 weeks) AF and AT. It is concluded that LL may not protect the atria from the initiation of AF as a result of rapid atrial pacing or a similar offensive stimulus. However, once the stimulus is terminated, there is a conversion from AF back to NSR or AT [23].

Studies of LA mechanical function: Though the primary goal of RF ablation of AF is to achieve NSR, the restoration of LA mechanical function is an important secondary goal. We have evaluated the LA mechanical function pre and post linear lesion creation using standard transthoracic echocardiography and pulsed Doppler techniques. Two groups of 6 dogs were studied: 1) Normal = healthy dogs in NSR and 2) AF = dogs with chronic AF for 6 months due to rapid atrial pacing for 57±14 days. In both groups, long LL were created in the LA and RA with an expanding loop catheter. Rhythm: NSR was restored with LL in the 6 AF dogs. In 10/12 dogs overdriveable reentry type AT was inducible after ablation. However, all dogs maintained NSR 6 months post ablation.

LV and valvular function: LV function was preserved in both sets of dogs. Moderate mitral regurgitation was present in 50% of the AF dogs before ablation. At 6 months post ablation 2 of 5 AF dogs had only mild MR.

LA systolic area: LA systolic area was significantly larger before ablation in the AF group (12 ± 1.7 vs. 10 ± 1.3 cm^2, $p<0.032$). The atria decreased in size and reached a plateau within 2 months post ablation. The atrial size was similar in both groups and was significantly smaller than before ablation.

Doppler Echocardiography: No active LA contraction was recorded in the AF group prior to conversion to NSR, but within 2 days post ablation active contraction was recorded (0.21 ± 0.24 m/s). A-wave amplitude was reduced 43% from 0.7 ± 0.2 m/s to 0.4 ± 0.08 m/s in the Normal dogs 2 days post ablation. Maximal atrial mechanical function was recorded within 2 months post ablation and was not statistically significant between the 2 groups. The equal recovery suggests that the chronic AF in this rapid pacing dog model is not a pathological injury to the atria but rather an electrical remodeling. After 6 months of recovery, there was no evidence of thrombus or intracardiac trauma.

Histopathology of the ring electrode loop catheter: The evaluation of AF ablation in this model was further extended into the histopathological characteristics of the lesions and chronic atrial function. The 4 mm ring type ablation catheter created LL that were composed of thin, dense, bead-like individual lesions protruding from both the endocardial and epicardial surfaces. These individual lesions fused into one contiguous rigid cord, which was sharply different from the surrounding tissue. The average size of each bead was 6 x 7 mm, with the maximal length of the lesion up to 16 cm. The lesions transected the atria dividing them into distinct regions, some of which were completely isolated. Histologically, the lesions were characterized by extensive cartilage formation, proliferation of connective tissue, fibrosis and the presence of chronic inflammatory cells on the epicardial site. Among these changes some interrupted areas of relatively healthy myocardium were observed. From the endocardial side, lesions were totally covered with endothelium, and there was no sign of clot formation. The long-term organization of the RF lesion includes fibrosis, extensive formation of cartilage, and proliferation of connecting tissue resulting in the formation of rigid transmural structures within the atria. Complete endothelization of lesions reduces the danger of thrombogenesis[24].

Gross and Histological of the 12mm coil electrode loop catheter: LA lesion dimensions in the AF and Normal groups included length = 19± 4, 17± 4 cm; diameter = 8± 0.9, 7± 1 mm; and total lesion area = 15± 4, 12± 3 cm^2 (p = NS between groups). A higher percentage of transmural and contiguous lesions were created in the AF dogs versus the Normal dogs (transmural = 91± 10% vs. 65± 22%; contiguous = 100±11% vs. 91±31%). Calcification was palpable in 30±24% vs. 53±37% of lesions in the AF and Normal groups, respectively. On histological exam, the lesions consisted primarily of fibrous tissue, but calcium was noted in 30-50% of the LL (Fig. 4).

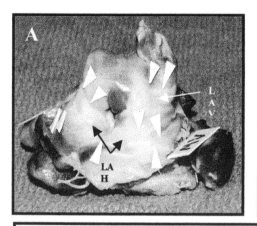
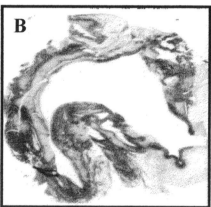

Figure 4. A. Sub PV encircling lesion (LAH) and vertical lesion bisecting the PV (LAV). B. Trichrome stain of the histological section taken from the sub PV lesion showing a contiguous and transmural fibrotic lesion.

Based on this data it was concluded: Significant acute reduction in LA mechanical activity was noted in the first week post ablation in all dogs. This finding is supportive of post ablation need for anticoagulation to prevent strokes. With this lesion set, LA mechanical activity recovery was completed 2 months post ablation, reaching 71%-80% of the pre-ablation state. These results were noted despite the lesion endocardial surface area of 12-15 cm^2 suggesting that the LA appendage, which was not ablated, may be the principal factor in the preservation of atrial contribution to transmitral flow[25-28].

In summary:

a. The loop catheter design is an effective tool to create long contiguous and transmural LL.

b. The design was modified to 12 mm coils which increased the efficiency of the system.

c. In multiple studies of the acute and chronic dog model in NSR and chronic AF we have proven that this catheter technology is capable of creating long (16-19 cm) LL and ablating AF with 83-90% efficacy rate.

d. Monitoring the local electrogram reduction of greater than 50% and temperature provide a measure of lesion contiguity and transmurality.

e. Incomplete lesions that are either nontransmural, noncontiguous, or both result in the formation of AT.

f. The most important lesions to ablate rapid pacing induced AF were LA lesions set were the total conversion to either NSR or AT occurred in 15/21 (73%), and only 6/21 (27%) RA lesion resulted in the conversion.

g. Linear lesion sets placed in both atria following the ablation of AF or in NSR were found to prevent rapid pacing induced AF from sustaining in 92% of the dogs.

h. Identification of highly Fx local electrical activity provides a mappable target for regionalized ablation, the majority of which is under the PVs.

i. Analysis of the LL 6 months later revealed that the lesions are completely endothelialized, and include fibrosis, extensive formation of cartilage, and proliferation of connecting tissue resulting in the formation of rigid transmural structures within the atria.

j. LA mechanical function revealed significant acute 43% reduction in LA mechanical activity in the first week post ablation in all dogs.

k. LA mechanical activity recovery was completed 2 months post ablation, reaching 71%-80% of the pre-ablation state, despite lesion endocardial surface area of 12-15 cm^2.

References

1. Haissaguerre M, Jais P, Shah DC, et al. Spontaneous initiation of atrial fibrillation by ectopic beats originating in the pulmonary veins. NEJM 1998; 339(10): 659-66.

2. Maloney JD, Milner L, Barold S, et al. Two-staged biatrial linear and focal ablation to restore sinus rhythm in patients with refractory chronic atrial fibrillation: procedure experience and follow-up beyond 1 year. PACE 1998; 21:2527-32.

3. Hsieh MH, Chen SA, Tai CT, et al. Double multielectrode mapping catheters facilitate RF catheter ablation of focal atrial fibrillation originating from pulmonary veins. J Cardiovasc Electrophysiol 1999; 10:136-44.

4. Fieguth HG; Wahlers T; Borst HG. Inhibition of atrial fibrillation by pulmonary vein isolation and auricular resection--experimental study in a sheep model. Eur J Cardiothorac Surg 1997; 11:714-21.

5. Cosio F, Lopez-Gil M, Arribas F, et al. Mechanisms of induction of typical and reversed atrial flutter. J Cardiovasc Electrophysiol 1998; 9: 281-91.

6. Nathan H., Eliakim M. The junction between the LA and the pulmonary veins: an anatomic study of the human heart. Circulation 1966; 34: 412-22.

7. Rexford C, Calhoun LM. The extent of cardiac muscle in the great veins of the dog. Anat Rec 1964; 150: 249-56

8. Avitall B, Gupta G, Millard S. Catheter Design for Interventional Electrophysiology. In Singer I, Barold S, Camm A (eds) : Non-pharmacological Therapy of Arrythmias for the 21st Century: The State of the Art. Armonk, NY, Futura Publishing Co, 1998.

9. Avitall B, Helms R, Koblish J, et al. The Creation of Linear Contiguous Lesions in the Atria with an Expandable Loop Catheter. JACC 1999; 33:972-84.

10. McRury ID, Panescu D, Mitchell MA, et al. Nonuniform heating during radiofrequency catheter ablation with long electrodes: monitoring the edge effect. Circulation 1997; 11: 4057-64.

11. Gupta G, Millard S, Urbonas A, et al. The Creation of Linear Lesions to Ablate Atrial Fibrillation: 12-mm Coil Electrodes vs. 4-mm Ring Electrodes. PACE 1998; 21: 57; 804.

12. Haines D. The biophysics of radiofrequency catheter ablation in the heart: The importance of temperature monitoring. PACE 1993; 16: 587-91.

13. Avitall B, Kotov A, Helms R. New Monitoring Criteria for Transmural Ablation of Atrial Tissues. Circulation 1996; 94: I-904.

14. Avitall B, Helms R, Kotov A et al. The Use of Temperature Versus Local Depolarization Amplitude to Monitor Atrial Lesion Maturation During the Creation of Linear Lesions in Both Atria. Circulation 1996; 94: I-904,

15. Avitall B, Helms R, Chiang W, Perlman B. Nonlinear Atrial Radiofrequency Lesions Are Arrhythmogenic: A Study of Skipped Lesions in the Normal Atria. Circulation 1995; 92: I-265.

16. Avitall B, Gupta G, Bharati S, Helms R, Kotov A. Atrial Fibrillation in the Chronic Dog Model: The Long Term Success and Failure. Circulation 1997; 96: I-382.

17. Avitall B, Kotov A, Helms R.W, et al. Transcatheter Ablation of Chronic Atrial Fibrillation in the Canine Rapid Atrial Pacing Model:Is the Cure Worse Than the Disease? JACC 1997; 29 (2)(Supplement A):32A.

18. Avitall B, Gupta G, Bharati S, et al. Are Transmural Contiguous Lesions Essential? Post Atrial Fibrillation Ablation: Lesion Morphology vs. Outcome. JACC 1998; 31 (2):4;367A.

19. Avitall B, Kotov A, Bharati S, et al. Mapping of Atrial Fibrillation: Directed Localized Ablation of Fractionated Local Electrical Activity Confers Conversion. Circulation 1997; 96 (8): I-382.

20. Avitall B, Hartz R, Bharati S, et al. The Correlation of Local Histology with Fractionated Local Electrical Activity During Atrial Fibrillation in

Patients Undergoing the Maze Procedure and Mitral Valve Replacement. PACE 1996; 19;725.

21. Avitall B,Bharati S,Kotov A, et al. Histopathologic Similarities Between the Human Mitral Disease Chronic Atrial Fibrillation and the Canine Rapid Pacing Model of Chronic Atrial Fibrillation. PACE 1997; 20 (2):1139.

22. Avitall B, Urbonas A, Millard S, et al. Ablation of Atrial Fibrillation in the Rapid Pacing Canine Model using a Multi-electrode Loop Catheter Ablation System: Atrial Dominance and Targets for Ablation. Circulation, submitted.

23. Avitall B, Urbonas A, Millard S, et al. Do Linear Lesion Provide Protection from Induction of Atrial Fibrillation? PACE 1999; 22 (4):893.

24. Avitall B, Kotov A, Bharati S, et al. Long Term Remodeling of the Atria After Atrial Fibrillation Ablation with Multiple Long Atrial Linear Lesions. PACE 1997;20 (2): 19;1054.

25. Avitall B, Helms R, Chiang W, et al. The Impact of Transcatheter Generated Atrial Linear Radiofrequency Lesions on Atrial Function and Contractility. PACE 1996;19:698.

26. Avitall B, Urbonas A, Gupta G, et al. Intra-atrial ultrasound Pre and Post Linear Lesions:Alterations in Atrial Mechanical Function. Circulation 98 (17): 1998.

27. Urbonas A, Urboniene D, Gupta G, et al. Time Course of Atrial Rhythm and Mechanical Recovery Following the Creation of Linear Lesions in the Left and Right Atria in Normal Dogs vs. Chronic Atrial Fibrillation Model Dogs. PACE 1998; 21 (2): 963.

28. Avitall B, Urbonas A, Urboniene D, et al The Time Course of Left Atrial Mechanical Recovery Post Linear Lesions: Normal Sinus Rhythm versus a Chronic Atrial Fibrillation Dog Model. Circulation, submitted.

18.
PATHOLOGY OF ATRIAL FIBRILLATION—ULTRASOUND VERSUS RADIOFREQUENCY

Saroja Bharati, M. D

Maurice Lev Congenital Heart and Conduction System Center, The Heart Institute for Children, Hope Children's Hospital, Christ Hospital and Medical Center, Oak Lawn, IL, University of Illinois at Chicago and Rush Medical College, Chicago, IL

Introduction

Today radiofrequency ablation is the method of choice to treat all types of cardiac arrhythmias in all age groups. This is being done without significant damage to the AV node and the AV bundle, thereby preventing the need for implantation of a permanent pacemaker.[1-15] However, procedure related complete AV block either transient or permanent may occur rarely.[16-20] Likewise, recurrence of arrhythmias have been reported.[21] In general, the quality of life has been demonstrated to improve significantly following RF ablation for all types of supraventricular arrhythmias.[14, 22-24] However, RF ablation of intractable drug resistant arrhythmias, such as atrial flutter and fibrillation remain a challenge in the clinical management of patients.[14] The problems following RF ablation for atrial flutter and/or fibrillation are: Pacemaker dependency following AV node ablation, ventricular tachycardia and sudden death. Although atrial fibrillation and atrial flutter may originate from multiple sites of both atria, selective RF ablation of arrhythmias originating from focal areas in atrial fibrillation has been attempted rarely.

In this discussion we compare the pathological findings in atrial fibrillation ablation in the chronic dog model by RF energy with the pathological findings following circumferential ablation of pulmonary vein ostia with a new ultrasound ablation catheter to see if the latter technique can be applied in the human.[25-31]

Pathology following transmural contiguous lesions in atrial fibrillation ablation by RF energy:

Pathologically, atrial fibrillation ablation by RF in the canine produces tremendous scar tissue formation with extensive cartilage formation of the ablative site. In addition, considerable fatty infiltration, focal fibrosis elsewhere in the atria, myocardial disarray and chronic inflammatory cells to a varying degree are present in and around the targeted areas.

From Ovsyshcher IE. *Cardiac Arrythmias and Device Therapy: Results and Perspectives for the New Century.* Armonk, NY: Futura Publishing Company, Inc., © 2000

Clinically, there was cardiomyopathy and congestive heart failure in the canine model with or without recurrence of atrial fibrillation in some.[25-30]

Pathology of circumferential ablation of pulmonary vein ostia with a new ultrasound catheter

Acute experiments in the canine model produces hemorrhage, necrosis and chronic inflammatory cells in and around the pulmonary venous ostia. Chronic experiments in the canine produces increase in fibrous tissue with total replacement of smooth muscle fibers by connective tissue with some increase in elastic tissue. In addition, the adjacent left atrial myocardium at its junction with the pulmonary veins reveal mild fibrosis. There is occasional mild cartilage formation of the left atrium and stenosis of the pulmonary veins with thrombosis in one.[31]

The pathological lesions following circumferential ablation of pulmonary vein ostia with an ultrasound ablation catheter in a chronic canine model has the following advantages over RF ablation of atria and/or pulmonary vein.

1.   The lesions are focal affecting mostly the targeted area.

2.   Lesions are less severe in nature.

3.   Cartilage formation if present is less severe.

4.   Thrombosis of the pulmonary veins producing stenosis— rare.

All of the above pathological features observed in a limited number of chronic canine model following circumferential ablation of pulmonary vein ostia with a new ultrasound ablation catheter suggests that this procedure may be used to ablate focal arrhythmic foci in atrial fibrillation in the human.

References

1.   Bharati S, Lev M: Pathologic Observations of Radiofrequency Catheter Ablation of Cardiac Tissue in Radiofrequency Catheter Ablation of Cardiac Arrhythmias: Basic Concepts and Clinical Applications. S.K. Stephen Huang (ed): Armonk, NY, Futura Publishing Co, 1994; pp. 41-81

2.   Huang SK, Bharati S, Graham AR, et al.: Closed chest catheter desiccation of the atrioventricular junction using radiofrequency

energy - A new method of catheter ablation. J Am Coll Cardiol 1987; 9:349-58.

3.   Huang SK, Bharati S, Lev M, et al.: Electro- physiologic and histologic observations of chronic atrioventricular block induced by closed-chest catheter desiccation with radiofrequency energy. PACE, 1987; 10:805-816.

4.   Huang SK, Graham AR, Bharati S, et al.: Short-and Long-term Effects of Transcatheter Ablation of the Coronary Sinus by Radio Frequency Energy. Circulation 1988; 78:416-427.

5.   Marcus FI, Blouin LT, Bharati S, et al.: Production of chronic first degree atrioventricular block in dogs, using closed-chest electrode catheter with radiofrequency energy - Electrophysiologic and Pathologic Correlations. Journal of Electrophysiology 1988; 2:315-326.

6.   Bharati S, Lev M: Histopathologic changes in the heart including the conduction system after catheter ablation. PACE 1989; 12:159-169.

7.   Langberg J, Bharati S, Lev M, et al.: Catheter ablation of accessory pathways using radiofrequency energy in the canine coronary sinus. JACC 1989; 13: 491-96.

8.   Ring ME, Huang SKS, Bharati S, et al.: Catheter Ablation of the Ventricular Septum With Radiofrequency Energy. American Heart Journal 1989; 117:1233-1240.

9.   Bharati S, Lev M: The Morphology of the AV Junction and Its Significance in Catheter Ablation. Editorial. PACE 1989; 12:879-882.

10. Huang SKS, Bharati S, Graham AR, et al.: Chronic Incomplete Atrioventricular Block Induced by Radiofrequency Catheter Ablation. Circulation 1989; 80:951-961.

11. Lee MA, Huang SKS, Bharati S, et al.: Transcatheter radiofrequency ablation in the canine right atrium. Journal of Interventional Cardiology 1991; 4:125-133.

12. Marcus FI, Blouin LT, Bharati S, et al.: Dissociation of Atrioventricular Conduction and Refractoriness Following Application of Radiofrequency Energy to the Canine Atrioventricular Node: Acute and Chronic Observations. PACE 1992; 15:1702-1710.

13. Gamache C, Bharati S, Lev M, et al.: Histopathologic Study Following Catheter Guided Radiofrequency Current Ablation of the Slow Pathway in a Patient with AV Nodal Reentrant Tachycardia. PACE 1994; 17:247-251.

14.   Morady, F: Radio-frequency ablation as treatment for cardiac arrhythmias. N Engl J Med 1999; 7:534-44.

15.   Pitzalis, M, Luzzi, G, Anaclerio, et. al.: Radiofrequency catheter ablation of atrio-ventricular accessory pathways. Rev Port Cardiol 1998; 17:15-22.

16.   Gaita, F, Riccardi, R, Calo, L: Importance and implications of the occurrence of AV block following radiofrequency ablation. Editorial, Heart 1998; 6:534-5.

17.   Singh, B, Sudan, D, Kaul, U: Transient complete atrioventriculr block following radiofrequency ablation of left free wall accessory pathway. J Interv Card Electrophysiol , 1998; 2:305-307.

18.   Seidl, K, Hauer, B, Zahn, R, et. al.: Unexpected complete AV block following transcatheter ablation of a left posteroseptal accessory pathway. PACE 1998; 21:2139-42.

19.   Liu, J, Dole, L: Late complete atrioventricular block complicating radiofrequency catheter ablation of a left posteroseptal accessory pathway. PACE 1998; 21:2136-2138.

20.   Elhag, O, Miller, H: Atrioventricular block occurring several months after radiofrequency ablation for the treatment of atrioventricular nodal re-entrant tachycardia. Heart 1998; 79:616-618.

21.   Vassilikos, V, Ho, SY, Wong, CY, et. al.: Recurrence of accessory pathway conduction after successful radiofrequency ablation: Histological findings. J Interv Card Electrophysiol 1997; 4:311-315.

22.   Manolis, A, Katsivas, A, Lazaris, E, Vassilopoulos, C, Louvros, N: Ventricular performance and quality of life in patients who underwent radiofrequency AV junction ablation and permanent pacemaker implantation due to medically refractory atrial tachyarrhythmias. J Interv Card Electrophysiol 1998; 2:71-76.

23.   Anselme, F, Saoudi, N, Poty, et. al.: Radiofrequency catheter ablation of common atrial flutter:significance of palpitations and quality-of-life evaluation in patients with proven isthmus block. Circulation 1999; 4:534-40.

24.   Wellens, H: Catheter ablation of cardiac arrhythmias. Editorial, Circulation 1999; 99:195-197.

25.   Avitall B. Kotov A, Bharati S et. al.: Transcatheter ablation of chronic atrial fibrillation in the canine rapid atrial pacing model: Is the cure worse than the disease? (Abstract) J Am Coll Cardiol 1997; 29:A-32A.

26.   Kotov A, Bharati S, Helms RW: The chronic atrial fibrillation canine model: A new approach to increase yield and efficiency. (Abstract) J Am Coll Cardiol 1997; 29:471A.

27.   Avitall B, Kotov A, Bharati S, et. al. : Long Term Remodeling of the Atria After Atrial Fibrillation Ablation with Multiple Long Atrial Linear Lesions. (Abstract) PACE 1997; 20:1054.

28.   Avitall B,, Gupta GN, Bharati S, et. al. : Atrial Fibrillation Ablation in the Chronic Dog Model: The Long Term Success and Failure. (Abstract) Circulation 1997; 96:282.

29.   Avitall B, Kotov A, Bharati S, et. al.: Mapping of Atrial Fibrillation: Directed Localized Ablation of Fractionated Local Electrical Activity Confers Conversion. (Abstract) Circulation 1997; 96: I-382.

30.   Avitall B, Gupta GN, Bharati S, et. al.: Are Transmural Contiguous Lesions Essential? Post Atrial Fibrillation Ablation: Lesion Morphology vs. Outcome. (Abstract) J Am Coll Cardiol 1998; 31:367A-368A.

31.   Wilber, DJ, Arruda, M, Bharati, S, et al.: Circumferential Ablation of Pulmonary Vein Ostia with an Ultrasound Ablation Catheter: Acute and Chronic Studies in a Canine Model. (Abstract) Circulation 1999, 100: I-373.

19.

TEMPORARY INTERNAL ATRIAL DEFIBRILLATION IN PATIENTS WITH AF: CONCLUSIONS FROM THE USE OF THE LATEST TECHNOLOGY.

Panos E. Vardas, MD, PhD, Emmanuel M. Kanoupakis MD, Emmanuel G. Manios, MD.

Cardiology Department, University Hospital, University of Crete, Heraklion, Greece.

Introduction

Atrial fibrillation is an arrhythmia associated with more hospital admissions than any other cardiac disorder. Its prevalence in the general population is approximately 2 %, with incidence increasing with advancing age, reaching 10 % in patients over 70[1,2]. Generally, atrial fibrillation is a poorly tolerated disorder due to the unpleasant side effects like feelings of tachycardia or irregularity. Reduced ventricular filling as a result of loss of atrial contraction may result in fatigue and reduced exercise tolerance[3]. It is also known that high, irregular ventricular rate can lead progressively to the development of tachycardiomyopathy with symptoms and signs of heart failure[4]. Beyond the haemodynamic results, atrial fibrillation is one of the most usual causes of the creation of thromboembolic events[5]. Specifically, the danger is five-fold in subjects with non rheumatic atrial fibrillation and eighteen - fold in the rheumatic group[6]. Therefore, notwithstanding the reservations which have been registered from time to time, with reference to the restoration of this frequent arrhythmia, all the aforementioned important health risks confirm the need for restoration of sinus rhythm.

For years anti-arrhythmic medication has formed the basic therapeutic approach to this aim. The efficacy rate of restoration from atrial fibrillation to sinus rhythm is between 40 and 70 %[7-11]. Apart from this, the problems which arise during their use are normally the undesirable side effects, with that of the increased risk of proarrhythmia as first and foremost[12].

The next step in converting the arrhythmia is electrical defibrillation. In 1962 Lown et al first examined the method in which shocks are delivered transthoracically in an attempt to defibrillate the atria[13]. Using an electrical charge ranging from 100 - 360 Joules, the external cardioversion has a success rate of 61 - 90%.

For those patients for whom external defibrillation of atrial fibrillation had failed and medications were unable to make arrhythmia

From Ovsyshcher IE. *Cardiac Arrythmias and Device Therapy: Results and Perspectives for the New Century.* Armonk, NY: Futura Publishing Company, Inc., © 2000

bearable, new alternative techniques based on catheters which allow internal cardioversion of atrial fibrillation have been developed in recent years, with greater effectiveness and safety.

Animal studies

Mirowski and Mower performed the earliest studies on internal atrial defibrillation in 1974[14]. This and other reports probed the feasibility of catheter based atrial defibrillation in animal models[15-17]. Using shocks delivered between the right atrium and a skin patch or endocavitary shocks with energies less than 5 J cardioversion was achieved, with a high success rate. Cooper et al[18] systematically evaluated various electrode configurations and shock waveforms in the sheep model of atrial fibrillation, suggesting that an electrode configuration that encompasses both the right and left atrium will have lower defibrillation thresholds. Biphasic shocks were delivered between the right atrial appendage and the coronary sinus, and cardioversion was achieved with thresholds of 1.4 ± 0.3 J.

Human studies

Early studies in humans with transvenous leads were less optimistic. Nathan et al[19] suggested that transvenous cardioversion of various supraventricular arrhythmias would not have a great success rate despite considerable discomfort with the shock. Levy et al[20] described a method of high energy transvenous atrial defibrillation in humans, delivering shocks between a proximal pole of a catheter in the right atrium and a back plate. They successfully defibrillated 9 out of 10 patients with atrial fibrillation, resistant to external electrical cardioversion and similar results were reported by Kumagai et al[21].

In 1992, the internal cardioversion of atrial fibrillation began to gain an advantage as, in a randomised trial which compared classical external atrial defibrillation with 300 - 360 J to internal atrial defibrillation with 200 - 300 J revealed success rates of 67 % and 91 % respectively[22]. In addition to being acutely more efficacious, internal cardioversion can also convert patients in whom external cardioversion has failed.

Internal low - energy cardioversion

Although these studies indicated that catheter based atrial defibrillation is feasible in humans, they did not establish thresholds, relatively well- tolerated by patients, for achieving defibrillation. It was however, already known from the 1980's in experimental models[15,16], that the restoration of atrial fibrillation is possible with low energy levels, if the electrical field is closer to, or within, the atria. So, for example, less than 1 J delivered between paddle electrodes on the left and right atrial epicardial surfaces were enough for the restoration of patients with atrial fibrillation induced artificially during cardiopulmonary bypass[23].

Alt et al[24] were among the first who applied the intracardiac low-energy atrial defibrillation in 14 patients with substantially enlarged atria and a history of persistent atrial fibrillation. With the one catheter in the right atrium and the other in coronary sinus or in the pulmonary artery, the average energy, that was used was 3.7 ± 1.7 J and the success rate was 91 %. Extremely encouraging was the fact that internal atrial defibrillation proved effective in patients with chronic atrial fibrillation, who had been resistant to external high energy cardioversion[25-28]. These results were confirmed in a large prospective study which compared the low-energy intracardiac cardioversion and conventional external cardioversion in 187 consecutive patients with chronic atrial fibrillation and the restoration rate was 93% and 79% respectively with mean energy for successful cardioversion 5.8 ± 3.2 J for the internal and 313 ± 71 J for the external cardioversion group[29].

Critical factors related to the efficacy of temporary internal atrial defibrillation seem to be electrode configuration. According to the critical mass hypothesis, the most effective electrode system would be one that is able to encompass the most fibrillation tissue between the electrodes. The creation of an homogenous electrical field which embraces both atria can allow the application of energy to the right atrium and near the left atrium whether in the coronary sinus or in the left pulmonary artery and should result in increased myocardial field strength and decreased energy loss. This could also explain something that has been noticed in various studies i.e. that the application of high or low energy between the heart and the skin or between electrodes that do not include the left atrium does not have especially good efficacy rates. In addition to this, the specific electrode configuration also faces other kinds of problems like, for example, those encountered in obese patients or patients with hyperextension of the lungs and thorax, where the increased transthoracic resistance leads to unsuccessful external restoration.

More recently, advanced systems with balloon-guided single lead catheters have appeared[30]. The proximal and distal high-energy electrode array for internal defibrillation consists of six rings. When the catheter is advanced in the heart, the distal array is positioned in the left pulmonary artery and the proximal is in contact with the lower lateral right atrial free wall. In a comparative evaluation of this system, with the conventional two catheters it seems that the placement time is reduced by 25 % , and the fluoroscopy time is reduced by 48 %. On the contrary, there was no difference either in the amount of energy (8.4 $\pm$ 3 vs 7.2 $\pm$ 3 J) used nor in the possible complications, while the primary success rate was as high (94 % vs 93 %)[30].

Important advantages of the new technology are the possibility of haemodynamic monitoring from the distal edge of the catheter (Swan-Ganz type), a fact that could be used in its placing, without fluoroscopy even in areas beyond the laboratory, like intensive care units[31]. The sensing and pacing possibilities presuppose safety in this method as, although the rate and kind of bradycardiac complications of cardioversion in patients suffering from atrial fibrillation are not exactly known, there are enough patients who require pacemaker support after the cessation of arrhythmia[32]. Furthermore, knowing more today about the changes of the electrophysiological properties of the atrium (atrial remodelling) after the restoration of atrial fibrillation, the atrial overdrive pacing (which is available with the new systems) can certainly suppress the ectopic contractions which are the cause of early recurrences of arrhythmia[33,34].

Safety

If we exempt the fact that temporary internal low energy cardioversion of atrial fibrillation is an invasive method which requires catheterisation in patients who are usually taking anti-coagulants, the safety of the method remains very high[35]. Mechanical complications in high energy endocavitary shocks are generally related to barotrauma, which does not occur with lower energies, just as subendocardial necrosis is not evident, a fact supported by the observation that CK does not show significant changes. Of course, the application of any kind of energy that exceeds the pacing threshold is a forerunner of malignant ventricular arrhythmias. Such proarrhythmic phenomena are not evident if the shocks are synchronized to the R wave with a minimum RR interval of 500 ms, conditions which are available with the new systems, while the supportive pacing which also encompasses protections from possible bradycardiac phenomena in patients with longstanding atrial fibrillation whose sinus node function is undetermined.

Tolerability

The determinants of discomfort caused by intracardiac electric discharges are not entirely known. Different factors from the kind of shock waveform, the placement of the electrodes to the psychological conditions can affect the feeling of pain from the shocks. From the bibliography it is evident that voltages between 100 - 180 V, equivalent to

0.5 - 1 J, can be tolerated without sedation[35]. Of course, the average of 7-8 J which is required for low energy cardioversion is much higher than the pain threshold, but with mild sedation seems well tolerated[36], and certainly bears no relationship with the deep sedation that is necessary for the high energy used in external fibrillation cases.

Our center's experience agrees with that of the bibliography as far as the efficacy and safety of temporary internal cardioversion in patients with chronic atrial fibrillation. Specifically, we evaluated the system of single catheter in 36 patients with a mean arrhythmia duration of 18 ± 13 months. Successful restoration of sinus rhythm was achieved in 32 patients (89 %) with an average energy of 7.5 ± 1.3 J. In three patients it was necessary to employ supportive pacemaking after the restoration, while the average fluoroscopy time was 13.2 ± 9.1 minutes. In none of the cases was there an noticeable increase in the myocardial enzymes compared with those before the procedure, while two cases showed haematoma in the right groin without specific results.

Conclusions

Internal cardioversion of chronic atrial tachycardia is possible, effective and safe, using biphasic shocks and transvenous biatrial electrodes requiring very low energies. These methods can be applied easily and simply, while some facilities the newer systems possess, may very well make this the method of first choice, for the restoration of atrial fibrillation.

There are several acute settings in which low energy internal cardioversion may be indicated like in atrial fibrillation that involves diagnostic electrophysiological studies and catheter ablations, and where the use of anti-arrhythmic medication may make the procedure difficult. This is also the case in intensive care units, in post operative or post myocardial patients and, in patients for whom general anesthesia may be hazardous or contraindicated. It is also important that the application of these techniques in cases of atrial fibrillation resistant to conventional methods has been shown in a number of studies.

As a first choice method it can be applied in all those cases, in which it is highly unlikely, that the patient will respond to external cardioversion (like obese patients or those with chronic pulmonary obstructive disease). Finally the experience which is gained from these techniques has important implications for the clinical development of implantable atrial defibrillators for patients with paroxysmal atrial fibrillation.

References

1. Kannel WB, Abbott RD, Savage DD, et al. Epidemiologic features of chronic atrial fibrillation: the Framingham study. N Engl J Med 1982:306;1018-22.
2. Davidson E, Weinberger I, Rotenberger Z, et al. Atrial fibrillation: cause and time of onset. Arch Inter Med 1989:149;457-9
3. Ueshima K, Myers J, Ribis I, et al. Hemodynamic determinants of exercise capacity in chronic atrial fibrillation. Am Heart J 1993:125;1301-5.
4. Shinbane J, Wood M, Jensen N, et al. Tachycardia – induced cardiomyopathy: A review of animal models and clinical studies. J Am Coll Cardiol 1997:29;709-15.
5. Kistler JP. The risk of embolic stroke: another piece of the puzzle. N Engl J Med 1994:331;1517-9.
6. Wolf P.A., Dawber TR, Thomas HE Jr, et al. Epidemiologic assessment of chronic atrial fibrillation and the risk of stroke: the Framingham study. Neurology 1978:28;9973-977.
7. Bianconi L, Boccadamo R, Pappalardo A, et al. Effectiveness of intravenous propafenone for conversion of atrial fibrillation and flutter of recent onset. Am J Cardiol 1989: 64; 335-341.
8. Gosselink AT, Grijns HJ, Van Gelder IC, et al, Low – dose amiodarone for maintenance of sinus rhythm after cardioversion of atrial fibrillation or flutter. JAMA 1992:267;3289-93.
9. Bianconi L Mennuni M, Lukic V et al. Effects of oral propafenone administration before electrical cardioversion of chronic atrial fibrillation: a placebo controlled study. J Am Coll Cardiol 1996:28;700-6
10. Tieleman RG, Gosselink AT, Grijns HJ, et al. Efficacy, safety and determinants of conversion of atrial fibrillation and flutter with oral amiodarone. Am J Cardiol 1997:79;53-7.
11. Kochiadakis GE, Igoumenidis NE, Parthenakis FI, et al. Amiodarone versus Propafenone for cardioversion of chronic atrial fibrillation: results of a randomized controlled study. J Am Coll Cardiol 1999:33;966-71.
12. Falk RH. Proarrythmia in patients treated for atrial fibrillation or flutter. Ann Intern Med 1992:117;141-50.
13. Lown B, Perlroth MG, Kaidbey S et al. Cardioversion of atrial fibrillation. N Engl J Med 1962:269;325-31.
14. Mirowski M, Mower MM, Langer AA. Low-energy catheter cardioversion of atrial tachyarrhythmias. Clic Res 1974:22;290.

15. Dunbar DN, Tobler HG, Fetter J, et al. Intracavitary electrode catheter cardioversion of atrial tacharrhythmias in the dog, J Am Coll Cardiol 1986:7;1015-27

16. Kumagai K, Yamanouchi Y, Tashiro , et al. Low energy synchronous transcatheter cardioversion of atrial flutter/fibrillation in the dog. J Am Coll Cardiol 1990:16;497-501

17. Powell AC, Garan H, McGovern BA, et al. Low energy conversion of atrial fibrillation in the sheep. J Am Coll Cardiol 1992: 20; 707-771.

18. Cooper RA, Alferness CA, Smith WM, et al. Internal cardioversion of atrial fibrillation in sheep. Circulation 1993:87;1673-86.

19. Nathan AW, Bexton RS, Spurrell RAJ, et al. Internal transvenous low energy cardioversion for the treatment of cardiac arrhythmias. Br Heart J 1984:52;377-84.

20. Levy S, Lacombe P, Cointe R, et al. High energy transcatheter cardioversion of chronic atrial fibrillation. J Am Coll Cardiol 1988:12;514-518.

21. Kumagai K, Yamanouchi Y, Hiroki T, et al. Effects of transcatheter cardioversion on chronic lone atrial fibrillation. PACE 1991:14;1571-75.

22. Levy S, Lauribe P, Dolla E, et al. A randomized comparison of external and internal cardioversion of chronic atrial fibrillation. Circulation 1992:86;1415-1420.

23. Keane D, Boyd E, Anderson D, et al. Comparison of biphasic and monophasic waveforms in epicardial atrial defibrillation. J Am Coll Cardiol 1994:24;171-6.

24. Alt E, Schmitt C, Ammer R, et al. Initial experience with intracardiac atrial defibrillation in patients with chronic atrial fibrillation. PACE 1994: 17;1067-1078.

25. Sopher SM, Murgatroyd FD, Slade AKB, et al. Low energy internal cardioversion of atrial fibrillation resistant to transthoracic shocks. Heart 1996:75;635-8.

26. Schmitt C, Alt E, Plewan A, et al. Low energy intracardiac cardioversion after failed conventional external cardioversion of atrial fibrillation. J Am Coll Cardiol 1996: 28;994-999.

27. Levy S, Ricard P, Lau C, et al. Low energy cardioversion of spontaneous atrial fibrillation. Immediate and long-term results. Circulation 1997: 96; 253-259.

28. Levy S, Ricard P, Lau C, et al. Multicenter low-energy transvenous atrial defibrillation (XAD). Trial results in different subsets of atrial fibrillation. J Am Coll Cardiol 1997:29; 750-755.

29. Alt E, Ammer R, Schmitt C, et al. A comparison of treatment with low-energy intracardiac cardioversion and conventional external cardioversion. Eur Heart J 1997:18;1796-1804.

30. Alt E, Ammer R, Lehmann G, et al.Efficacy of a new balloon catheter for internal cardioversion of chronic atrial fibrillation without anaesthesia. Heart 1998:79;128-132.

31. Plewan A, Valina C, Herrmann R, et al. Initial experience with a new balloon–guided single lead catheter for internal cardioversion of atrial fibrillation and dual chamber pacing. PACE 1999:22(Pt II);228-232.

32. Prakash A, Saksena S, Mathew P, et al. Internal atrial defibrillation: effects on sinus and atrioventricular nodal function and implanted cardiac pacemakers. PACE 1997:20;2434-41.

33. Wijffels MCEF, Kirchhof CJHJ, Dorland R, et al. Atrial fibrillation begets atrial fibrillation. A study in awake chronically instrumented goats. Circulation 1995: 92;1954-1968.

34. Tieleman RG, Van Gelder IC, Grijns HJ, et al. Early recurrence of atrial fibrillation after electrical cardioversion: a result of fibrillation induced electrical remodelling of the atria? J Am Coll Cardiol 1998: 31;167-173.

35. Murgatroyd FD, Slade AKB, Sopher SM, et al. Efficacy and tolerability of transvenous low energy cardioversion of paroxysmal atrial defibrillation in humans. J Am Coll Cardiol 1995: 25;1347-1353.

36. Santini M, Pandozzi C, Toscano S, et al. Low energy intracardiac cardioversion of persistent atrial fibrillation. PACE 1998:21;2641-50.

20.
THE IMPLANTABLE ATRIAL DEFIBRILLATOR: INDICATIONS AND RESULTS.

Massimo Santini, MD, FACC, Renato Ricci MD, Claudio Pandozi MD,
Maria Carmela Scianaro, MD, Salvatore Toscano MD,
Giuliano Altamura MD.
Department of Cardiology, San Filippo Neri Hospital, Rome, Italy.

Introduction

Atrial Fibrillation (AF) is the most common arrhythmia in clinical practice. The prevalence of AF is approximately 2% in an unselected adult population and increases with each decade of life, approximating 10% in patients older than 75 years[1,2]. The arrhythmia is associated to substantial morbidity and mortality. Several nonpharmacologic strategies have been developed to treat recurrent drug-refractory AF, including cardiac pacing, catheter ablation techniques, surgical procedures and Atrial Defibrillator implantation. Two different devices have been introduced for clinical implantation: the Atrioverter METRIX (InControl Inc, Redmond, USA) and the Dual Defibrillator JEWEL AF (Medtronic Inc., Minneapolis, USA).

The Atrioverter METRIX

The Atrioverter is based on a three-lead system, including two leads implanted in the right atrium lateral wall and into the coronary sinus to deliver low-energy atrial shock (up to 300 or 600 volts, according to the model 3000 or 3020) and a ventricular lead to synchronize the shock and to allow post-shock back-up ventricular pacing. Atrial shock can be released automatically or activated by the patient or the physician. The device has been evaluated[3] in 51 patients, 40 Male and 11 Female, mean age 56±8 years, with drug refractory atrial fibrillation recurring from once a week to once a quarter, without heart failure and with left ventricular ejection fraction ≥ 40%. Stated the need of having very low atrial defibrillation threshold at implant, only 54% of selected patients were actually implanted. Patients were followed for 259±138 days. During the follow-up 3719 shocks were delivered, 3049 during testing and 670 on spontaneous episodes. Shock synchronization was programmed on R waves with pre-shock RR interval ≥ 500 msec. The specificity detection on sinus rhythm was 100%; the sensitivity detection on AF was 92.3%. No pro-arrhythmic effects or inappropriate shocks were observed. 41 patients experienced at least 1 episode of AF during the follow-up (5.6 on average, range 1-26). The success rate of atrial shocks was very high (96%). Atrial Defibrillation Threshold (ADFT) at

From Ovsyshcher IE. *Cardiac Arrythmias and Device Therapy: Results and Perspectives for the New Century.*
Armonk, NY: Futura Publishing Company, Inc., © 2000

implant was 1.5±0.7 J for model 3000 and 2.7±1.1 J for model 3020. 3-month ADFT did not change significantly (1.8±0.6 J and 2.7±0.5 J respectively). Early recurrence of AF was observed in 62 episodes (27%) and in 21 patients (51%). Taking into account arrhythmia early recurrences, the overall success rate decreased to 74%. In figure 1 an appropriately detected episode of AF stored in the device memory is represented. Both right atrium–coronary sinus and right ventricle–coronary sinus electrograms confirm AF diagnosis.

Figure 1: AF episode stored in the Atrioverter memory.

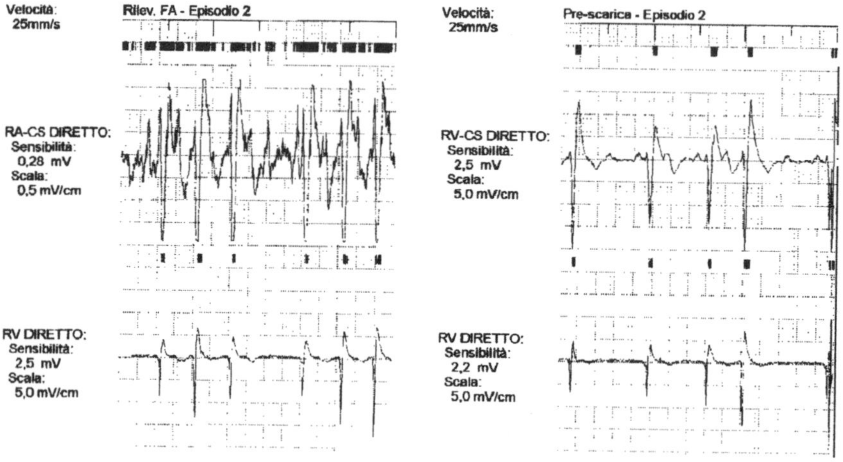

The Dual Defibrillator JEWEL AF

The dual defibrillator combines dual chamber ICD features with the capability of automatically detecting and treating atrial tachycardia (AT) and AF. Available atrial therapies include Anti-Tachy-Pacing (ATP) (Ramp, Burst+, 50-Hz Burst) and Low-Energy Cardioversion. According to that, the device can be used in preventing AF by pacing and in treating AF both by painless ATP therapies or by atrial shock. A two lead configuration (right atrium and double coil right ventricle) or a three lead configuration (inserting an extra coil into the coronary sinus) can be utilized. Considering the availability of ventricular therapies for ventricular tachycardia or fibrillation the device can be safely implanted also in patients with heart failure and/or at risk of life-threatening arrhythmias. Furthermore, patients candidate to ICD implantation for ventricular tachyarrhythmias who usually show a very high incidence of AF-AT (up to 40-50% during the life-span of the ICD[4,5] can be treated for both atrial and ventricular arrhythmias.

Atrial or dual chamber pacing can play a major role in preventing AF, mainly in patients with sinus bradycardia[6,7]. New pacing algorithms such as Atrial Rate Stabilization (ARS), Switchback Delay or Consistent Atrial Pacing (CAP)[8] can increase the antiarrhythmic benefit of atrial pacing. Reduction of premature atrial beats, short-long atrial cycle prevention, reduced dispersion of conduction and refractoriness, maintenance of high degree of exit block from subsidiary atrial pacemakers can be considered the main mechanisms responsible for AF prevention[9]. Alternative atrial pacing techniques, such as biatrial pacing[10], dual site right atrial pacing[11] or interatrial septum pacing[12] could be implemented in the next future to improve the overall clinical outcome[13].

Personal experience with the dual defibrillator
To evaluate the effectiveness of the dual defibrillator in detecting and treating spontaneous atrial arrhythmias and to evaluate the incidence of such arrhythmias in ICD patients, we have enrolled in a prospective study 39 patients, 32 Male, 7 Female, mean age 65 ± 10 years. 21 patients had ischaemic heart disease, 9 idiopathic dilated cardiomyopathy and 9 other heart diseases. Mean left ventricular ejection fraction was $39\pm9\%$. 18 patients had AT/AF before implantation. In 4 patients recurrent drug-refractory AF was the only indication to ICD implantation. A two lead configuration (right atrium and double coil right ventricle) was utilized. All patients had their device programmed in DDD pacing mode with automatic mode switching algorithm switched on. The detection setting was 170-300 msec for Atrial tachycardia (AT) and 100-250 msec for AF. The duration of sustained AF/AT required to initiate therapy was programmed 5 minutes for ATP therapies and 1 hour for shock therapies. ATP therapies were automatically activated in all patients. AT treatment step up protocol included A-Burst+, A-Ramp and A-50 Hz Burst Pacing. AF ATP therapy included A-50 Hz Burst Pacing. Atrial cardioversion was automatically activated in patients who chose this option. The energy delivered was selected taking into account the atrial defibrillation threshold measured during implantation (A-shock energy twice ADFT). The programmed shock pathway was can + superior vena cava (SVC) > right ventricle (RV), with tilt 50%. A-defibrillation was synchronized to a non-refractory ventricular event and aborted in presence of high ventricular rate. In the other patients in-hospital manual shock using the implanted device was performed as soon as possible after AF onset. The patients were evaluated 1 month after the implantation and every three months. At each follow-up session a detailed analysis of data stored in the device memory was performed. Available data for each treated atrial

episode included the summary of the episode, the therapy sequence, a 6-second pre-therapy atrial electrogram, a marker chain before electrogram onset and before episode termination. Treated and non-treated atrial episodes stored in the ICD memory were analyzed and correlated with patient referred symptoms. Marker chains and stored electrograms were used to verify appropriate detection of atrial tachyarrhythmias and efficacy of delivered therapy by two independent observers.

Results

The mean follow-up was 8±7 months (range 1-24). ADFT at implant was 5.4±3.3 J (range 2-16 J). During the follow-up, 219 sustained and 4400 unsustained atrial episodes were detected. 112 sustained episodes were clinically classified as AT (51%), 102 as AF (47%) and 5 (2%) as sinus rhythm. The detection positive predictive value was 98%. Inappropriate detection was due to far field atrial oversensing in only one patient. The problem was solved by reducing atrial detection sensitivity.

Figure 2: Effective 50-Hz burst on AF

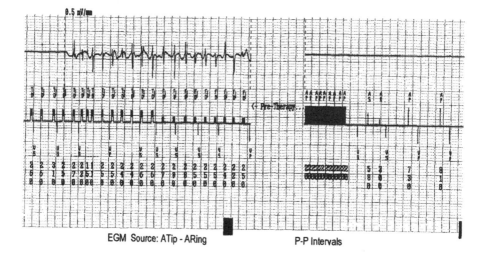

The therapy success rates were: 1)AT: ATP=85% (90/106), atrial shock=100% (6/6); 2)AF: 50-Hz Burst=19% (14/72), atrial shock=63% (19/30). Mean delivered energy was 17.3±6.9 J in effective shocks and 10.4±8.3 J in ineffective shocks. Ineffective atrial shocks were related to measured delivered energy less than twice ADFT in 55%, exactly twice ADFT in 27% and high ADFT (>27 J) in 18%. Excluding atrial shocks in which measured delivered energy was less than twice ADFT, the overall efficacy of atrial shock on AF increased to 79%. ATP efficacy strongly correlated with the median AA interval at arrhythmia onset, showing the best results in treating atrial arrhythmias with atrial cycles between 220 and 280 msec. In figure 2 effective 50-Hz burst on AF is drawn. In figure 3 automatic atrial shock on AF restores sinus rhythm.

Figure 3: Effective automatic atrial shock on AF.

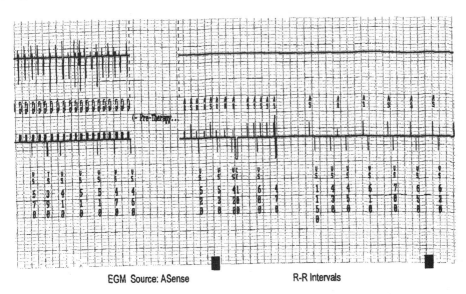

EGM Source: ASense   R-R Intervals

Discussion

Clinical experience with the implantable atrial defibrillator has added new information in the challenging issue of treating drug refractory AF. The first point is the growing role which can be played by ATP therapies. In our experience in patients with prior documented AF, about 50% of sustained atrial episodes start as AT and can be treated successfully by ATP (85% in our study population). Moreover, 50-Hertz Burst had mild (19%), but unexpectedly valuable, efficacy on AF, as confirmed by others[14]. According to that, more data are needed about atrial activity at arrhythmia onset to optimize ATP programming (delay and therapy sequences). AF prevention by atrial pacing can increase the overall benefit of painless therapies available in last generation devices. Atrial shock is effective in restoring sinus rhythm, but open issues persist. Shock efficacy on AF is strongly dependent on delivered energy level. In our study population the low success rate was mainly due to the episodes in which the measured delivered energy was less than or exactly the same as twice the ADFT values. Others had success rate > 90% by programming the device at the maximum programmable energy (27 J)[14]. The success rate is also depending on lead configuration, since the three-lead system is usually associated to lower ADFT if compared to the two-lead system. However, the coronary sinus lead adds complexity to the implant procedure and can be responsible for system-related increased morbidity during the follow-up[15]. At the moment, the cost-benefit ratio of third lead implantation needs further investigation. Patient tolerance of atrial shocks is crucial in the evaluation of quality of life and overall cost-benefit ratio of implanted device. Discomfort from low energy shocks seems related to energy delivered, shock waveform and lead configuration[16]. However, the number of shocks delivered to treat a single episode and psychological components can play a key role[17]. It is not unusual to find patients who perceived severe discomfort after internal shocks at very low energy[18].

Early cardioversion of AF is expected to prevent atrial remodelling and to facilitate persistence of sinus rhythm and prevention of early recurrence of AF[19]. According to that, the overall burden of AF should decrease during the follow-up of patients implanted with atrial defibrillator. This concept has been confirmed only by preliminary findings[20] and needs further investigation in large prospective trials. Similarly, the impact of atrial defibrillator in prevention of stroke and progression to chronic AF should be tested in clinical studies.

Patient selection

Guidelines to select candidates for the implantable atrial defibrillator are matter of debate[21]. Patients with sinus bradycardia and recurrent paroxysmal AF could be successfully treated by dual chamber pacing, mainly if combined with overdrive algorithms, alternative pacing sites and ATP therapies, which are going to be implemented in the next pacemaker generation. In patients with drug refractory persistent AF, already treated with internal or external cardioversion, atrial or dual defibrillator implantation may be indicated, mainly if the arrhythmia recurrence is between 1 week and three months[22]. In patients with heart failure and/or coronary artery disease ventricular back-up should be suggested. Finally, patients with conventional indication to ICD implantation and prior AF or at risk of AF should receive a dual defibrillator.

References:

1. Kalman JM, Tonkin AM: Atrial fibrillation: epidemiology and the risk and prevention of stroke. PACE 1992;15:1332-1346.
2. Wolf PA, Abbott RD, Kannel WB: Atrial fibrillation as an independent risk factor for stroke: The Framingham study. Stroke 1991;22:983-988.

3. Wellens HJJ, Lau CP, Luderitz B, et al.: Atrioverter: an implantable device for the treatment of atrial fibrillation. Circulation 1998;98:1651-1656.

4. Schmitt C, Montero M, Melichercik J: Significance of supraventricular tachyarrhythmias in patients with implanted pacing cardioverter defibrillators. PACE 1998;17:295-302.

5. Grimm W, Flores B, Marchlinski F: Electrocardiographically documented unnecessary, spontaneous shocks in 241 patients with implantable cardioverter defibrillators. PACE 1992;15:1667-1673.

6. Santini M, Alexidou G, Ansalone G, et al: Relation of prognosis in sick sinus syndrome to age, conduction defects and modes of permanent cardiac pacing. Am J Cardiol 1990;65:729-735.

7. Andersen HR, Nielsen JC, Thomsen PEB, et al: Long-term follow up of patients from a randomised trial of atrial versus ventricular pacing for sick-sinus syndrome. Lancet 1997;350:1210-6.

8. Ricci R, Santini M, Puglisi A, et al: Intermittent or continuous overdrive atrial pacing significantly reduces paroxysmal atrial fibrillation recurrences in brady-tachy syndrome (Abstract). Eur Heart J 1999;20(Suppl):218.

9. Josephson ME, Schibgilla VH: Non-pharmacological treatment of supraventricular arrhythmias. Eur Heart J 1996;17:26-34.

10. Daubert C, Mabo P, Berder V, et al: Atrial tachyarrhythmias associated with high degree interatrial conduction block. Prevention by permanent atrial resynchronization. Eur J C P E 1994;4:35-44.

11. Saksena S, Prakash A, Hill M: Prevention of recurrent atrial fibrillation with chronic dual-site right atrial pacing. J Am Coll Cardiol 1996;28:687-694.

12. Padeletti L, Porciani MC, Michelucci A, et al: Interatrial septum pacing: a new approach to prevent recurrent atrial fibrillation. J Interventional Cardiac Electrophysiology 1999;3:35-43.

13. Prakash A, Delfault P, Giorgberidze I, et al: Interventional therapeutic procedures in patients with preexisting dual site right atrial pacing system for refractory atrial fibrillation. Am J Cardiol 1998;81:1274-1277.

14. Sulke N, Bailin SJ, Swerdlow CD: Worldwide clinical experience with a dual chamber implantable cardioverter defibrillator in patients with atrial fibrillation and flutter (abs.). Eur Heart J 1999;20(Abs Suppl):114.

15. Gallik DM, O'Connor ME, Warman E, Swerdlow CD: Optimal defibrillation pathway for an implantable atrial defibrillator without a coronary sinus lead (abs). PACE 1999;22:505.

16. Ammer R, Alt E, Ayers G, et al: Pain threshold for low energy intracardiac cardioversion of atrial fibrillation with low or no sedation. PACE 1997;20:230-236.

17. Santini M, Pandozi C, Gentilucci G, et al: Intra-atrial defibrillation of human atrial fibrillation. J Cardiovasc Electrophysiol 1998;9:S170-S176.

18. Nathan AW, Bexton RS, Spurell RA, Camm J: Internal low energy cardioversion for the treatment of cardiac arrhythmias. Br Heart J 1984;52:377-384.

19. Wijffels MCEF, Kirchhof CJHJ, Dorland R, Allessie MA: Atrial fibrillation begets atrial fibrillation: a study in awake chronically instrumented goats. Circulation 1995;92:1954-1968.

20. Timmermans C, Wellens HJJ, for the Metrix investigators: Effect of device-mediated therapy on symptomatic episodes of atrial fibrillation (abs). J Am Coll Cardiol 1998;31:331A.

21. Heisel A and Jung J: The atrial defibrillator: a stand-alone device or part of a combined dual chamber system? Am J Cardiol 1999;83:218D-226D.

22. Jung W, Luderitz B: Implantable atrial defibrillator: quo vadis? PACE 1997;20:2141-2145.

Part IV.

Pacing for AF Prevention

21.
PREVENTION OF ATRIAL FIBRILLATION BY PACING

J. Claude Daubert, MD, Gilles Revault d'Allonnes, MD, Dominique Pavin, MD, Philippe Mabo, MD.

Departement de Cardiologie & Maladies Vasculaires, Centre Cardio-Pneumologique, Hopital Pontchaillou - CHU, Rennes, France

Introduction

Pacing techniques can be used to terminate and prevent recurrence of paroxysmal atrial tachycardia. For many years anti-tachycardia pacing has been widely used for the acute treatment of re-entrant tachycardia, including a fully excitable gap in the reentry circuit, atrial flutter in particular. The use of pacing in prevention of arrhythmia has on the contrary developed more slowly because of its theoretical complexity and technical hardware and software resources required to implement the theoretical design (pacing systems, algorithms). But the major advances achieved in the last few years have provided clear hope that cardiac pacing will soon be available to effectively and efficiently prevent atrial flutter and atrial fibrillation (AF). However, the exact standing of preventive pacing in relation to other non pharmacological approaches, especially catheter-ablation techniques and the atrial defibrillator, has to be clarified.

How can cardiac pacing work to prevent atrial fibrillation ?

Different electrophysiological mechanisms may account for the antiarrhythmic effect of atrial pacing: i) Rate-control to prevent the arhythmogenic consequences of bradycardia and of erratic heart rate, especially the dispersion of refractoriness. This effect, very simple to obtain, may be of particular importance to treat arrhythmias that are directly related to bradycardia, especially the so-called "vagally mediated atrial tachyarrhythmias"[1]. This effect can also be of interest for the prevention of tachyarrhythmias in the Brady-tachy syndrome, despite the random (or apprently random) alternating of bradycardia and tachycardia episodes; ii) Overdrive suppression of atrial premature beats, especially through suppression of automatic foci, may contribute to prevent initiation of AF. It has been know for many years that temporal dispersion or recovery of excitability in the atrium and in the ventricle is a function of heart rate[2] and that the incidence of ectopic beats is itself a function of the basic rate, at least in the ventricule[3]. It has been clearly demonstrated that overdrive pacing, either permanent (possibly sensor-driven) or dynamic with the induction of minimal increment atrial overdriving after every atrial premature complex, significantly reduces the incidence of atrial premature beats. However, the exact role of atrial extrasystoles in arrhythmias initiation is still a matter of debate[1]. There is no clear evidence yet that extrasystole suppression may significantly contribute to preventing AF; iii) Supression of compensatory pauses. The deleterious consequences of the so-called

From Ovsyshcher IE. *Cardiac Arrythmias and Device Therapy: Results and Perspectives for the New Century.* Armonk, NY: Futura Publishing Company, Inc., © 2000

"long-short cycle" or "short-long-short cycle" phenomena are known to promote the initiation of life-threatening ventricular tachyarrhythmia[6,7]. The same has not been clearly shown to occur at the atrial level, except in the special case of vagally-mediated atrial tachyarrhythmia. Theoretically, the electrophysiological consequences of this phenomenon can be prevented by rate-smoothing algorithmes but the effectiveness of such techniques in preventing arrhythmias is not known ; iv) Multiple-site atrial pacing may contribute to preventing arrhythmia by different mechanisms. By correcting asynchrony and the uneven activation resulting from organic or functional conduction blocks, multiple-site pacing may prevent the occurrence of macroreentry. Multiple-site pacing may also work by increasing the coupling interval of the premature beart in the abnormal substrate. This can be achieved by pre-exciting the reentry area or by selecting one or more pacing sites antidromic to the premature beat activation[8]; v) Inhibition of atrial tissue by sub-threshold stimulation has been hypothesized as a way to prevent refractory atrial tachyarrhythmia[9]. However, this concept is still at the planning stage and has not found any practical application so far; vi) Finally, a number of experimental reports and Allessie et al's study in particular[10] suggest that any treatment that effectively prevents or at least significantly decreases the rate of arrhythmia recurrence participates in a remodelling process of the electrophysiologic substrate which subsequently enhances the preventive effect of the original treatment. This hypothesis can be applied to cardiac pacing as to other therapeutic approaches.

Clinical implications
Different forms of arrhythmia from different etiologies can be potentially prevented by atrial pacing. Some indications have already been validated, others are being evaluated, and others still are merely at the blueprint stage. But regardless of indications, there is an urgent need for prospective and randomized studies to evaluate the true clinical relevance of this therapeutic method. The technical resources presently available to achieve arrhythmia prevention are mainly the following three: i) Standard, single-site atrial pacing with a single-chamber atrial pacemaker or an atrial-based dual-chamber device. In that respect, the role of rate responsiveness and of the atrial pacing site have to be discussed; ii) Multiple-site atrial pacing with different possible configurations and finally iii) specific pacing algorithms to suppress atrial premature beats.

Arrhythmia prevention with single-site atrial pacing
Rate control by single site atrial pacing has been used for many years in arrhythmia prevention[11]. Of the various clinical indications that have been investigated, two can be considered as validated, i.e., the syndrome of "vagally mediated atrial tachyarrythmias" and the prevention of chronic AF (and related complications) in the Brady-tachy syndrome and one is still purely speculative, i.e., the prevention of paroxysmal lone AF (not related to one of the two above mentioned syndromes).

- Syndrome of "vagally-mediated atrial tachyarrhythmias"

This syndrome, described be Coumel in 1978[1], is characterized by AF or paroxysmal flutter syndromes prone to recurrence and occurring in young subjects with apparently healthy hearts. Each episode, recorded with a Holter device, is preceded by a gradual sinus rhythm reduction. With this background of gradual bradycardia, arrhythmia proper usually occurs together with a longer cycle following atrial extrasystole. This model of "bradycardia-dependant" arrhythmia constitutes an outstanding opportunity to assess the preventive effect of isolated anti-bradycardia pacing. The shared experiment performed by Labiboisiere hospital was reported by I. Denjoy et al in 1997[12]. It involved 20 highly symptomatic patients not responding to anti-arrhythmic drug treatment. Atrial single-chamber or dual-chamber pacemaker was implanted and set to a baseline frequency between 70 and 90 bpm. After a mean follow-up of 6 years, 17 patients (85%) were asymptomatic and had suffered no recurrence of arrhythmia, althrough that result could only be achieved in 16 of them by maintaining low-dose anti-arrhythmic monotherapy.

- Prevention of chronic AF and related complications in the brady-tachy syndrome.

The brady-tachy syndrome constitutes a very different situation because bradycardia and tachycardia episodes alternate in an apparently random manner. The natural history of that syndrome is still little known because it was soon overshadowed by very wide indications for cardiac pacing. It is known to carry a very high risk of evolution towards chronic AF in the mid- or longer term[13]. The question remains whether cardiac pacing is capable or not to prevent recurrence of paroxysmal AF and evolution toward permanent AF. That question may never be answered fully because no prospective ranzomized study on the long-term effects of pacing or absence of pacing in that indication has ever been conducted. In fact, the only valid piece of information abailable relates to the non-natural history of the syndrome, i.e., the history of patients primarily treated by permanent cardiac pacing. In the last 10 years, a number of retrospective studies have compared the long-term effects of ventricular (VVI) and atrial (AAI) single-chamber pacing methods. The results from these studies[14-16] suggested that atrial pacing very significantly reduces the incidence of chronic AF. Compiling the results from all these studies revealed that the average annual incidence is 1.5% in patients with AAI pacing whereas it is eight times higher (12%) in patients with VVI pacing. Meanwhile, certain studies have demonstrated a significant reduction of the incidence of thrombo-embolic events and higher survival rate in groups of patients with atrial single-chamber pacing. These preliminary results have been confirmed by those of a prospective randomized study published by Andersen in 1994[17] and 1997[18]. In that trial, 225 patients with symptomatic sinus node dysfunction and normal AV conduction were randomized to receive either an atrial single-chamber pacemaker (n=110) or a VVI unit (n=115). follow-up, based on very simple parameters, lasted 5.5±2.4 years on average. The results showed a significant reduction in the AAI group in the risk of evolution towards chronic AF (9% vs 22%; p=0.004) and in the incidence of AF present at 1 follow-up visit or more (23.6% vs 34.8%; p= 0.012). In the same way, the incidence of thrombo-embolic events was significantly reduced (11.8% vs 22.6%; p=0.023). There was a significant reduction in cardiovasculaire mortality (17% vs 33.9%; p=0.006) and a significant trend to a lower global mortality rate (35.5% vs 49.6%; p=0.045). In the echocardiographic substudy, the same group[19] showed that clinical benefit from atrial pacing was paralleled with a significant limitation in the time-progression of left atrial dilatation and of left ventricular systolic dysfunction. Finally the preliminary results of the PAC-A-TACH study[20] were recently reported. In that trial, 198 pts, mean age 72 years, with the brady-tachy syndrome were equally randomized to receive a DDDR pacemaker (n=100) or a VVIR unit (n=98). Patients were followed a median 23.7 months and monitored for recurrent atrial tachyarrhythmias. At the end of follow-up, 9% of pts in the DDDR group and 44% in the VVIR group were crossed over to the other pacing mode (p<0.0001). The major reason for cross-over was recurrent atrial tachyarrhythmias in the DDDR group and pacemaker syndrome (28%) and recurrent arrhythmias (13%) in the VVIR group. Surprisingly there was no significant difference between the two groups in the 1-year incidence of atrial tachyarrhythmia recurrences (48% in DDDR vs 43% in VVIR), but the survival rate was significantly better in the atrially paced patients thant in the ventricularly paced patients (96.8 % vs 93.2% ; p=0.007). Despite the somewhat discordant results of these prospective studies, it appears possible to conclude that permanent atrial or atrial-based paicng, by comparison with the conventional VVI mode, reduces the long-term incidence of chronic AF and of thrombo-embolic events in patients chronically implanted for sick sinus syndrome, and especially for bradycardia-tachycardia syndrome. So ventricular pacing has to be definitively abandoned in that indication.

- Prevention of "lone" paroxysmal AF with atrial pacing.

What about the prevention of paroxysmal AF ? The reply is quite simple : we knowed most nothing about it. There is a simple explanation for our ignorance : until recent years, no reliable diagnostic instruments were available to identify and quantify these sometimes very transient and often asymptomatic arrhythmias. It is now reasonable to expect that this probem will be solved in the near future thanks to the Holter functions of the most sophisticated and modern pacemakers, including continuous intracardiac ECG monitoring through implanted electrodes. Excellent correlations with surface Holter have been reported by Garrigue and Cazeau[21] with the range of Chorus 6234 and Chorus RM 7034 pacemakers (ELA Recherche, France). These novel diagnostic instruments have now been validated and there remains to undertake prospective, randomized studies to compare the effects of atrial pacing with those of no stimulation, so as to determine whether or not cardiac pacing is capable of preventig paroxysmal AF episodes or at least to reduce the nomber and duration of such episodes.

The "Atrial Pacing for Paroxysmal Atrial Fibrillation Peri Ablation" study tried recently to answer that question. The PA3 trial was a multicentric Canadian trial that was designed to determine the effect of atrial-based pacing on the frequency of recurrent paroxysmal AF. Patients identified for ablation received a DDDR pacemaker three months before a planned AV nodal ablation. During this 3-months period they were randomly assigned to one of two pacing modes that effectively result in either atrial pacing (DDIR 70 bpm) or no pacing (DDI 40 bpm). After AV nodal ablation, they were randomly assigned to either DDDR or VDD pacing mode and then crossed-over to the other pacing mode at 6 months. The pacemakers used were capable of mode-switching and also count the nomber of mode-switches, thus enabling the investigators to determine the frequency with which AF has recurred. During the first part of the protocol[22] no significant difference was observed for the primary and secondary endpoints of the study (time to first recurrence of sustained paroxysmal AF? time interval between successive episodes of PAF...) between the two groups. The only significant difference concerned the PAF episodes burden that was significantly greater during atrial pacing than with no pacing (1.00 vs 0.32 hr/day; $p < 0.016$). The preliminary results of the second part of the study (comparison DDDR vs VDD post-ablation) were recently presented and went exactly in the same way[23]. So we do not have any evidence at that time that conventional atrial pacing may contribute to prevent recurrences of drug-refractory PAF in patients without associated bradycardia, at least over the short term period.

- *Role of rate responsiveness in arrhythmia prevention with single-site atrial pacing.*

By smoothing heart rate, especially during strain and rest, and by "capping" (sometimes permanently) the spontaneous atrial activity, rate responsiveness could have additional preventive effect in atrial arrhythmia, AF in particular. Published results[24-26] are not convincing but perhaps that is due to insufficient means. The concept should certainly be reconsidered in the light of modern assessment techniques, in particular by using pacemakers featuring powerful diagnostic functions.

- *Role of pacing site.*

Permanent atrial leads (screw-in leads or passive "J" shaped atrial leads positioned in the right atrial appendage) are conventionally placed in the high right atrium. However, recent electrophysiologic data suggest that alternative pacing sites could result in an increased effectiveness of permanent atrial pacing to prevent arrhythmia and the initiation of AF in particular. In 17 patients with history of palpitations but without any documented episode of AF or atrial flutter,

Papageorgiou et al.[27] carried out programmed atrial pacing at two different pacing sites, the high right atrium (HRA) and the distal coronary sinus (DCS). AF inducibility and intra-atrial conduction delay at four different sites (HRA, His bundle area, posterior triangle of Kock, and DCS) were studied. AF could be reproducibly induced in 8 patients with HRA pacing, but in none with DCS pacing. During HRA stimulation, patients with AF inducibility exhibited significantly longer conduction in the posterior triangle of Koch and markedly broader local electrogram than with CS pacing. In a complemenary study[28] the same authors showed that DCS pacing could suppress the propensity of atrial premature beats originating from HRA to induce AF by decreasing their prematurity at the posterior triangle of Koch and by preventing the possible occurrence of microreentry. These experimental data may have important practical implications for AF prevention. It should be of interest to compare the effects of long-term pacing at the two pacing (HRA and DCS) sites used alternately in the same patients. Modern lead technology today permits permanent pacing of the coronary sinus, either at the ostium by using screw-in leads inserted in the low posterior right atrium[29] or into the median or the distal part of CS through specifically designed coronary sinus leads[30]. An other technical possibility to pace permanently the interatrial septum was described by Spencer et al in 1997[31] with inserting a screw-in lead in the anterior and superior part close to Bachman's bundle (BB) area. This new pacing modality was aimed to provide a more symetrical activation of the two atria while preserving the normal craniocaudal sequence. Prospective randomized studies are now ongoing to compare the effects of BB pacing and of conventional high right atrial pacing for AF prevention in patients with a conventional indication to pace[32]. Preliminary results seem encouraging.

- Role of multisite pacing.
Multisite atrial pacing is a novel and promising concept for the prevention of recurrent and drug-refractory atrial tachyarrhythmias. Two different technical approaches have been described so far. Biatrial synchronous pacing was introduced by our group in 1990[33]. Dual site right atrial pacing has been proposed more recently by Saksena et al[29]. The two techniques differ in two major points :
* the pacing sites. In our technique, the leads are placed in the upper right atrium, and in the median or distal part of the coronary sinus[30] for selectively pacing and sensing the left atrium. In Saksena's technique[29], the tip electrode of the second lead (screw-in lead) is fixed to the rim of the coronary sinus ostium in the low posterior right atrium, which is known to be a key area for arrhythmogenesis in patients with AF;
* the pacing mode. In our technique, the two atrial leads are connected to the atrial port of a bipolar DDDR pacemaker (ELA Recherche, France) through a Y-bifurcated adaptor, and a special algorithm of "atrial resynchronization" is loaded into the RAM memory of the pacemaker. The algorithm triggers instantaneous atrial synchronous pacing after every atrial event sensed, either sinus beat or right

atrial extrasystole sensed by the right atrial lead, or left atrial premature beat sensed by the coronary sinus lead, thus mimicking AAT pacing mode at the atrial level. This results in an effective and permanent resynchronization of the electrical activity wihtin the atrium. In Saksena's technique[29] the device is a standard DDDR pacemaker. So simultaneous pacing in the two atrial sites is only possible on paced atrial cycles, and there is no pacing at any site on the atrial cycles sensed nor well as during spontaneous sinus rhythm as on atrial extrasystoles. To compensate for this major technical limitation, Saksena et al.[29] proposed to permanently overdrive the intrinsic atrial rate by programming a basic pacing rate at 80-90 bpm, by systematically using sensor-driven pacing, and by giving cardiodepressor drugs to slow down the intrinsic heart rate. Irrespective of their technical characteristics, the two pacing modes have nearly identical electrophysiologic effects. In a recent study Prakash et al.[34] have shown that dual site right atrial pacing and biatrial pacing identically reduced P wave duration and homogenized local activation times in the crista terminalis (34 ± 15 vs 37 ± 20 ms) and coronary sinus ostium (21 ± 20 vs 19 ± 15 ms) regions, by comparison with spontaneous sinus rhythm and single site atrial pacing (upper right atrium, coronary sinus ostium, and distal coronary sinus). Data from other acute electrophysiological studies go in the same way[35]. Biatrial synchronous pacing was primarily evaluated in patients with evidence of high degree intraatrial conduction delay on surface ECG and during intracardiac mapping studies[33,36-38]. A pilot experiment using the most advanced technology in "triple chamber" pacemakers (algorithm of "atrial resynchronization"; highly sophisticated Holter functions including intracardiac ECG storage permitting reliable diagnosis and counting of arrhythmia episodes)has recently been reported[38]. This prospective non-randomized study included 86 patients whose mean age was 66 years, most of whom (75%) had an associated structural heart disease such as hypertrophic or dilated cardiomyopathy in particular. Selection criteria were: a) P wave duration >120 ms in addition to a significantly prolonged (<100 ms) interatrial conduction time (measured from the upper right atrium to the distal coronary sinus); b) a long history, on average 5 ± 4 years, of multiple recurrences of atrial tachyarrhythmia with at least two documented episodes during the preceding 6 months and drug failure (mean 2.7 ± 1.8 failed drugs, including amiodarone). Atrial flutter was observed in 56 patients, but most of the documented episodes (40 patients) corresponded to atypical forms whith slow, fragmented and low-voltage atrial waves. Endocardial mapping studies, performed in 9 patients with this particular form of flutter, provided in all cases arguments consistent with a left atrial reentry circuit or at least with the involvement of the left atrium in the circuit. Episodes of type I atrial flutter were documented in only 22 % of patients. Atrial flutter and AF were observed alternately in 52 patients. Finally, arrhythmia was characterized by its evolution in a permanent form only in 40 % of patients, requiring electrical cardioversion to restore normal sinus rhythm. Arrhtymia prevention was the sole indication for pacemaker implantation in 34 patients. Sinus node disease or high degree atrioventricular block, a classic indication for permanent pacing, was associated in the other 52 patients. The mean duration of follow-up time following pacemaker implantation was 33 ± 28 months, ranging from 6 to 109 months. P wave duration decreased from a mean value of 187 ± 29 ms before implantation to 106 ± 14 ms (p<0.0001) during biatrial pacing. At the end of follow-up 55 patients (64%) still remained in sinus rhythm. 28 patients (32.6%) had no documented recurrence, and 27 patients had one or more recurrences in paroxysmal and/or persistent form. In responder patients, drug treatment could be significantly reduced with a mean number of 1.4 ± 0.6 drugs at end follow-up as compared with 1.7 ± 0.5 during the pre-implantation period (p=0.01). The other 31 patients evolved towards chronic AF after a mean follow-up of 36 months. When comparing responder and non-responder patients in uni- and multivariate analysis, we found only one predictive factor of positive response, i.e. a P wave duration <160 ms prior to biatrial pacing implantation during normal sinus rhythm.

These preliminary results could be considered as consistent with a probable effect of biatrial pacing to prevent recurrent and drug-refractory atrial tachyarrhythmias in patients with intraatrial doncuction delay. These results led our group to undertake a prospective randomized, corssover and multicenter study aimed at validating this new concept. Inclusion in the SYNBIAPACE study started on late 1995 and was completed on Decembre 1997. The study consisted on an intra-patient comparison of three different pacing modes according to a dual crossover design over 3 month periods: a) "inhibited" or no atrial pacing (DDD-40 bpm); b) standard DDD pacing (70 bpm) at a single high right atrial site; and c) biatrial synchronous pacing (DDTA-70 bpm). The primary end point was time to first arrhythmia recurrence as documented by the pacemaker Holter function including intracardiac ECG storage. Forty-three patients (mean age 64 ± 12 years), mean P wave duration during normal sinus rythm (148 ± 31 ms) completed the overall protocol. Results showed no statistically significant differences in the three pacing modes, neither for the primary end point nor for the total time spent in atrial arrhythmia during the 3 months period (Tab. I). Whitin the limits of that protocol (small nunmber of highly selected patients; short follow-up time ; deliberate abstention from overdire pacing to assess the effects of atrial resynchronization alone, etc), the SYNBIAPACE study showed only a trend (NS) in favor of biatrial synchronous pacing. So the concept of atrial resynchronization to prevent atrial arrhythmias in patients with intraatrial conduction delay is still being to validate. Further studies including larger populations, and probably aimed at assessing the effects of combining biatrial and overdrive pacing are needed.

Table I

	Inhibited	Standard DDD	DDTA
Time to first recurrence (days)	39 ± 22	37 ± 22	62 ± 24
Total time spent in AA (days)	5 ± 13	7 ± 16	4 ± 18

The clinical experience with dual site right atrial pacing is still limited. Delfaut et al.[39] have recently reported the long-term results (28 ± 11 months) of a series of 30 patients (mean age 69±12 years), who were chronically implanted with a dual site right atrial DDDR pacemaker. Inclusion criteria were: i) a long history (mean duration 42±50 months) of symptomatic recurrent (at least two documented episodes during the past 3 months), and drug-refractory (mean number of antiarrhythmic drugs 3.6±1.7) atrial tachyarrythmias, ii) AF and/or atrial flutter, and b) a conventional indication for permanent cardiac pacing principally sinus node dysfunction or drug-induced bradycardia. The study protocol consisted of an initial prospective but non-randomized sequential crossover comparison of dual site right atrial pacing and single site right atrial pacing whether at the high right atrium or at the coronary sinus ostium, during periods of 3 to 6 months. After completing the crossover phase, the patients were definitively reprogrammed in dual site right atrial mode. Follow-up was principally based on the monitoring of symptomatic AF recurrences. When compared with no pacing during the 3 months pre-implant period, the two atrial pacing modes significantly increased the rate of freedom from symptomatic AF recurrences (0% with no pacing vs 62% with single site right atrial pacing and 89 % with dual site right atrial pacing; p<0.0001) and the arrhythmia free interval (9±10 days with no pacing vs 143±10 days with single site right atrial pacing and 195± 96 days with dual site right atrial pacing; p<0.0001). The two atrial pacing modes showed a significantly greater benefit with dual site right atrial pacing for the arrhythmia free interval (p<0.005). During the single site right atrial pacing period, no significant differences were observed between the subgroups of patients who were paced at the high right atrium and those paced at the coronary sinus ostium. In the long-term study with a mean follow-up time of 28±11 months, 14 patients (46.6%) did not experience any recurrent episode of symptomatic AF, 11 patients (36.6%) had at least one recurrence but remained atrially paced, and 5 patients (16.6%) were in chronic AF. The total rate of freedom from symptomatic AF was 78% at 1 year, and 56% at 3 years. In the patients who remained atrially paced at the end of follow-up, the mean number of antiarrhythmic drugs per patient was not significantly reduced as compared with the pre-implantation period.

__In summary__ these preliminary data show that overdrive atrial pacing in combination with antiarrhythmic durgs markedly reduce recurrent AF in patients with a conventional indication for permanent cardiac pacing, and provide some arguments in favor of a complementary preventive effect of dual site right atrial pacing as compared with single site pacing. However these results have to be confirmed in prospective, multicenter and randomized studies. The DAPPAF trial is now ongoing in the United States. This study is a ranzomized, crossover comparison of dual site atrial pacing, single site (high right atrium) pacing, and a support pacing control period (DDI or VDI at 50 bpm) done in 6 month intervals. Inclusion criteria are history of paroxysmal and drug-refractory AF and bradyarrhythmic indication for pacing. Inclusion is expected to be completed in 1999.

Overdrive suppression of atrial premature beats.

From many years specially designed algorithms have been proposed for the suppression of atrial extrasystoles by overdrive pacing. This old concept has recently been reevaluated by Murgatroyd et al.[40] by using a new algorithm loaded into the RAM memory of a DDD pacemaker (ELA Recherche, France). This algorithm causes the basic pacing rate to increase fractionally after each atrial premature complex. After a plateau period, the pacing rate is allowed to fall again gradually. The algorithm so determines a pacing rate that suppresses a majority of atrial premature beats. The algorithm also contains an element of smoothing in that it prevents post-extrasystolic compensatory pauses. The algorithmic effects were studied in 34 chronically implanted patients with frequent atrial extrasystoles and recurrent episodes of atrial tachyarrhythmia. The algorithm was programmed for automatic ON-OFF switching every two hours. Comparing the effects of switching "ON" and "OFF" by 24-h ambulatory ECG and by interrogating the pacemaker Holter functions elicited a significant decrease in the total number of atrial extrasystoles and of salvos with the algorithm being active. It was also noted that in all patients with frequent AF episodes during the study period, less episodes occurred when the algorithm was programmed as "ON". These preliminary data suggest that such algorithms could contribute to arrhythmia prevention in association with single-site or multiple-site atrial pacing. However, the exact role of atrial extrasystoles in AF initiation remains controversial[41] and additional data are needed to assess the true impact of atrial extrasystole suppression on preventing the initiation of AF or other types of atrial tachyarrhythmia.

In conclusion, we can reasonably assume that, in the near future, permanent atrial pacing will have an important role in the prevention of highly recurrent and drug-refractory atrial tachyarrhythmias. However, it is unlikely that atrial pacing per se, so sophistacated as the technology may be (multiple-site pacing, specialized algorithms...), will ensure complete and permanent protection. Therefore the future of implantable devices for this indication will probably require the development of new multifunction systems capable not only to significantly reduce the rate of arrhythmia recurrences by preventive pacing, but also to terminate the few recurrent episodes with ATP, or more probably, defibrillation functions.

REFERENCES

1. Coumel P., Attuel P., Lavallee J.P. et al. Syndrome d'arythmie auriculaire d'origine vagale. Arch Mal Coeur 1978; 71:645-56.

2. Han J., Millet D., Chizzinotti B., et al. Temporal dispersion of recovery of excitability in atrial and ventricle as a function of heart rate. Am Heart J 1966; 71: 481-7.

3. Han J., Detraglia J., Millet D., Moe G.K. Incidence of ectopic beats as a function of basic rate in the ventricle. Am Heart J 1966; 72:632-9.

4. Murgatroyd F.D., Curzen N.P., Aldergather J., et al. Clinical features and drug therapy in patients with paroxysmal atrial fibrillation: results of the CRAFT multi-center database. J Am Coll Cardiol 1993; 21:380A (abstract).

5. Capucci A., Santarelli A., Boriani G., et al. Atrial premature beats coupling interval determines lone paroxysmal atrial fibrillation onset. Int J Cardiol 1992; 36:87-93.

6. Denker S., Lehmann M.H., Mahmud R., et al. Facilitation of ventricular tachycardia induction with abrupt changes in ventricular cycle lengh. Am J Cardiol 1984;53:508-15.

7. Leclercq J.F., Maison-Blanche P., Cauchemez B., et al. Respective role of sympathetic tone and of cardiac pauses in the genesis of 62 cases of ventricular fibrillation recorded during Holter monitoring. Eur Heart J 1988; 9:1276-83.

8. Mehra R. How might pacing prevent atrial fibrillation? In "Nonpharmacological management of atrial fibrillation" FD Murgatroyd & AJ Camm Eds., Futura Publishing Company Inc., Armonk, 1997, pp: 283-308.

9. Prystowsky EN., Windle J.R. Inhibition in the human heart: a review. Eur J CPE 1994; 1:21-6.

10. Wijffels M.C.E.F., Kirchholf C.J.H.J., Dorland R., et al. Atrial fibrillation begets atrial fibrillation: a study in awake chronically instrumented goats. Circulation 1995; 92:1954-68.

11. Moss A.J., Rivers R.J. Jr, Griffin L.S.C., et al. Transvenous left atrial pacing for the control of recurrent ventricular fibrillation. NEJM 1968; 278:928-33.

12. Denjoy I., Leenhardt A., Thomas O., et al. Prevention of vagally mediated atrial tachyarrhythmia by permanent atrial pacing. In "Prevention of tachyarrhythmia with cardiac pacing". JC. Daubert, EN Prystowsky, A. Ripart, Eds. Futura 1997; pp. 87-97.

13. Shaw D.B., Holman R.R., Gowers J.L. Survival in sino-atrial disorder (sick sinus syndrome). Br Heart J 1988; 116:16-22.

14. Sutton R., Kenny R.A. The natural history of sick sinus syndrome.PACE 1986;9: 1110-14.

15. Rosenqvist M., Brandt J., Schuller H., et al. Long term pacing in sinus node disease : the effects of stimulation mode on cardiovascular morbidity and mortality. Am Heart J 1988 ;116:16-22.

16. Santini M., Alexiou G., Ansalone G., et al. Relation of prognosis in sick sinus syndrome to age, conduction defects and modes of permanent cardiac pacing. Am J Cardiol 1990; 65:729-35.

17. Andersen HR., Theusen L., Bagger J., et al. Prospective ransomized trial of atrial versus ventricular pacing in sick sinus syndrome. Lancet, 1994; 344:1923-8.

18. Andersen HR., Nielsen JC., Thomsen PE. et al. Long-term follow-up of patients from a ransomized trial of atrial versus ventricular pacing for sick sinus syndrome. Lancet, 1997;350:1210-16.

19. Nielsen JC., Andersen HR., Thomsen PE. et al. Heart failure and echocardiographic changes during long-term follow-up of patients with sick sinus syndrome randomized to single chamber atrial or ventricular pacing. Circulation 1998; 97:987-95.

20. Wharton JM., Sorrentino RA., Campbell P. et al. Effect of pacing modality on atrial tachyarrhythmia recurrence in the tachycardia-bradycardia syndrome: preliminary results of the Pace Atrial Tachycardia Trial. Circulation 1999; 98:I-494A.

21. Garrigue S., Cazeau S., Ritter P., et al. Incidence des arythmies atriales chez les patients stimules au long cours en mode double chambre. Apport des fonctions Holter du stimulateur. Arch Mal Coeur 1996; 89:873-82.

22. Gillis AM., Wyse G., Connolly SJ., et al. Atrial pacing periablation for prevention of paroxysmal atrial fibrillation. Circulation 1999; 99:2553-8.

23. Gillis AM., Connoly SJ., Dubuc M.,et al.Comparison of DDDR vs VDD pacing post total AV node ablation for prevention of atrial fibrillation. PACE 1999; 22:801.

24. Kato R., Terasawa T., Gotoh T., et al. Antiarrhythmic efficacy of atrial demand (AAI) and rate responsive atrial pacing. In M. Santini, M. Alliegro (eds) Progress in Clinical Pacing. Excerpta Medica, Amsterdam, 1988:15-24.

25. Heywood G., Katristis D., Ward J., et al. Atrial rate adaptative pacing in sick sinus syndrome: Effects on exercise capacity and arrhythmias. Br Heart J 1993;69: 174-8.

26. Santini M., Ricci R., Puglisi A., et al. Antiarrhythmic effects of DDD-DDIR pacing in sick sinus syndrome with chronotropic incompetence. PACE 1995;18: 848A.

27. Papageorgiou P., Monaham K., Boyle N. Site-dependant intra-atrial conduction delay. Relationship to initiation of atrial fibrillation. Circulation 1996; 94: 384-9.

28. Papageorgiou P., Anselme F., Monaham K., et al. Coronary sinus pacing prevents induction of atrial fibrillation. (abstract). JACC 1996; 27:313A.

29. Saksena S., Prakash A., Hill M., et al. Prevention of recurrent atrial fibrillation with chronic dual-site right atrial pacing. JACC 1996; 28:687-94.

30. Daubert C., Leclercq C., Le Breton H., et al. Permanent left atrial pacing with specifically designed coronary sinus leads. PACE 1997; 20:2755-64.

31. Spencer WH., Zhu DW., Markowitz T., et al. Atrial septal pacing: a method for pacing both atria simultaneously. PACE 1997; 20:2739-45.

32. Bailin SJ., Adler SW., Giudici MC., et al. Bachman's bundle pacing for the prevention of atrial fibrillation : initial trends in a multi-center randomized prospective study. (abstract). PACE 1999; 22:727.

33. Daubert C., Mabo P., Berder V., et al. Arrhythmia prevention by permanent atrial resynchronization in patients with advanced interatrial block. (abst) Eur Heart J 1990; 11:237.

34. Prakash A., Delfaut P., Krol RB., et al. Regional right and left atrial activation during single- and dual-site atrial pacing in patients with atrial fibrillation. Am J Cardiol 1998; 82:1197-204.

35. Wen-Chung R., Shih-Ann C., Ching-Tai T., et al. Effects of different atrial pacing modes on atrial electrophysiology, implicating the machanism of biatrial pacing in prevention of atrial fibrillation. Circulation 1997; 96:2992-6.

36. Daubert C., Mabo P., Berder V., et al. Atrial tachyarrhtymias associated with high degree interatrial conduction block. Prevention by permanent atrial resynchronization. Eur JCPE 1994; 4:35-44.

37. Daubert C., Gras D., Berder V., et al. Resynchronisation atriale permanente par la stimulation biatriale synchrone pour le traitement preventif du flutter auriculaire associee a un bloc inter-auriculaire de haut degre. Arch Mal Coeur 1994; 87: 1535-46.

38. Daubert C., Pavin D., Victor F., et al. In "Atrial flutter and fibrillation: from basics to clinical applications".Saoudi N.,SchoelsW., El-Sherif N. eds. Futura 1998:293-315.

39. Delfaut P., Saksena S., Prakash A., et al. Long-term outcome of patiens with drug-refractory atrial flutter and fibrillation after single and dual-site atrial pacing for arrhythmia prevention. J Am Coll Cardiol 1998; 39:1902-8.

40. Murgatroyd FD., Nitzche R., Slade AKB., et al. A new pacing algorithm for overdrive suppression of atrial fibrillation. PACE 1994; 17:1966-71.

41. Murgatroyd FD. Modes of onset of spontaneous episodes of atrial fibrillation : implications for the prevention of atrial fibrillation by pacing. In "Prevention of tachyarrhythmias with cardiac pacing". JC. Daubert, EN Prystowsky, A. Ripart (eds), Futura, 1997; pp. 53-65.

22.
PRACTICAL AND TECHNICAL ASPECTS OF BIATRIAL PACING

Andrzej Kutarski MD, PhD

University Medical Academy, Lublin, Poland

Resynchronising atrial pacing modes stays more and more popular and present indications for them can be divided into three groups:

1. Prevention of atrial arrhythmias. Classical RAA pacing is effective in 70-80% pts with BRT syndrome and in bradycardia dependent AF (for example vagal AF)[1], but in pts with inter- and intra-atrial conduction disturbances (IACD) it prolongs interatrial conduction time. Simultaneous pacing of earliest and latest activated areas of atria during sinus rhythm and premature atrial contractions restores synchronicity of atrial depolarisation/repolarisation and decreases dispersion of repolarisation[2-5]. Clear indications for resynchronising atrial pacing where not established but they are applied usually in pts with: **a)** frequent recurrence of atrial arrhythmias – (daily, weekly), **b)** IACD ($P_{II, III}$ over 120 ms) and total atrial activation time (from onset P_{II} to end A_{OE} or CS) over 150 ms), and **c)** unsuccessful antiarrhythmic therapy

2. Hemodynamic indications. Hemodynamic consequences of IACD in pts with dual chamber pacing system were described as "pacemaker syndrome in DDD pacing " and proper AV delay programmability was possible during Doppler's mitral flow evaluation only. BiA pacing/sensing in atrial channel provides to synchronous atrial contraction and allows safe programming of even ultra- short AV delay; it is especially important in pts with congestive cardiomyopathy[4,7].

3. Avoidance of ventricular capture (and AV node ablation necessity) in pts paced for HCM. In a lot of pts with HCM (with left ventricle outflow tract obstruction) coexists different degree of IACD; usually AV conduction remains normal. Standard DDD pacing system offers satisfied ventricular pacing during the rest. Exercises (catcholamines) improve AV conduction and provide to sinus capture of ventricles; programming of too short AV creates risk of "pacemaker syndrome in DDD pacing" and ablation of AV node was proposed solution. Safe programming even of ultra short AV delay is possible and easy when both of atria are paced simultaneously.

Till now, especial pacemakers for BiA pacing, containing additional channel for left atrial pacing are not available and only standard pacers have to be used. There are three main problems of BiA pacing: **a)** rela-

From Ovsyshcher IE. *Cardiac Arrythmias and Device Therapy: Results and Perspectives for the New Century.* Armonk, NY: Futura Publishing Company, Inc., © 2000

tively high frequency (over 10%) CS lead dislocation, **b)** often high pacing threshold (PTh) values and/or **c)** high energy requirement for synchronous pacing of both atria.

BIATRIAL PACING SYSTEMS – DIFFERENT ADVANTAGES AND DISADVANTAGES

There are a lot of possibilities of atrial leads connections which offer significantly different sensing / pacing conditions and each one of them presents extremely specific advantages and disadvantages. The question: "how to connect atrial lead for BiA pacing?" remains still actual.

I) In the "classical" split bipoles configuration proposed by Daubert for biatrial[8] and later by Ceazeau & Ritter for biventricular[7] pacing, cathode paces usually right and anode left atrium where pacing thresholds (PTh) are usually high. Pacing between two electrodes

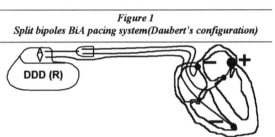

Figure 1
Split bipoles BiA pacing system(Daubert's configuration)

DDD (R)

joined by the "Y" connector in series and connected to atrial or ventricular BP part was named as "split BP pacing configuration" by Barold[4] (figure 1). It permits for excellent sensing both of atria and excellent resynchronising pacing (if AAT program is applied) even during sinus rhythm and during premature ectopic beats originating from right or left atrium as well[6]. Disadvantages of this configuration (electrodes connected in series) remain high global impedance and secondary to them – relatively high PTh[2,9-11]. CS is paced with anodal current however it is known since early 70-ies that anodic stimulation is worse in comparison to cathodic one[12]. Recently Stokes and Kay presented current knowledge on differences of cathodal and anodic electrophysiological effects[13,14]: 1) higher pacing threshold during anodic pacing; 2) special arrhythmogenic anodic current properties; its possible because "the threshold of anodic stimulation with electrodes of equal size is lower than that for cathodic stimulation in the strength-interval curve at shorter pulse widths"[13,14]; 3) tip corrosion caused by anodal potential is less important now.

II) Frequent problems with proper left atrial (LA) pacing observed with us in patients with classical Daubert's pacing system convinced us to the question: if the change in right atrium (RA) and CS leads polarity and cathodal CS pacing can really improve conditions of CS pacing[9,10]?

Comparison of Acute pacing conditions in 12 pts	RA threshold V/0,5 ms	RA energy	CS prox. threshold V/0,5 ms	CS prox. Energy	CS dist. threshold V/0,5 ms	CS dist. Energy
Cathodic pacing (UP)	0,53	0,56	2,40	6,67	4,94	8,72
Anodic pacing (UP)	1,03	1,07	3,45	7,95	6,28	10,22

Our long-term experience with modified split BP configuration indicated better functionality of this pacing system[9].

Cathodic RA	No of records (patients): 13
Anodic CS	No problems: 7 (54%)
"Classical"	Problems with pacing/sensing/resynchronisation: 6 (46%)
Cathodic CS	No of records (patients): 49
Anodic RA	No problems: 42 (86%)
"Inverted"	Problems with pacing/sensing/resynchronisation: 7 (14%)

Pacing conditions showed to be better using our modified SBP configuration[9].

Pacing Parameters	Pacing conditions on pacing with our modified SBP configuration — Lead connection		after operation	Period of observation — 1 month	Period of observation — 2 months	Period of observation — 3 months
Pacing Threshold (V)	Cathode - RA Anode-CS "Classical"	No.	11	6	2	1
		average	5,6	4,3	3,8	3,9
	Cathode - CS Anode - RA"Inverted"	No.	52	27	15	6
		average	4,9	5,0	4,8	3,4
Energy Consumption (µJ)	Cathode – RA Anode-CS "Classical"	No.	11	6	2	1
		average	33,8	16,8	22,1	19,0
	Cathode - CS Anode - RA"Inverted"	No.	49	26	15	6
		average	22,2	23,8	21,0	12,4

Both of described split BP BiA pacing systems (Fig. 1 and 2) can be characterised by having good sensing conditions, being well guard against muscular interference; thanks to summing-up of impedance (splitted electrodes) offer lower energy consumption but on the other hand if the global resistance is too high (approaching 1600 Ohm) the lost of LA capture becomes more evident and energy consumption gives rising tendency due to high current output and increased current drain for the pacemaker voltage doubler. These systems prefer low /moderate impedance leads and high impedance related pacing problems can be predicted if high impedance lead was previously implanted to RA. Additional, not examined until now disadvantage of this pacing con-

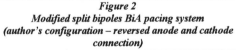

Figure 2
Modified split bipoles BiA pacing system
(author's configuration – reversed anode and cathode connection)

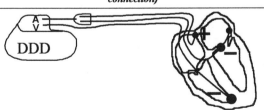

figuration seems to be pacing of the one of the atria using anodic current; pro-arrhythmic effect of anodic current (possibility of pacing during relative refractory period)[13-14]. Possibility of ventricular pacing if electrode is located in the distal part of CS and if high output values are programmed have to be taken into consideration.

III) Some years ago Cazeau et al. proposed different lead connection for multisite cardiac pacing – dual unipolar configuration (Fig.3). Leads are connected parallel and together to the cathode of the pacemaker atrial port using unipolar-unipolar Y-connector (DUP)[4,15]. DUP BiA pacing configuration offers worse atrial

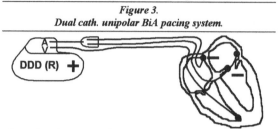

Figure 3.
Dual cath. unipolar BiA pacing system.

sensing conditions due to real unipolar sensing of both atria; pectoral myopotentials can be sensed if too high sensitivity is programmed. Global resistance and PTh values are relatively low but energy consumption is significantly higher than using SBP configuration[4,11,16,17]. In cases of high LA PTh capacity of standard pacemaker can be not sufficient to guarantee the programmed high voltage output[15]. The main advantage of DUP configuration seems to be avoidance of anodic pacing and risk of its proarrhythmic effect.

IV) Pacing condition in previously described pacing configurations are strongly depended from global impedance (lead connected in series or parallel). OLBI system was constructed for RA wall pacing from the rings of floating electrode. Two separate capacitors system are used to obtain two separate impulses (opposite polarisation increases the penetration of them). In fact this system gives us two independent - from each other - pacing circuits and permits to use two unipolar leads for simultaneous pacing of two places of heart in unipolar configuration (figure 4)

We compared the utility of the three presented above systems (SBP, DUP and OLBI) for BiA pacing / sensing and we focused especially on sensing conditions and energy consumption. In 12 pts with brady-tachy- (BRT) syndrome during implantation of BiA pacing system we compared (with ERA 300B) using different connections[11,16].

Lead connections	RA-tip of UP lead CS-tip of BP lead			RA-tip of UP lead CS-ring of BP lead		
Pacing configuration	OLBI	SBP	**DUP**	OLBI	SBP	DUP
Amplitude A (mV)	2,8	2,0	1,5	2,4	2,7	1,9
Threshold (V)	**3,30**	**5,55**	**6,04**	**1,83**	**3,91**	**2,31**
Resistance (ohm)	796,8	787,2	344	589,1	622,2	214
Energy (uJ)	**8,04**	**7,3**	**15,7**	**6,03**	**5,9**	**10,5**

Utility of ring of BP CS lead permits to decrease PTh during pacing with

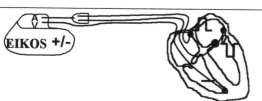

Figure 4
Biatraial pacing using DDD pacemaker with OLBI sytem in atrial channel

all configurations but differences of energy consumption are not spectacular. BiA OLBI™ pacing offers lowers PTh; energy consumption is comparable to SBP configuration and significantly lower than during DUP BiA pacing. Independence from global resistance is the most important advantage of OLBI™ pacing system. It seems to be solution for pts with impedance related problems during BiA pacing[11,16]. It presents full independence of both atrial circuits from impedance of each one (due to separation of these atrial circuits the impedance neither does not sum nor do not divide). Utility and advantages of this system

seems to show the direction towards real three-chamber pacemaker construction.

V) Inspired with Daubert's and Saksena's promising results we started with BiA pacing three years ago using standard leads and pacemakers[5]. "Y" connec-

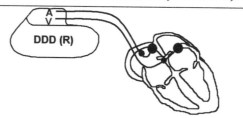

Figure 5
The oldest one (1988) Markewitz-Osterholzer BiA pacing system for recipient-donors atria resynchronisation)

tors were not available in our market in this time and we decided to implant resynchronising systems described in 1988 by Markewitz and Osterholzer[18] (Fig.5) for resynchronisation of donor and recipient atria in pts after orthotopic heart transplantation and sinus node insufficiency. The lead implanted to atrial remnant was connected with atrial port and

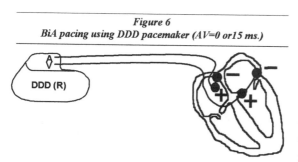

Figure 6
BiA pacing using DDD pacemaker (AV=0 or15 ms.)

the other one implanted to right atrium (RA) of transplanted heart – to ventricular port of DDD pacemaker. The recipient atrium served as sensor and VDD (with short AV delay) program enabled restoration of chronotropic function of transplant if only recipient sinus function was preserved[18].

VI) Review of literature suggests that nobody tried to use both of channels of standard DDD pacemaker for BiA pacing during this time (Fig. 6). Our primary experience with this pacing system were very promising[2,5] and similar to other authors which later used it[6,8]. After necessary re-operation in post-operative period (19%) due to dislocation of leads, exit block surgical complications a lot of pts (80%) could be paced successfully during long term period[19]. The reasons of late re-operation during long-term period were related to specific disadvantages of this pacing system – atrial arrhythmias originating from atrium connected to ventricular channel of pacemaker (11%) and late occurrence of AV conduction disturbances. Moderately elevated PTh in CS do not create real problem and pacemaker output in CS connected channel can be programmed only slightly over threshold energy; simultaneous pacing of RAA with standard output safe margin prevents sudden breaks of pacing[19]. Advantages of BiA (DDD) pacing system: precious (separate for each atrium) output programming (energy saving), sensing both of atria separately in BP configuration (lower V amplitude sensing), maintenance of atrial pacing in case of dislocation/exit-block of CS lead and possibility of separate evaluation of CS pacing/sensing conditions (important for evaluation of a new models of CS designed leads). Main disadvantages of this pacing system are: impossibility of ventricular pacing if A-V block occur later and impossibility of resynchronisation of premature LA excitations if "standard" mode connection of leads was applied[2,5,19].

General and detail conclusions:

1. There is urgent requirement for special pacemaker designed for BiA pacing
2. Standard SSI, DDD pacemakers and different "Y" connectors enables simultaneous pacing of both atria but all lead connections systems shows specific disadvantages; strong dependence from global resistance decreases effectiveness of pacing and utility of ventricular channel for left atrial pacing closes the way for three-chamber pacing additionally.

    i.   Sensing conditions are better during BP (SBP and OLBI) than UP (DUP) configuration.

    ii. Utility of the ring of standard BP CS lead, in place of its tip enables significantly reduction of PTh and energy consumption.

    iii. DUP BiA pacing configuration shows to be the most energy consuming in spite of relatively lower PTh values; it can be explained by parallel connection of electrodes (resistors) and secondary the lowest global impedance.

    iv. Independence from global resistance seems to be the most important advantage of OLBI system. It seems to be the solution for patients with impedance related problems during BiA pacing. The advantages of this system seem to show the direction towards real three-chamber pacemaker construction. BiA pacing is very promising mode for suppression of atrial arrhythmias.

   v. BiA pacing using DDD pacemaker is the simplest solution but appearance of LA arrhythmias and the risk of AV conduction disturbances remain its main limitations.

3. Additional left atrial channel with possibility of separate output programming and BP pacing is the most desirable solution and consist challenge for biomedical technology.

References

1. Saksena S., Prakash A., Nandini M., Giorgberidze I. et al. Prevention of atrial fibrillation by pacing. In: Barold SS. Mugica J. (ed.): Recent Advances in Cardiac Pacing. Goals for the 21st Century. Armonk NY, Futura Publishing Company Inc. 1998: 101-114.
2. Kutarski A., Poleszak K., Oleszczak K., Koziara D., Widomska-Czekajska T. Biatrial and coronary sinus pacing – long term experience with 246 patients. Progress Biomed Research 1998; 3: 114-120
3. Daubert C., Mabo P., Berder V., Gras D. Atrial flutter and interatrial conduction block: preventive role of biatrial synchronous pacing? In: Waldo A., Touboul P. (ed.) Atrial flutter. Advances in Mechanism and management. Futura Publishing co. Armonk NY 1996; 331-346
4. Barold SS., Cazeau S., Mugica J., Garrigue S., Clementy J. Permanent multisite pacing. PACE 1997; 20: 2725-2729
5. Kutarski A., Oleszczak K., Koziara D, Poleszak K. Permanent biatrial pacing - the first experiences. PACE 1997; 20: 2308 (abstr.)
6. Daubert C., Leclercq C., Pavin D. et al. Biatrial synchronous pacing. A new approach to prevent arrhythmias in patients with atrial conduction block. In Daubert C. Prystovsky E. Ripart A. (ed.): Prevention of Tachyarrhythmias with Cardiac Pacing. Armonk, New York; Futura Publishing Company Inc. 1997: 99-123
7. Cazeau S., Ritter P., Bakdach S., Lazarus A., Limousin M., Henao L., Mundler O., Daubert J., Mugica J. Four chamber pacing in dilated cardiomyopathy. PACE. 1994; 17: 1974-1979
8. Daubert C., Gras D., Leclerq Ch., Baisett M., Victor F., Mabo Ph. Biatral synchronous pacing: a new therapeutic approach to prevent refractory atrial tachyarrhythmias. JACC, 1995; 25: 230 (abstr).

9. Kutarski A., Oleszczak K., Schaldach M., Koziara D., Poleszak K., Widomska-Czekajska T. Cathode or anode in coronary sinus in patients with Daubert's biatrial pacing system. HeartWeb 1999; 4: article No. 99030001

10. Kutarski A., Oleszczak K., Baszak J., Schaldach M., Poleszak K., Koziara D., Widomska-Czekajska T. Cathode or anode in coronary sinus (CS) in pts with Daubert's BiA pacing system? Arch Mal Coeur Vaiss 1998; 91III: 337 (abstr.)

11. Kutarski A., Schaldach M., OLBI stimulation in biatrial pacing? A comparison of acute pacing and sensing conditions for split bipolar and dual cathodal unipolar configurations. Progr Biomed Res 1999; 4: 236-240

12. Preston T.A. Anodal stimulation as a cause of pacemaker – induced ventricular fibrillation. Am Heart J 1973; 86: 366 (abstr.)

13. Stokes K.B. Kay G.N. Artificial electric cardiac stimulation. In Ellenbogen KA, Kay GN, Wilkoff BL (ed.): Clinical Cardiac Pacing, Philadelphia, United States, W.B Saunders Company, 1995: 3-37.

14. Kay G.N. Basic aspects of cardiac pacing. In: Ellenbogen K. (ed.) Cardiac Pacing. Blackwell Scientific Publications. Boston, 1992: 32-119

15. Limousin M. Current limitations of multisite pacing technnmology. Arch Mal Coeur Vaiss 1998; 91III: 246 (abstr.)

16. Kutarski A., Schaldach M., OLBI stimulation for biatrial pacing? A comparison of acute pacing/sensing conditions with split bipoles and dual cathodal unipolar configuration. PACE 1999; 22 II: 12 (abstr.)

17. Kutarski A., Oleszczak K., Wojcik M. Split bipoles or dual cathodal UP configuration for permanent biatrial pacing? A comparison of output requirement and sensing conditions. Pace 1999; 22 II: 155 (abstr.)

18. Markewitz A., Osterholzer G., Weinhold C., Authuber M., Keinkes BM. Recipient P wave synchronised pacing of the donnor atrium in a heart transplanted patient: A case study. PACE 1988; 11: 1402-1403

19. Kutarski A., Widomska-Czekajska T., Oleszczak K., Wojcik M., Poleszak K. Clinical and technical aspects of permanent BiA pacing using standard DDD pacemaker – long term experience in 47 patients. Progr Biomed Res. 1999; 4: 394-404

23

MULTISITE ATRIAL PACING FOR THE PREVENTION OF RECURRENCE OF ATRIAL FIBRILLATION: OPTIMISTIC AND PESSIMISTIC VIEWS.

Panos E. Vardas, MD, PhD, Emmanuel G. Manios, MD, Emmanuel N. Simantirakis, MD

Cardiology Department, University Hospital, University of Crete, Heraklion, Greece.

Introduction

Permanent pacing for the prevention of atrial fibrillation (AF) in patients who are at a high risk for this arrhythmia is a relatively new concept. Single site atrial pacing has been found in several retrospective studies[1-3] to be associated with a lower incidence of AF when it is compared with that of ventricular pacing. Results from recent prospective randomized trials indicate that patients with sick sinus syndrome benefit from atrial pacing. However, single site atrial pacing offers no clear improvement in the incidence of AF in other groups of paced bradyarrhythmic patients.[4-7] Thus single site atrial pacing cannot be considered as a treatment for the prevention of recurrent AF.

Recently multisite atrial pacing has been suggested as an alternative pacing treatment to prevent recurrences of AF. The rationale for biatrial pacing and also for dual-site right atrial pacing is derived from the premise that intraatrial and interatrial conduction delays are essential to the reentrant mechanisms that underline AF[8,9]. It has been thought that multisite atrial pacing resynchronizes atrial electrical activity and attenuates conduction delays and thus it may prevent AF induction[10]. This hypothesis has been tested in acute studies, with inducible arrhythmia, and in long-term trials.

The acute studies

Acute studies offered a careful observation of clinical electrophysiological parameters in the atria during uni- and bifocal atrial pacing and an assessment of the inducibility of AF under these conditions. Papageorgiou et al,[11] showed the importance of site-dependent intraatrial conduction delays for the initiation of AF. Prakash et al,[12] mapped the regional atrial activation, with high right atrial premature beats in dual-site right atrial pacing modes, and found a significant reduction in AF inducibility in dual site mode as compared to that from a single high right atrial site. Yu et al,[13] showed that premature stimulation in the high right

From Ovsyshcher IE. *Cardiac Arrythmias and Device Therapy: Results and Perspectives for the New Century.* Armonk, NY: Futura Publishing Company, Inc., © 2000

atrium causes a greater delay in conduction to the His bundle area, right posterior septum and distal coronary sinus than does premature atrial stimulation in the distal coronary sinus. These authors also showed that when the high right atrium and distal coronary sinus were driven simultaneously the conduction delay caused by premature stimulation in the high right atrium was significantly reduced.

Furthermore the previous groups in other studies found that either biatrial pacing or dual-site right atrial pacing can reduce the inducibility of AF. [14,15]

This however is the optimistic aspect of these studies. A careful observer could find a number of weakpoints in these studies. Such weakpoints are the method of arrhythmia induction and the type and number of patients who are studied.
The protocol for AF inducibility did not have a crossover design in any of the three studies, since unifocal pacing was evaluated before bifocal in every case. It is possible that this sequence influenced the inducibility of AF. It is also possible that the number of extrastimuli also affected the sensitivity of the evaluation, since in some cases one extrastimulus was used and in others three. In a recent study which was carried out in our department, 75 patients were randomised into two groups and the inducibility of AF or atrial tachycardia following the delivery of up to two ectopic beats was examined. In the first group the ectopic beats were administered during single site high right atrial pacing and in the second group during biatrial pacing from high right atrium and coronary sinus. We found no difference in AF inducibility between unifocal right atrial pacing and biatrial pacing.[16]

The Papageorgiou and Yu studies involved patients with no organic heart disease, indeed the former included patients with no clear history of AF. Also, the number of patients studied was small, as Papageorgiou et al acknowledged.

Apart from the above, it should be noted that it is not known whether acute studies are of relevance to patients with spontaneous AF or whether they can predict responders and non-responders to long term biatrial pacing.

Long-term studies of multisite pacing
The clinical effectiveness of this method for the prevention of AF relapses could be demonstrated in long-term clinical studies.

Indeed, permanent multisite atrial pacing has been applied in an increasing number of patients who have already completed quite a long follow - up period. At the same time, more properly designed prospective, randomized studies have been aimed at an assessment of the therapeutic effect of multisite pacing in patients with a chronic history of atrial arrhythmias. Let us examine whether the available data gives us sufficient reason to be enthusiastic.

Let the start be made with the results of the latest randomized, prospective, crossover SYNBIAPACE study. This study showed a trend towards a reduction in the incidence of atrial arrhythmias during biatrial pacing, as compared to DDD mode, at 70 and 40 bpm, without a clear benefit.[17]

The results of another prospective but non-randomized study have recently been published. According to the findings of this study 32.6% of patients remained in sinus rhythm, while in another 31% medication reduced the incidence of relapse, compared to the period before the application of pacing.[18]

However, smaller studies, also recent, did not confirm these observations. Neugebauer et al,[19] found that episodes of AF were not prevented after biatrial pacing in 12 patients with symptomatic paroxysmal AF or persistent AF, with documented interatrial conduction delays. However, these patients responded better to antiarrhythmic drugs after biatrial pacing. Another prospective, randomized, single-blinded study,[20] showed that there was a significant reduction in the overall duration of AF with either right or biatrial pacing, when compared with the unpaced control period. When right atrial pacing was compared with biatrial pacing no difference could be demonstrated in either the duration or the frequency of AF episodes.

In the case of dual-site right atrial pacing, on a chronic basis, we must rely on the findings of smaller studies, since the results of randomized, prospective studies, such as the Dutch DRAPPAF study are not yet available.

In a prospective, crossover, non-randomized study,[21] which compared the efficacy of single- and dual-site right atrial pacing for the prevention of AF in 30 patients with paroxysmal arrhythmia, 56% of patients remained in sinus rhythm for three years. After following the same protocol as Saksena's team in our own center we were able to present our joint results. After following 40 patients over a period of 7-30 months we found that 53% of patients remained in sinus rhythm without drugs; when those receiving medication were included the percentage rose to 87%[22]. Finally, Lau et al,[23] recently presented the findings of the NIPP-AFF study, for 15 patients with dual-site right atrial pacing and taking sotalol. Compared to high right atrium pacing, dual-site atrial pacing was associated with a prolonged time to AF recurrence and a reduced time in AF.

Given the high incidence of AF during the immediate postoperative period in patients who undergo cardiac surgery, biatrial pacing has been tried as a non-pharmacological therapy. The main findings are again conflicting. Daoud et al,[24] and Orr et al,[25] reported that simultaneous right and left atrial pacing significantly reduced the incidence of AF following open heart surgery to 17.9% and 10%, respectively. In contrast, Gerstenfeld et al,[26] in a first report from a study of 61 patients, found no significant difference in the proportion of patients developing AF after coronary artery bypass grafting, whether atrial pacing alone, biatrial pacing or no pacing was applied. However, it is interesting that the same authors recently reported findings from 98 patients in which biatrial pacing appeared to have a beneficial effect. A recent study by Lee et al,[27] cast further doubt on the value of biatrial pacing in postoperative cardiac bypass patients, showing that medication significantly reduced the incidence of AF compared to placebo (12% versus 34%) to a degree comparable or superior to that achieved by biatrial pacing.

Conclusions

Can we therefore be optimistic that multisite atrial pacing could provide the solution to the problem of paroxysmal atrial fibrillation, or should we temper our enthusiasm?

The aforementioned evidence does not undoubtedly prove the usefulness of the method, since it originates from studies with limited statistical power which are often not suitably randomized. Furthermore it does not allow us to select the patients who could benefit nor the cost benefit relationship of this kind of therapy. However, enough of the evidence is encouraging and allows us to continue our efforts. Even in the event that multisite atrial pacing proves non-applicable, our knowledge and experience of atrial fibrillation will have been enriched.

References

1. Feuer JM, Shandling AH, Messenger JC. Influence of cardiac pacing mode on the long term development of atrial fibrillation. Am J Cardiol 1989: 64; 1376 -1379
2. Stangl K, Seitz K, Wirtzfeld A, et al. Differences between atrial single chamber pacing (AAI) and ventricular single chamber pacing (VVI) with respect to prognosis and antiarrhythmic effect ion patients with sick sinus syndrome. PACE 1990: 13; 2080-2085

3. Rosenqvist M, Brandt J, Schuller H. Long term pacing in sinus node disease: effects of stimulation mode on cardiovascular morbidity and mortality. Am Heart J 1988:116; 16-22

4. Andersen H, Thuesen L, Bagger J, et al. Prospective randomized trial of atrial versus ventricular in sick sinus syndrome. Lancet 1994:344; 1523-1528

5. Lamas GA, Orav EJ, Stambler BS, et al. Quality of life and clinical outcomes in elderly patients treated with ventricular pacing as compared with dual-chamber pacing. N Engl J Med 1998: 338; 1097-1104

6. Gillis AM, Kerr CD, Connolly SJ, et al. Identification of patients most likely to benefit from physiologic pacing in the Canadian trial of physiologic pacing. PACE 1999: 22; 728.

7. Skanes AC, Krahn AD, Yee R, et al. Physiologic pacing reduces progression to chronic atrial fibrillation. PACE 1999: 22;728.

8. Simpson R, Foster JR, Gettes LS. Atrial excitability and conduction in patients with interatrial conduction defects. Am J Cardiol 1982: 50; 1331-1337

9. Bayes de Luna A, Cladellas M, Otter R, et al. Intraatrial conduction block and retrograde activation of left atrium and paroxysmal supraventricular tachyarrhythmias. Eur Heart J 1988: 9; 1112-18

10. Daubert C, Berder V, Mabo P, et al. Arrhythmia prevention by permanent atrial resyncronization in advanced interatrial blocks.(abstr) Circulation 1990:91(suppl III);181

11. Papageorgiou P, Monahan K, Boyle NG, et al. Site-dependent intra-atrial conduction delay: Relationship to initiation of atrial fibrillation. Circulation 1996: 94; 384-389.

12. Prakash A, Delfaut P, Krol RB, et al. Regional right and left atrial activation patterns during single- and dual-site atrial pacing in patients with atrial fibrillation. Am J Cardiol 1998: 15;1197-1204

13. Yu WC, Chen SA, Tai CT, et al. Effects of different atrial pacing modes on atrial electrophysiology: Implicating the mechanism of biatrial pacing in prevention of atrial fibrillation. Circulation 1997: 96; 2992-2996.

14. Prakash A, Saksena S, et al. Acute effects of dual-site right atrial pacing in patients with spontaneous and inducible atrial flutter and fibrillation. J Am Coll Cardiol 1997: 29;1007-1114.

15. Papageorgiou P, Anselme F, Kirchhof CJ, et al. Coronary sinus pacing prevents induction of atrial fibrillation. Circulation 1997; 96: 6, 1893-1898.

16. Manios EG, Igoumenidis NE, Kochiadakis GE, et al. Inducibility of atrial tachyarrhythmia in patients with lone atrial fibrillation. PACE 1999: 22; 843.

17. Mabo P, Daubert JC, Bohour A. Biatrial synchronous pacing for atrial arrhythmia prevention: The SYNBIAPACE study. PACE 1999: 22; 755.

18. Revault d' Allones G, Victor F, Pavin D, et al. Long term effects of biatrial synchronous pacing to prevent drug refractory atrial tachyarrthnias: A pilot study. PACE 1999: 22; 755

19. Neugebauer A, Mende M, Kolb HJ, et al. Long term results of synchronous biatrial pacing for prevention of symptomatic atrial fibrillation. PACE 1999: 22; 875.

20. Levy T, Walker S, Rochelle J, et al. Evaluation of biatrial pacing, right atrial pacing, and no pacing in patients with drug refractory atrial fibrillation. Am J Cardiol 1999: 8; 426-429.

21. Delfaut P, Saksena S, Prakash A, et al. Long-term outcome of patients with drug-refractory atrial flutter and fibrillation after single- and dual-site right atrial pacing for arrhythmia prevention. J Am Coll Cardiol 1998: 32; 1900-8.

22. Prakash A, Vardas P, Delfaut P, et al. Multicenter experience with single site and dual site atrial pacing in refractory atrial fibrillation. (Abstr) PACE 1997;20(Suppl)1074

23. Lau CP, Tse HF, Yu CM, et al. Dual site right atrial pacing in paroxysmal atrial fibrillation without bradycardia (NIPP-AF study). PACE 1999: 22;804.

24. Daoud EG, Riba A, Strickberger A, et al. Simultaneous right and left atrial epicardial pacing for prevention of post open-heart surgery atrial fibrillation. PACE 1999: 22; 707

25. Orr WP Tsui S, Stafford PJ, et al. Synchronised bi-atrial pacing for the prevention of atrial fibrillation after coronary artery bypass surgery. PACE 1999: 22;755.

26. Gerstenfeld EP, Khoo M, Martin R, et al. Effectiveness of bi-atrial pacing for reducing atrial fibrillation after coronary artery bypass graft (GABG) surgery. PACE 1999: 22;754.

27. Lee SH, Chang CM, Hung CR, et al. Intravenous amiodarone is effective in preventing atrial fibrillation after coronary artery bypass grafting. PACE 1999: 22; 718.

24

PACING AND DEFIBRILLATION FOR THE PREVENTION AND TERMINATION OF ATRIAL FIBRILLATION.

Philip Spurrell, MRCP, Neil Sulke, MD FACC.

Department of Cardiology, Eastbourne General Hospital, Eastbourne, UK.

Introduction

Atrial fibrillation is not just a single disorder but a multitude of entities. It is this diversity that may in part explain its resistance to medical intervention. As a consequence of this diversity different therapeutic interventions may have differing effects upon AF prevention and termination. Patient selection is therefore crucial.

Table 1	Paroxysmal AF		Persistent AF	Permanent AF
Triggers	+++	+	+	++
Promoters	+	+++	+	++
Perpetuators	+	+	++(+)	+++

The relative contribution of triggers, promoters and perpetuators (Table 1) in a patient with atrial fibrillation may provide a guide as to which interventions are likely to be beneficial.

Table 2	Drug	Pacing	Cardioversion	RF Ablation	Surgery
Triggers	II	Overdrive	No	Focal	No
Promoters	?	Pre-excitation	Reversed Remodelling	Area	No
Perpetuators	Ic,III	Entrain-ment	Yes	Catheter Maze	Maze/ Corridor

Table 2 shows possible pharmacological and device-based therapy as well as surgical interventions that can be used against various mechanisms of atrial fibrillation. We will discuss the use of pacemakers and atrial defibrillators in the treatment of different forms of atrial fibrillation, in this chapter. (Table 1 & 2 adapted from M.Allessie).

PAROXYSMAL AF

Single Site Pacing

A large number of retrospective studies have demonstrated that atrially based pacing in patients with Sick Sinus Syndrome reduces progression to atrial fibrillation as well as a reduction in thromboembolic complications when compared to ventricular pacing[1-3]. A large prospective study in 225 patients with sick sinus syndrome also demonstrated a beneficial effect of atrial pacing compared to ventricular pacing with significantly higher

From Ovsyshcher IE. *Cardiac Arrythmias and Device Therapy: Results and Perspectives for the New Century.* Armonk, NY: Futura Publishing Company, Inc., © 2000

survival, less atrial fibrillation, fewer thromboembolic complications and less heart failure[4].

Various groups are currently assessing the benefits of atrial septal pacing as standard right atrial appendage pacing is sometimes a source of delayed interatrial conduction. Atrial septal pacing with active fixation has been shown to be safe, reliable and stable with subsequent reduction in the P wave durations[5,6]. Currently data is only available on small patient numbers but has demonstrated a significant reduction in arrhythmic episodes compared to pre-implant, but not within patient trials[6].

Multi-site Pacing

Recent studies have assessed the effects of multi-site pacing in patients with symptomatic drug refractory atrial fibrillation. Patients with marked inter-atrial conduction block and prolonged surface P wave duration (resulting in delayed and abnormal activation of the left atrium) may predispose to atrial tachyarrhythmias including atrial flutter and atrial fibrillation. The technique involves simultaneous pacing of the high right atrium and distal coronary sinus. In this patient population 84% of patients were free of atrial arrhythmias over a mean follow-up period of 34 months[7].

Multisite, uni-atrial pacing (high right atrium and coronary sinus os) is technically easier and has been shown to confer an additional benefit over single site pacing alone. Current clinical experience has shown 78%, 63% and 56% of patients were free of AF recurrences at 1, 2, and 3 years respectively in a non-crossover study design[8].

Currently larger prospective randomised studies including SYNBIAPACE, DAPPAF, PIPAF and DRAPPAF are underway. Preliminary results from SYNBIAPACE have recently been released. This study of three phases of three months compared a control phase of DDD pacing at 40bpm, single site pacing at 70bpm and biatrial pacing at 70bpm. In 43 patients, results show no statistical difference between the three pacing modes but there was a trend in favour of biatrial pacing[9].

Levy and colleagues have compared a control group of right atrial pacing at 40bpm with standard right atrial pacing and biatrial pacing[10]. There was a significant improvement seen in biatrial pacing over the control group in the 19 patients assessed but no additional advantage over standard right atrial pacing. It is possible that there is a subgroup of patients who may benefit from biatrial pacing but this has yet to be defined.

Overdrive Pacing

Two studies have reported benefit from atrial overdrive pacing in patients with vagally mediated paroxysmal atrial fibrillation (Coumel's Syndrome)[11,12]. This patient group is not representative of most patients with paroxysmal atrial fibrillation and caution is required when extrapolating these favourable results to the population as a whole.

22 patients with sick sinus syndrome had atrial overdrive pacing for 65% of the study period. After one month this resulted in 'complete suppression of AF' in 14 patients and a reduction in AF load in the remainder[13]. Currently more sophisticated algorithms achieving >95% atrial overdrive pacing are under evaluation, in longer-term studies with better Holter monitoring[14].

Prevention of Triggers

Studies assessing ambulatory ECG recordings prior to the onset of paroxysmal AF episodes have demonstrated many potential triggers responsible for the induction of AF[15]. The Vitatron AF Therapy Study and ELA PIPAF study are currently in progress assessing the effects of preventative atrial pacing upon these and total AF burden.

In our centre, which is participating in the Vitatron study, we have scrutinised over 150 detailed onset reports from 25 patients with paroxysmal AF. A variety of different onset mechanisms were seen in our patient population and also within the same patient. Only 20% of these episodes were of sudden onset i.e. no discernible trigger seen. This suggests that a large percentage of triggers may be amenable to preventative atrial pacing.

Preventative pacing algorithms under assessment include atrial overdrive pacing, suppression of PACs, prevention of pauses post PAC and prevention of post exercise rate drop. Data on the effects of these algorithms on AF burden, quality of life and patient acceptance is not yet available. Further algorithms are under development, most crucially post termination arrhythmia recurrence suppression, the commonest trigger in many patients.

PERSISTENT AF

Anti-tachycardia Pacing

Waldo's group has demonstrated the ability to entrain and terminate certain forms of atrial flutter with rapid atrial pacing[16]. Previous theories suggested that in persistent atrial fibrillation there was no excitable gap within which to capture and terminate atrial fibrillation. However Allessie's group and others have demonstrated that such an excitable gap although small, does exist, and that certain areas of the atrium can be entrained with rapid atrial pacing[17,18]. However in these studies no termination of AF could be achieved.

Small studies have demonstrated varying degrees of success in patients with paroxysmal AF and to a lesser degree with persistent AF[19-23]. One study assessing the efficacy of rapid atrial pacing of various durations and at several sites was also unable to terminate atrial fibrillation[22]. Interestingly the control period of sub-threshold rapid atrial pacing did result in one episode of termination demonstrating that this was spontaneous rather than pacing induced.

The Jewel AF study has demonstrated a success rate for termination of atrial fibrillation with 50Hz burst pacing of 40% in a population of patients with an Implantable Atrial and Ventricular Defibrillator[23]. However in our subgroup of patients with persistent AF only, we have seen no termination of atrial fibrillation in 22 in-hospital assessments and have shown that 50Hz burst pacing may be proarrhythmic resulting in episodes of ERAF (early recurrence of atrial fibrillation) following cardioversion.

Implantable Atrial Defibrillators

External transthoracic cardioversion of atrial fibrillation has been well established since it was first described in 1962. This technique is capable of restoring sinus rhythm in approximately 80% of patients. However between 50 and 70% of patients have reverted back to atrial fibrillation within one year. These figures can be improved with the addition of antiarrhythmic drugs but exposes the patient to the potential side effects and proarrhythmic effects that are associated with these drugs[24]. For these reasons attention has turned towards the possibility of an implantable atrial defibrillator. The ideal device would be capable of reliably detecting atrial fibrillation and consistently achieving safe and successful defibrillation using a painless shock.

The most effective endocardial lead configuration involves shock delivery between a right atrial electrode and a distal coronary sinus electrode[25]. This brackets the largest amount of atrial tissue between the electrodes resulting in atrial defibrillation thresholds of 2 to 12 Joules. Work with different waveforms and sequential shocks is underway to reduce defibrillation energy requirements still further[26,27]. Unfortunately, endocardial defibrillation cannot yet be achieved with energy levels that are painless.

Previous studies have suggested that delivery of energies above 0.1 Joule cause discomfort or pain[28,29]. Some data suggests that high and low defibrillation energies are perceived by patients to be equally painful. In addition a repeated shock is perceived as more painful regardless of its energy. This highlights the importance of achieving sinus rhythm with a single shock, or better still with painless pacing therapies. However sedative drugs can dramatically improve tolerability[30].

The first implantable atrial defibrillator (Metrix device, In Control Inc, Redmond, USA) consists of a three lead system with right atrial and distal coronary sinus shocking coils and a ventricular lead to allow R wave synchronisation and post shock ventricular pacing. It is capable of delivering shocks to a maximum of 6J. This device has been shown to be safe with no incidence of ventricular proarrhythmia following over 5000 atrial defibrillation shocks. Automatic atrial defibrillation or magnet activation by patient or physician is programmable.

Serial increase in post-shock sinus rhythm duration has been seen in some patients treated with repeated endocardial defibrillation[31,32]. This supports the concept of 'sinus rhythm begets sinus rhythm' in patients with persistent AF. Thus sinus rhythm should be restored as rapidly as possible to avoid adverse electrophysiological remodelling. In order to achieve this the device would be programmed to deliver automatic shocks within minutes of AF onset. This would seriously affect device tolerability.

The first implantable atrial and ventricular defibrillator, the Jewel AF (Medtronic Inc, Minneapolis, USA) is under evaluation. In addition to atrial defibrillation, which can be automatic or patient-activated, the device can provide anti-tachycardia pacing for atrial tachyarrhythmias, (atrial ramp and burst) as well as 50Hz burst pacing. Tiered therapy can be programmed separately for atrial tachycardias, atrial fibrillation and ventricular tachycardias in addition to ventricular defibrillation for VF. The rate stabilisation function also prevents pauses post PACs. The device can deliver a defibrillation shock of up to 27J.

Our group of 14 patients with persistent AF has currently delivered over 60 out-of-hospital patient activated atrial defibrillation shocks at an output of 27J with 100% success rate for attainment of sinus rhythm. Atrial defibrillation shocks are well tolerated by the patients with the aid of sedation. (A small group has been performing some shocks without any form of sedation at all). An on-going randomised study of 3 sedation regimes including opiate analgesia plus benzodiazepine versus anxiolytic alone versus analgesic alone is nearing completion with anxiolytic apparently preferred.

Hybrid Therapies

The use of several modalities of treatment in a single patient may provide additional benefits over single therapy alone[33]. This concept of hybrid therapy may take the form of varying combinations of ablation, pacing (including preventative and antitachycardia pacing), atrial defibrillators and drugs. Certain combinations may prove to be synergistic for specific types of AF. This new avenue of therapy offers exciting opportunities for the future treatment of AF.

Conclusion

Atrial fibrillation is not a single entity and therapy is unlikely to be straightforward as the disorder develops. A combination of therapies is the way forward and certainly with the advances in device therapy in the last few years, and the promise of rapid evolution in future technology, effective treatment if not cure of this common arrhythmia is now a reality.

References

1. Rosenqvist M, Brandt J, Schuller H. Long-term pacing in sinus node disease: effect of stimulation mode on cardiovascular mortality and morbidity. Am Heart J 1988;116:16-22
2. Hesselson A, Parsonnet V, Bernstein A et al. Deleterious effect of long -term single chamber ventricular pacing in patients with sick sinus syndrome: hidden benefits of dual chamber pacing. J Am Coll Cardiol 1992;19:1542-1549
3. Sgarbossa E, Pinski S, Maloney J et al. Chronic atrial fibrillation and stroke in paced patients with sick sinus syndrome: relevance of clinical characteristics and pacing modalities. Circulation 1993;88:1045-1053
4. Andersen R, Nielsen J, Thomson P et al. Long-term follow-up of patients from a randomised trial of atrial versus ventricular pacing for sick sinus syndrome. Lancet 1997;350:1210-1216
5. Katsivas A, Manolis A, Lazaris E et al. Atrial septal pacing to synchronize atrial depolarization in patients with delayed interatrial conduction. PACE 1998;21(11 pt2):2220-2225
6. Padeletti L, Porcianni M, Michelucci A et al. Interatrial septum pacing: a new approach to prevent recurrent atrial fibrillation. J Interv Card Electrophysiol 1999;3(1):35-43
7. Daubert C, Mabo P, Berder V et al. Atrial tachyarrhythmias associated with high-degree interatrial conduction block: Prevention by permanent atrial resynchronization. Eur J Cardiac Pacing Electrophysiol 1994;4(1):35-44

8. Delfaut P, Saksena S, Prakash A et al. Long-term outcome of patients with drug-refractory atrial flutter and fibrillation after single- and dual-site right atrial pacing for arrhythmia prevention. J Am Coll Cardiol 1998;32:1900-1908

9. Daubert C, D'Allonnes G, Mabo P. Multisite atrial pacing to prevent atrial fibrillation. Proceedings of the International Meeting on Atrial Fibrillation. Bologna, Italy. Sept 1999.

10. Levy T, Walker S, Rochelle J et al. Evaluation of bi-atrial, right atrial pacing and no pacing, in patients with drug refractory atrial fibrillation. Am J Cardiol (Accepted for publication)

11. Coumel P, Friocourt P, Mugica J et al. Long-term prevention of vagal atrial arrhythmias by atrial pacing at 90/minute: Experience with 6 cases. PACE 1983;6:552-560

12. Attuel P, Pellerin D, Mugica J et al. DDD pacing: An effective treatment modality for recurrent atrial arrhythmias. PACE 1988;11:1647-54

13. Garrigue S, Barold S, Cazeau S et al. Prevention of atrial arrhythmias during DDD pacing by atrial overdrive. PACE 1998;21(9):1751-1759

14. Murgatroyd F, Nitzsche R, Slade A et al. A new pacing algorithm for overdrive suppression of atrial fibrillation. Chorus Multicentre Study Group. PACE 1994;17(11 ptII):1966-1973

15. Murgatroyd F. Modes of onset of spontaneous episodes of atrial fibrillation: Implications for the prevention of atrial fibrillation by pacing. In Daubert C et al (ed): Prevention of tachyarrhythmias with cardiac pacing. Armonk, NY, Futura Publishing Co,1997, pp 53-65

16. Waldo A, Maclean W, Karp R et al. Entrainment and interruption of atrial flutter with atrial pacing: studies in man following open heart surgery. Circulation 1977;56:737-745

17. Kirchof C, Wijffels M, Allessie M. Pace termination of atrial fibrillation. Olsson S, Allessie M, Campbell R (Editors): Atrial fibrillation: Mechanisms and Therapeutic Strategies, Futura Publishing Co, 1994.

18. Pandozi C, Bianconi L, Villani M et al. Local capture by atrial pacing in spontaneous chronic atrial fibrillation. Circulation 1997;95(10):2416-22

19. Haffajee C, Stevens S, Mongeon L et al. High frequency atrial burst pacing for termination of atrial fibrillation. PACE 1995;18(ptII):804

20. Jung W, Wolpert C, Spehl S et al. A prospective randomized comparison of high-frequency burst pacing with antitachycardia ramp pacing for termination of induced atrial tachycardias. J Am Coll Cardiol 1998;31(2, suppl A):357A-358A

21. Giorgberidze I, Saksena S, Mongeon L et al. Effects of high-frequency atrial pacing in atypical atrial flutter and atrial fibrillation. J Int Card Electrophysiol 1997;1(Suppl 2):111-123

22. Paladino W, Bahu M, Knight B et al. Failure of single- and multisite high-frequency atrial pacing to terminate atrial fibrillation. Am J Cardiol 1997;80(2):226-227

23. Sulke N, Bailin S, Swerdlow C. Worldwide clinical experience with a dual-chamber implantable cardioverter defibrillator in patients with atrial fibrillation and flutter. (Abstract) Eur Heart J 1999;20:699

24. Coplen S, Antman E, Berlin J et al. Efficacy and safety of quinidine therapy for maintenance of sinus rhythm after cardioversion. A meta-analysis of randomised controlled trials. Circulation 1990;82:1106-1116

25. Cooper R, Alferness C, Smith W et al. Internal cardioversion of atrial fibrillation in sheep. Circulation 1993;87(5):1673-86

26. Harbinson M, Allen J, Imam Z et al. Rounded biphasic waveform reduces energy requirements for transvenous catheter cardioversion of atrial fibrillation and flutter. PACE 1997;20(1 pt2):226-229

27. Cooper R, Plumb V, Epstein A et al. Marked reduction in internal atrial defibrillation thresholds with dual-current pathways and sequential shocks in humans. Circulation 1998;97(25):2527-2535

28. Murgatroyd F, Slade A, Sopher M et al. Efficacy and tolerability of transvenous low energy cardioversion of atrial fibrillation in humans. J Am Coll Cardiol 1995;25:1347-1353

29. Ammer R, Alt E, Ayers G et al. Pain threshold for low energy intracardiac cardioversion of atrial fibrillation with low or no sedation. PACE 1996;19(ptII):230-236

30. McNally E, Meyer E, Langendorf R. Elective countershock in unanaesthetized patients with use of an oesophageal electrode. Circulation 1966;33:124-127

31. Sulke N, Kamalvand K, Tan K et al. A prospective evaluation of recurrent atrial endocardial defibrillation in patients with recurrent atrial fibrillation. (abstract) Heart 1996;75(suppl):42

32. Timmermans C, Wellens H. Effect of device-mediated therapy on symptomatic episodes of atrial fibrillation. J Am Coll Cardiol 1998;31(2):331A

33. Lesh M, Kalman J, Roithinger F et al. Potential role of 'hybrid therapy' for atrial fibrillation. Semin Interv Cardiol 1997;2(4):267-271

Part V.

Implantable Cardioverter Defibrillator

25. IMPACT OF IMPLANTABLE DEFIBRILLATOR STUDIES ON CLINICAL PRACTICE

Seah Nisam, BSEE

Guidant Corporation, Zaventem, Belgium

Introduction

The implantable cardioverter defibrillator (ICD), introduced into clinical practice by Michel Mirowski and colleagues in 1980[1], quickly demonstrated its efficacy in rapid termination of life-threatening ventricular tachycardias and fibrillation (VT/VF)[2]. If the 1980s can be considered as the decade of major technological improvements in ICDs and their acceptance by the medical community, the 1990s will certainly be remembered as the decade highlighted by multiple large, prospective, randomized trials, comparing the impact on patient survival of ICD therapy compared to conventional medical therapy[3 4]. Four of these trials targeted patients with previous documented episodes of sustained VT/VF: Dutch cost-effectiveness study, Cardiac Arrest Study Hamburg (CASH), Antiarrhythmics Versus Implantable Defibrillators (AVID), Canadian Implantable Defibrillator Study (CIDS)[5 6 7 8].

Two additional large trials focused on patients with previous myocardial infarction, left ventricular disfunction, and nonsustained ventricular tachycardia (NSVT), but who had never presented with symptomatic, sustained VT/VF: Multicenter Automatic Defibrillator Implantation Trial (MADIT), Multicenter UnSustained Tachycardia Trial (MUSTT) [9 10]. Another study, the Coronary Artery Bypass Graft and defibrillator Patch (CABG-Patch)[11], did not show benefit for ICDs, but this trial differed significantly from all the above in that the patients had never had VT/VF – neither spontaneously nor induced – prior to the study. The details on these study protocols have been given in the cited publications, so will not be covered here. The results of these already completed randomized, prospective ICD trials are summarized in Figure 1. They show a generally 40-50% lower mortality for patients receiving ICD therapy, versus "conventional" medical management, usually amiodarone. The impact that these studies have had on the indications for ICDs will be the focus of our paper.

From Ovsyshcher IE. *Cardiac Arrythmias and Device Therapy: Results and Perspectives for the New Century.* Armonk, NY: Futura Publishing Company, Inc., © 2000

Comparison of all-cause Mortality in Randomized ICD Studies

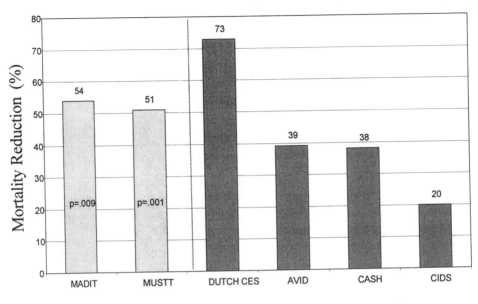

Primary Prevention Studies   Secondary Prevention Studies

Figure 1. The histograms report the reduction in all-cause mortality for ICD versus controls for each of the six indicated studies. "Primary prevention" refers to those trials conducted on patients without previous episodes of sustained VT/VF, and identified via the respective risk-stratification cascades; "Secondary prevention" covers the four trials on patients who had been resuscitated from sudden cardiac death or syncopal sustained VT/VF. *Reproduced, with permission from Ref. 12.*

ICD Indications and their Evolution

In order to get a better impression of the manner in which the above mentioned studies have changed medical practice, specifically the patient selection criteria for ICD therapy, we will first review how ICD guidelines have evolved over time. Table 1 provides an overview of this evolution as a function of clinical results and ICD studies.

Within the current (AHA/ACC/NASPE 1998) guidelines[13] listed in Table 1, the Class I indications 1-3 directly reflect the results of AVID, which were subsequently reinforced by the results reported from CASH and CIDS.

Indication 3, *syncope of undetermined origin,* is well supported by the CIDS study in which approximately one-sixth of the patients had been included for "unmonitored syncope." Indication 4, sometimes referred to in practice as the "MADIT indication," indeed reflects the results of that study. MUSTT, which was first reported *after* these Guidelines were published, reinforces the MADIT results. There are indications that the most important consequence of MUSTT will be the acceleration into clinical practice of *prophylactic* implantation of ICDs[14]. Many physicians still reluctant after MADIT to implement the lessons from that study have indicated that MUSTT's conclusive results will lead them to apply the MADIT/MUSTT screening cascade (Holter monitoring for the presence of NSVT, electrophysiologic studies to determine VT inducibility, and ICD implantation in the inducible patients.)

Discussion

Mortality from cardiovascular disease claims over half a million lives per annum, both in the U.S. and in Europe[15,16]. Deaths due to ventricular tachyarrhythmias account for approximately 50% of this mortality[17]. It is clear that these "epidemic" type numbers, for a condition for which the ICD has proven far more effective than any alternative, is the major explanation for the rapid and continuing expansion of ICD therapy, reaching in excess of 50,000 implanted patients during 1998[18,19]. Nevertheless, compared to the very large number of sudden cardiac deaths annually in the western world, it is evident that the opportunity for greatest expansion is still ahead. While some of these additional patients may come in the form of resuscitees due to improved cardiopulmonary resuscitation programs, the great majority will remain at risk until patient screening permits identification of - and *prophylactic* ICD therapy for – those at highest risk. The two large, prospective, randomized studies discussed above – MADIT and MUSTT – have already established a very clear screening cascade for identifying some of these patients: poor ventricular function, late after myocardial infarction, holter monitoring to identify those with NSVT, electrophysiological stimulation to identify the subgroup who are inducible, and in whom ICD implantation has been shown to be of significant benefit.

The impact of MADIT in terms of patient numbers was initially small, as the cardiology world was taken by surprise by its results, carefully awaiting confirmation from other, larger studies. Nevertheless, in just the third year after MADIT was published, it had led to approximately 5,000 patients receiving ICDs for that indication[14]. It is expected that MUSTT, a much larger and scientifically more rigorous study, but on a nearly identical patient population, and with nearly identical results as with MADIT (Table 2), will have a much larger and more immediate impact on clinical practice.

Table 1. Evolution in Guidelines for ICD implantation

Year	Indications for ICD implantation
1980	Resuscitated from at least two episodes of cardiac arrest, neither associated with acute MI, and one of which had to occur despite AARx treatment[1]
1982	One or more episodes of VF or hemodynamically unstable VT, not associated with acute MI (or other transient, reversible causes), but with evidence - from EP testing or Holter monitoring - of incomplete protection by AARx[2]
1986	Same, except relaxation of the requirement for initial inducibility and non-suppressibility following AARx[20]
1991	Class I Indications[21] (General consensus that ICD indicated): 1. ≥ 1 episodes of spontaneous sustained VT/VF in patients in whom EP testing and/or Holter monitoring could not be used to accurately predict efficacy of other therapies 2. Recurrent spontaneous sustained VT/VF, *despite* guided (by EP or Holter monitoring) AARx therapy 3. Spontaneous sustained VT/VF in case of a patient's non-compliance with - or intolerance of - AARx therapy 4. Patients with spontaneous sustained VT/VF, who remain persistently inducible at EP, while on "best" drug therapy or following VT surgery or catheter ablation Class II Indication (ICD an acceptable option, but no consensus): "Syncope of undetermined etiology in a patient with clinically relevant sustained VT or VF induced at EP study, in whom AARx therapy is limited by inefficacy, intolerance, or noncompliance"[21]
1998	Class I Indications[13] (General consensus that ICD indicated): 1. Cardiac arrest due to VT or VF, not due to a transient or reversible cause 2. Spontaneous sustained VT 3. Syncope of undetermined origin with clinically relevant, hemodynamically significant sustained VT or VF induced at EP study when drug therapy is ineffective, not tolerated, or not preferred 4. NSVT with coronary disease, prior MI, LV dysfunction, and inducible VF or sustained VT at EP study, that is not suppressible by a Class I AARx Class IIb Indication[13] (ICD an acceptable option, but no consensus): 1. Cardiac arrest presumed due to VF when EP testing is precluded by other medical conditions 2. Severe symptoms attributable to sustained VT/VF while awaiting cardiac transplantation 3. Familial or inherited conditions carrying a high risk for life-threatening VT/VF, such as long QT syndrome or hypertrophic cardiomyopathy 4. NSVT with coronary artery disease, prior MI, and LV dysfunction, and inducible sustained VT/VF at EP study 5. Recurrent syncope of unknown etiology in the presence of ventricular dysfunction and inducible VT/VF at EPS, when other causes of syncopy have been excluded

MI = myocardial infarction; AARx = antiarrhythmic drug;   EP = electrophysiological; VT/VF = ventricular tachycarcardia/ventricular fibrillation; NSVT = nonsustained ventricular tachycardia. (Table 1 reprinted with permission from Ref 12.)

One of the most compelling messages from the *two studies taken together* – as illustrated clearly from Table 2 – is that patients with depressed left ventricular function and NSVT *late after infarction* remain at unacceptably high risk of sudden cardiac death, despite being arrhythmically asymptomatic. The mean times from most previous MI in the MADIT and MUSTT cohorts were 27 and 39 months, respectively; yet the mortality in the control group patients was approximately 30% at two years. In both studies, the ICD treated patients had a better than 50% lower all-cause mortality compared to the control group (p < 0.009 in MADIT, p < 0.001 in MUSTT.) Two further important scientific contributions of MUSTT need to be mentioned: a) there was a *higher* use of beta-blockers in the control group than in the ICD-treated patients (51% vs 34%, p = 0.001)[22]. This shows clearly that the improved ICD results were not due to a "beta blocker imbalance," a criticism made of MADIT[23].

Table 2. MADIT & MUSTT
Freedom from All Cause Mortality (%)

Years	MADIT (n = 196)		MUSTT (n = 704)	
	ICD	Conv. Tx	ICD	No AARx
1	97	77	96	85
2	87	68	90	73
3	83	56	87	66
4	71	51	80	59
		(p = 0.009)		(p = 0.001)

Table 2. Probability of survival for the MUSTT and MADIT studies. The mortality reduction in MUSTT, for the ICD compared to *either* no antiarrhythmic drugs *or* electrophysiologically-guided antiarrhythmic drugs, was 51% (p < 0.001). The mortality reduction in MADIT for the ICD versus conventional therapy was 54% (p < 0.009).

b) The MUSTT study design included a "natural history" limb (the control group patients randomized to *no antiarrhythmic therapy)*, showing that such patients despite being asymptomatic are truly at high risk and that that risk is not the consequence of drug proarrhythmia.

Of the seven completed prospective, randomized ICD studies, we should not overlook the important lessons learned from CABG-Patch[11], the single deviant to results showing ICD superiority. The reasons for the neutral outcome in this trial have been previously reported[24,25,26]. Probably the most pertinent reason is that the patients studied in CABG-Patch - in contrast to the other six studies - had never had episodes of sustained VT, neither spontaneously nor induced. The important contribution of this study in better elucidating ICD indications is the demonstration that only patients with significant arrhythmic risk will benefit from ICD therapy. In that trial, the mortality during the two years following CABG surgery (excluding peri-operative mortality) was only 11%. While it may seem intuitively obvious, CABG-Patch poignantly shows that populations with such low risk generally do not need ICDs.

Conclusions

In a time when "evidence based medicine" has come to the forefront, it is quite logical that most of the guidelines for implanting ICDs adhere to the outcomes of prospective randomized clinical trials, comparing ICD therapy to pharmacological options. We have presented here the evolution in these guidelines, and their links to the seven completed ICD trials. MADIT and MUSTT are landmark studies, establishing the validity and need for *prophylactic* ICD therapy. These two studies not only demonstrate a greater than 50% survival benefit from ICD therapy; they also provide a very clear road map for identifying asymptomatic patients who are at high risk and benefit from ICD implantation: chronic coronary patients, with poor left ventricular function and NSVT. The impact of MADIT on clinical practice was initially slow, but still yielded some 5000 patients for ICDs in the third year (1998) after its publication. MUSTT strongly corroborates the MADIT findings, and its impact is expected to be much more profound and faster.

References

[1] Mirowski M, Reid P, Mower M, et al.   Termination of Malignant Ventricular Arrhythmias with an implanted Automatic Defibrillator in human beings. N. Engl. J. Med. 1980; 303:322-324.

[2] Mirowski M, Reid P, Winkle R, Mower M, Watkins L, Stinson E, Griffith L, Kallman C, Weisfeldt M. Mortality in patients with implanted automatic defibrillators. Ann Intern Med 1983; 98: 585-588.

[3] Nisam S, Thomas A, Mower M, Hauser R. Identifying patients for prophylactic automatic implantable cardioverter defibrillator therapy: Status of prospective studies. Am Heart J 1991; 122: 607-612.

[4] Bigger JT.   Primary Prevention of Sudden Cardiac Death using Implantable Cardioverter-Defibrillators. *From* Singer I, (ed.) Implantable Cardioverter-Defibrillator. Armonk, NY: Futura, Inc.; 1994:515-546.

[5] Wever E, Hauer R, Schrijvers G, van Capelle F, et al. Cost-effectiveness of implantable defibrillator as first-choice therapy versus electrophysiologically guided, tiered strategy in post-infarction sudden death survivors: a randomized study. Circulation 1996; 93:489-496.

[6] Kuck K-H, Cappato, R. Implantable heart defibrillator saves lives in patients with previous cardiac arrest. Oral presentation during "Hotline session: new-breaking clinical trials," at 47th annual scientific sessions of the American College of Cardiology meeting, Atlanta, GA. (Press Release, 30 March 1998).

[7] The Antiarrhythmic Versus Implantable Defibrillator (AVID) Investigators.   A Comparison of Antiarrhythmic-drug Therapy with Implantable Defibrillators in Patients Resuscitated from Near-fatal Ventricular Arrhythmias. N Engl J Med 1997; 337: 1576-83.

[8] Connolly, S. "Results from the Canadian Implantable Defibrillator Study (CIDS). Oral presentation during "Hotline session: new-breaking clinical trials," at 47th annual scientific sessions of the American College of Cardiology meeting, Atlanta, GA. (Press Release, 30 March 1998).

[9] Moss A, Hall J, Cannom D, Daubert J, Higgins S, Klein H, Levine J, Saksena S, Waldo A, Wilber D, Brown M, Heo M, for the MADIT Investigators. Improved survival with an implanted defibrillator in patients with coronary disease at high risk of ventricular arrhythmias. N Engl J Med 1996; 335: 1933-40.

[10] Buxton A. Results from the Multicenter UnSustained Tachycardia Trial (MUSTT). Oral presentation during "Hotline session: new-breaking clinical trials," at 48th annual scientific sessions of the American College of Cardiology meeting, New Orleans, LA March 8, 1999.

[11] Bigger JT, for the Coronary Artery Bypass Graft (CABG) Patch Trial Investigators.   Prophylactic use of implanted cardiac defibrillators in patients at high risk for ventricular arrhythmias after coronary artery bypass Graft Surgery. N Engl J Med 1997; 337: 1569-75.

[12] Nisam S. Clinical Results with Implantable Cardioverter Defibrillators. In Singer I.   Interventional Electrophysiology: 2nd Edition.   Lippincott Williams and Wilkins. 2000 (In Press).

[13] The ACC/AHA Task Force on Practice Guidelines.   ACC/AHA Guidelines for Implantation of Cardiac Pacemakers and Antiarrhythmia Devices. J of Am Coll Cardiol 1998; 31: 1175-1209.

[14] Wilber D, Nisam S. Survey of Prophylactic Defibrillator Implantation following MADIT Am J Cardiol 1999 (in Press).

[15] Pisa Z. Sudden Death: a worldwide problem. *In*: Kulbertus H, Wellens H, eds. Sudden Death. 3. The Hague/Boston/London: Martinus Hijhoff Publisher, 1980.

[16] Myerburg R, Kessler K, Castellanos A.   Sudden cardiac death: epidemiology, transient risk, and intervention assessment. Ann Intern Med 1993; 119: 1187-1197.

[17] Myerburg R, Interian A, Mitrani R, et al. Frequency of Sudden Cardiac Death and Profiles of Risk. Am J Cardiol 1997; 80 (5B): 10F-19F.

[18] Nisam S.   Can Implantable Defibrillators reduce non-arrhythmic mortality? J Intervention Cardiac Electrophysiol 1998; 2: 371-375.

[19] Cannom D.   A review of the cardioverter defibrillator trials.   Curr Opinions in Cardiol 1998; 13: 3-8.

[20] Mower M, Nisam S.   AICD Indications (Patients Selection):   Past, Present and Future. PACE 1988; 11: 2064-2070.

[21] Lehmann M, Saksena S.   NASPE Policy Statement: Implantable Cardioverter Defibrillators in Cardiovascular Practice: Report of the Policy Conference of NASPE. PACE 1991; 14: 969-979.

[22] Gold M, Rottman J, Wood M, Lehmann M, et al. The effect of clinical factors on the benefit of implantable defibrillators in the MUSTT trial. Circulation 1999; 100 (No 18): I-642 (Abstract).

[23] Friedmann P, Stevenson W. Unsustained ventricular tachycardia.   To treat or not to treat. Editorial. N Engl J Med 1996; 335: 1984-5.

[24] Domanski M, Exner D. Prevention of sudden cardiac death: a current perspective. J Electrocardiology 1999; 31: 47-53.

[25] Nisam S, Mower M. ICD Trials: an *extraordinary* means of determining patient risk? PACE 1998; 21: 1341-1346.

[26] Naccarelli G, Wolbrette D, Dell'orfano J, Patel H, Luck J. A decade of clinical trial developments in postmyocardial infarction, congestive heart failure, and sustained ventricular tachyarrhythmia patients. From CAST to AVID and beyond. J Cardiovasc Electrophysiol. 1998; 9: 864-891.

26.
DUAL CHAMBER IMPLANTABLE CARDIOVERTER DEFIBRILLATOR TECHNOLOGY

Marshall S. Stanton, M.D., and James E. Willenbring, B.S.E.E.

Medtronic, Inc., Minneapolis, USA

Introduction

As new implantable cardioverter defibrillators (ICDs) have been developed and introduced over the last fifteen years, they have advanced dramatically in effectiveness and the ease with which they can be implanted and managed. Many of these advancements have given physicians better tools to manage and improve both patients' survival and quality of life.

These advancements have included better defibrillation waveforms, less invasive lead systems, dramatic decreases in ICD size, improved diagnostic capabilities, and easy-to-use programming systems to help manage patients over time. Dual chamber ICDs represent one of the latest advances in technology for patients with life threatening ventricular arrhythmias. Single chamber ICDs, while being very effective at treating sudden death and ventricular tachycardia, are limited in areas that can have a dramatic effect on ICD patients' therapy and their quality of life. These limitations or drawbacks manifest themselves in the following areas:

- The type of bradycardia pacing therapy that can be delivered.
- The ability of the ICD to discriminate between true ventricular tachyarrhythmias and atrial fibrillation, atrial flutter, sinus tachycardia, and other supraventricular tachyarrhythmias.
- The types of tachyarrhythmia episode diagnostics that are stored.
- The potential for increased use of antiarrhythmic medications.
- The potential for device-device interactions if a patient has a separate pacemaker and ICD.

This present study has two objectives: (1) to identify how dual chamber ICD technology has been applied to address the single chamber ICD limitations, and (2) to identify unique limitations of dual chamber ICDs themselves.

Providing Hemodynamically Improved Bradycardia Pacing Therapy

In addition to traditional VVI pacing capability, newer ICDs can deliver rate-responsive pacing therapy for both chambers. ICD patients who require bradycardia pacing therapy may need the more physiologic pacing that dual chamber ICDs provide. Since many ICD patients have low ejection fractions,

From Ovsyshcher IE. *Cardiac Arrythmias and Device Therapy: Results and Perspectives for the New Century.* Armonk, NY: Futura Publishing Company, Inc., © 2000

those who are paced in VVI mode may experience pacemaker syndrome more frequently than other patients.[1] In addition, other studies have shown significant benefits of atrial pacing compared to VVI pacing, including increased survival, less atrial fibrillation, fewer thromboembolic complications, less heart failure, and a lower risk of AV block.[2]

Initial opinion upon introduction of dual chamber ICDs was that the number of ICD patients who would benefit from the dual chamber ICDs was limited. However, when examined further, the number of ICD patients that can benefit from more physiologic dual chamber rate-responsive pacing can be significant. One recent study looked at patients with definite, probable, and possible indications and showed that approximately half of ICD patients would probably benefit from dual chamber pacing modes.[3]

Discriminating Between Atrial & Ventricular Tachyarrhythmias
Single chamber ICDs are limited to analyzing ventricular rate and electrogram (EGM) information. The challenging rhythms for single chamber ICD detection algorithms are those with fast ventricular rates that fall within the ICD's ventricular tachycardia (VT) or ventricular fibrillation (VF) detection zones, but which actually are sinus tachycardia (ST) or atrial tachycardias with 1:1 conduction, atrial flutter (AFL), atrial fibrillation (AF), and other tachycardias like AV nodal reentrant tachycardia (AVNRT).

Each of the ICD manufacturers uses dual chamber information differently in the design of their detection algorithms. However, some key principles are important for any detection algorithm design:
- Improve specificity without compromising sensitivity to true VT/VF.
- Reduce the amount of blanking in both chambers (and cross-chamber blanking) to allow the ICD to sense as many intrinsic events as possible.
- Minimize delays to detecting VT and VF (especially when atrial and ventricular arrhythmias are occurring simultaneously).
- Allow for some oversensing and undersensing.
- Be simple to set and program.[4]

A summary of each manufacturer's method is presented below.

The Medtronic PR Logic™ detection algorithm uses a number of variables to differentiate atrial tachyarrhythmias and other SVTs from true ventricular tachyarrhythmias. The different criteria, modeled after ones that physicians use themselves to diagnose rhythms, are atrial (A) and ventricular (V) rates; the pattern of the P-waves relative to R-waves; A and V cycle length regularity; and AV dissociation. PR Logic combines these algorithm "building blocks" to make decisions about withholding therapy. As rhythms become more complicated, more of the building blocks are used to make an appropriate classification. For example, a simple, fast ventricular rhythm with few or no P-waves doesn't engage the dual chamber algorithm. This situation uses the basic rate and duration detection from single chamber ICDs.

More complicated rhythms with a single P-wave for most R-waves (e.g., sinus tachycardia, AVNRT) use not only rate, but also the pattern of where the P-waves fall relative to each R-wave. To classify a rhythm pattern, PR Logic divides each ventricular interval into three different zones: P-waves falling very close to each R-wave are classified as junctional, those falling in the beginning half of each ventricular interval are classified as retrograde, and those falling in the second half of each ventricular interval are classified as antegrade. In general, PR Logic withholds therapy for consistent, single atrial events that fall in the antegrade zone (sinus tachycardia) and junctional zone (AVNRT), and allows VT detection for single P-waves falling primarily in the retrograde zone.

The most complicated rhythms are the ones with multiple P-waves for each R-wave (AF, AFL). In these situations, PR Logic analyzes combinations of A and V rates, patterns for rhythms where one exists (e.g., AFL with 2:1 conduction), regularity of A and V cycle lengths, and AV dissociation (see example of this in Figure 1). Some of the most important rhythms to ensure that there is clear classification are AF or AFL occurring simultaneously with VT or VF. These also use almost all of the PR Logic building blocks.

Since it is important for the ICD's atrial sensitivity to be set to detect atrial fibrillation, PR Logic also has a specialized function that looks for far-field R-wave (FFRW) oversensing to avoid classifying sinus tachycardia as 2:1 atrial flutter. However, if FFRW sensing is intermittent, this can lead to a false positive detection of VT. Despite the underlying intricacy of this algorithm, PR Logic is easily programmed with three on/off switches that control the types of tachycardias that the algorithm looks for (atrial flutter/fibrillation, sinus tachycardia, and junctional tachycardias), and a rate parameter that allows physicians to limit PR Logic to certain rate ranges.

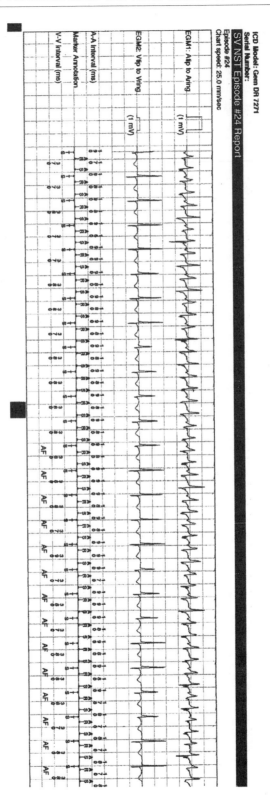

Figure 1. Example of the Medtronic PR Logic™ detection algorithm withholding ventricular detection during a spontaneous episode of 2:1 atrial flutter. The top channel is a bipolar atrial electrogram, the middle a bipolar ventricular electrogram, and the bottom a marker channel with atrial intervals on top and ventricular intervals on bottom. The rapid ventricular response to this patient's atrial flutter was fast enough to fall in the device's VT detection zone since the ICD was programmed to a tachycardia detection interval of 400 ms (150 bpm). The "TS" marker indicates the ICD sees a ventricular interval within the VT zone. The "AF" marker shows where the ICD is withholding VT detection because the pattern, rate, regularity, and AV dissociation criteria conclude that the fast ventricular rhythm is due to an atrial flutter. Paper speed = 25 mm/s.

The Guidant Atrial View™ dual chamber detection algorithm takes a different approach to discriminating true VT from rapidly conducted atrial arrhythmias. It builds upon its single chamber detection methods (including Onset and Stability) by adding rate comparisons between the atrium and the ventricle (Vrate>Arate) and determining if the atrial rate has exceeded an AF rate threshold.

After an arrhythmia has met the basic single chamber rate and duration criteria, Atrial View characterizes the onset of the ventricular rate as sudden or gradual using the single chamber Onset criteria (from intervals at the beginning of the episode), the regularity of the ventricular rate as stable or unstable (using the single chamber Stability criteria), and determines whether the atrial rate has exceeded the AF rate threshold. Atrial View then applies each criterion to decide if detection should be withheld. If the ventricular rate is greater than the atrial rate by more that 10 beats per minute (bpm), the algorithm overrules the other criteria and allows VT detection to occur. One difficulty with this algorithm is an 86 ms cross-chamber atrial blanking period that occurs after each sensed R-wave. Some atrial flutter rhythms may be inappropriately treated because every other P-wave falls within this blanking period and therefore the algorithm cannot see the fast atrial rate.[5]

ELA's PARAD+™ dual chamber detection algorithm relies upon an initial screen of ventricular stability and then looks for AV association and sudden onset. Once a sustained ventricular rhythm occurs in the VT detection zone, the algorithm declares the rhythm AF if less than a programmed percentage of the ventricular intervals are stable (nominally 75%). If the ventricular rhythm is stable, then P-R interval histograms are analyzed to determine if there is AV association. The rhythm is called associated if more than a programmed percentage (nominally 75%) of P-R intervals are stable. VT is detected if no association is seen and the current ventricular interval is no more than 63 ms longer than the previous interval average. If association is detected, the PARAD+ algorithm continues to analyze the P-R interval data to determine if the rhythm conducts 1:1 (e.g. sinus tachycardia) or >1:1 (e.g., 2:1 atrial flutter). If seen as a >1:1 rhythm, the rhythm is classified as atrial flutter and VT therapy is withheld. If classified as 1:1, the PARAD+ algorithm does two final checks. The first looks at whether the ventricular rate had a gradual onset so it can classify the rhythm as sinus tachycardia and withhold VT therapy, and the second looks at the chamber of origination for 1:1 rhythms with a sudden onset. If the origin of onset turns up to be ventricular, then VT detection occurs; otherwise, a 1:1 SVT (e.g., AVNRT) is diagnosed and VT therapy is withheld.

The Biotronik SMART Detection™ algorithm uses some similar character-istics as the ELA algorithm, but begins analysis by classifying rhythms into three groups: (1) V. rate > A. rate (which is classified as VT immediately), (2) A. rate > V. rate, and (3) 1:1 conducted rhythms. In the second group (A. rate > V. rate), the SMART algorithm detects SVT and withholds ther-apy if either the ventricular rate is unstable (AF) or if the ventricular rate is stable but the algorithm detects N:1 AV conduction (e.g., 2:1 AFL); other-wise it detects VT. For the third group (1:1 rhythms), SVT is detected and therapy withheld for two types of rhythms: one that has stable atrial and ventricular rates and a gradual onset (sinus tachycardia), and the other with an unstable ventricular rate but stable PR intervals. For all other 1:1 rhythms, VT is detected.

Providing Better Tachyarrhythmia Episode Diagnostics

In the electrophysiology lab, diagnosing complex tachyarrhythmias with multiple channels of ECG and intracardiac electrograms (EGMs) is routine. Unfortunately, single chamber ICDs provide only ventricular EGM informa-tion. This can limit a physician's ability to determine if the tachyarrhythmia episode was detected and treated appropriately. Many single chamber ICDs offer far-field EGM channels that provide a broader view of what is occur-ring (and also may show atrial signals). However, the lack of a clear atrial EGM channel is a disadvantage. With the dual chamber ICD's atrial lead signal, episode diagnostics start to approach what electrophysiologists are familiar working with in their lab.

Requiring Fewer Antiarrhythmic Medications

As part of on-going management of single chamber ICD patients, physicians prescribe antiarrhythmic medications to (among other reasons):

- Reduce the occurrence of AF/SVT episodes, and therefore reduce the chance of inappropriate shocks being delivered for those episodes.
- Control patients' fast ventricular response to atrial fibrillation or flutter so the ICD does not inappropriately shock this rhythm.
- Control patients' maximum sinus rate if they can increase their rate through exercise into their VT detection zone.

Since some dual chamber ICD detection algorithms help avoid inappropriate therapies better than single chamber ICD algorithms, we hypothesize that the need to use antiarrhythmic medications is less, and therefore fewer dual chamber ICD patients use these medications.

Decreasing Interactions Between Separate Devices

One of the more obvious benefits of dual chamber ICDs is the ability to implant a combined, single system in patients instead of a separate pacemaker and ICD. By reducing the amount of hardware, the patient and physician can benefit from shorter, easier implant procedures, fewer complications during long-term follow-up, and easier patient/device management.

During implants in patients with two separate devices it is typical to conduct complex (but necessary) testing for interactions between the two devices to ensure that the ICD functions are not compromised by the pacemaker, and vice versa.[6] The interactions include pacemaker output interfering with ICD sense amplifiers or detection algorithms (which may often be caused by the pacemaker seeing ventricular tachyarrhythmias as noise and shifting into a noise reversion mode that changes the pacemaker output to asynchronous pacing[7]), pacemaker mode or polarity changes post-ICD shock (dedicated bipolar pacemakers are typically required), and pacemaker undersensing during VF or post-ICD shock. This testing is mainly done at implant, but may be performed periodically during long-term follow-up. Lead placement with two separate devices is also more complicated; the required bipolar sensing leads need to be placed with their sensing vectors at a 90-degree angle from each other. Since dual chamber ICD circuitry is built to prevent these interactions, these ICDs have no need for this testing. In addition, there should be fewer pocket and vascular access issues at implant with only one device and two leads to place. During longer-term follow-up, having only one device and fewer leads in a dual chamber ICD system should reduce the potential for system complications and simplify follow-up.

Unique Limitations of Dual Chamber ICDs

With all of its benefits, dual chamber ICDs have some unique limitations or drawbacks of their own. These include issues related to atrial leads; over- and undersensing; how ICDs avoid interactions between tachyarrhythmia detection and high pacing rates; increased cost; and decreased longevity.

For ICD patients who would not have received a separate pacemaker, the additional atrial lead for their dual chamber ICD may result in a slightly more complex implant and more complications during follow-up. One manufacturer has an ambulatory test that looks for lead impedances out of normal operating ranges and then sounds a tone to indicate the patient should contact their physician. These features can potentially detect problems not only with atrial pacing electrodes, but also with ventricular pacing and high voltage electrodes. The ambulatory measurement and notification system reduces the chance that a patient with a lead issue could go undetected, and therefore unprotected, until the next scheduled follow-up.

Dual chamber ICDs use very high sensitivity in the atrium to appropriately detect and classify atrial fibrillation. Sometimes this causes the atrial lead to oversense far-field R-waves, which can negatively affect the ability of the ICD's dual chamber detection algorithm to correctly classify rhythms and withhold therapy appropriately. Some algorithms are designed to handle consistent FFRW sensing, but appropriate atrial lead position can be important to ensure correct atrial sensing and rhythm classification.

In patients who had separate pacemakers and ICDs, care needed to be taken to ensure that the upper pacing rate of the pacemaker could not be detected as VT by the ICD. In dual chamber ICDs, the devices themselves impose restrictions on their programmable ranges for upper rates and detection intervals to avoid this problem. In addition to this, though, the ICD must have enough of each ventricular interval "open," or not blanked, for it to sense the onset of a VT or VF. Combinations of high pacing rates (which decrease each ventricular cycle length) and the required blanking intervals after every paced event contribute to a smaller sensing window for VT and VF. In some dual chamber ICDs, automatic software limitations prevent devices from being programmed in ways that could cause undersensing of VT and VF. In other ICDs, you must remember to provide for an adequate safety margin when programming upper rates to ensure that VT and VF detection are not compromised. In either situation, patients who need higher upper pacing rates and who also have slow VT cycle lengths may find that the upper rates of their bradycardia pacing therapy need to be limited to ensure safe VT and VF detection.

The new technology of dual chamber ICDs comes at a higher price than single chamber ICDs. The ICD itself is a higher price, and the additional atrial lead adds to the cost. This is typically less than what would be charged for a patient receiving a separate pacemaker and ICD, but is more than the cost for a simple, single chamber ICD. Another cost-related consideration is the longevity of the ICD. A patient who needs full-time bradycardia pacing support will reduce the longevity of their dual chamber ICD substantially. Estimated longevities vary among manufacturers, but these factors may influence a physician's decision to use a dual chamber ICD.

Conclusions

This analysis shows that the advanced bradycardia pacing therapy, new detection algorithms, and more comprehensive diagnostic storage capabilities of dual chamber ICDs stand to help many ICD patients receive appropriate bradycardia pacing therapy, fewer inappropriate shocks, and reduce the interactions in patients with a separate ICD and pacemaker. The potential drawbacks of this new technology include slightly more complicated implants and device follow-up, some potential issues with over- and undersensing, faster drain of the ICD battery if pacing in both chambers, and increased cost.

References

1. Hayes DL, Rasmussen MJ, Friedman PA, et al.: Pacemaker syndrome in patients receiving ICDs. PACE 1998; 21:A406.
2. Andersen HR, Nielsen JC, Thomsen PE, et al.: Long-term follow-up of patients from a randomized trial of atrial versus ventricular pacing for sick-sinus syndrome. Lancet 1997; 350:1210-1216.
3. Best PJ, Hayes DL, Stanton MS: The potential usage of dual chamber pacing in patients with implantable cardioverter defibrillators. PACE 1999; 22(Pt 1): 79-85.
4. Olson WH: Dual chamber sensing and detection for implantable cardioverter-defibrillators. In Singer I, Barold SS, Camm AJ (eds): Nonpharmacological Therapy of Arrhythmias for the 21st Century. Armonk, NY, Futura Publishing Co, 1998: pp. 385-421.
5. Kühlkamp V, Dörnberger V, Mewis C, et al.: Clinical experience with the new detection algorithms for atrial fibrillation of a defibrillator with dual chamber sensing and pacing. J Cardiovasc Electrophysiol 1999; 10:905-915.
6. Glikson M, Trusty JM, Grice SK, et al.: A stepwise testing protocol for modern implantable cardioverter-defibrillator systems to prevent pacemaker — implantable cardioverter-defibrillator interactions. Am J Cardiol 1999; 83: 360-366.
7. Glikson M, Trusty JM, Grice SK, et al.: Importance of pacemaker noise reversion as a potential mechanism for pacemaker-ICD interactions. PACE 1998; 21:1111-1121.

27.
DUAL CHAMBER ICDs: SHOULD THIS BE THE STANDARD OF CARE FOR ALL ICD PATIENTS?

Jay N Gross, MD, Stanislav Weiner, MD

Division of Cardiology, Montefiore Medical Center, Albert Einstein College of Medicine. Bronx, NY, USA

ICDs were in clinical use for over a decade before VVI pacing was incorporated into these devices. During the subsequent five years, advances in ICD therapy occurred at a breath-taking pace, with the development of perfected transvenous technology, device miniaturization, tiered therapy, enhanced therapy specificity, and stored electrograms (EGM) capabilities. Perhaps the most important recent technological advance in the field is the advent of the dual chamber ICD (DDD-ICD), which merges the most sophisticated features of pacemaker and antitachycardia therapy.

Ironically, even after 20 years of DDD pacemaker use, the precise role of dual chamber pacing remains uncertain, with studies demonstrating a discrepancy between perceived advantage and objective benefit.[1] Thus, the need to carefully examine the application of DDD-ICD technology to a population whose primary indication for therapy is malignant ventricular tachyarrhythmias appears obvious.

The Role of Pacing in ICD Patients

Significant proportions of ICD recipients have concomitant bradyarrhythmias, with a reported prevalence of class I ACC/AHA pacemaker indications that vary from 5 to 29%.[2] Up to 80% of these patients are thought to benefit from dual chamber pacemakers.[3] De novo implantation of two separate devices in this patient population today is no longer acceptable, given the availability of fully capable pacing ICDs and the well recognized risks of potentially fatal device-device interactions.[4] Most patients with preexisting pacemakers who develop the need for an ICD can now be "upgraded" with a hybrid of an old pacing lead and new ICD device/lead hardware.

In addition to native disease, many ICD patients are at risk for iatrogenic sinus node dysfunction or AV conduction abnormalities. Most drugs, used as adjunctive therapy to reduce the incidence of ventricular arrhythmias and resultant ICD shocks, have significant negative chronotropic and dromotropic properties. The use of supplemental drug

From Ovsyshcher IE. *Cardiac Arrythmias and Device Therapy: Results and Perspectives for the New Century.* Armonk, NY: Futura Publishing Company, Inc., © 2000

therapy is quite common, as was demonstrated in the AVID trial, where greater then 50% of patients[5] in the ICD arm received adjunctive antiarrhythmic therapy. Furthermore, the ever-increasing use of β-adrenergic blockers in patients with ventricular dysfunction is likely to further exacerbate bradyarrhythmias in the ICD population. The role of dual chamber pacing for optimization of hemodynamics in select subsets of ICD patients is less uniformly accepted, but may be important in the setting of hypertrophic obstructive cardiomyopathy or dilated cardiomyopathy with prolonged atrioventricular conduction.[6,7]

Atrial Sensing: Enhancement of Tachyarrhythmia Detection and Discrimination

ICDs are designed to be exquisitely sensitive for the detection of malignant ventricular arrhythmias. This inevitably leads to a degree of non-specificity, resulting in a reported inappropriate shock rate of 14%.[8] Individualized adjustments of detection rates and durations, and use of algorithms that assess suddenness of onset, tachycardia stability, and electrogram morphology can prevent most inappropriate detection and therapy. Adjuvant pharmacological therapy for suppression or control of supraventricular arrhythmias is also frequently effective.

Though hard to precisely quantitate, a significant number of patients continue to have arrhythmia discrimination difficulties. In these patients, analysis of atrial EGM activity facilitates more effective tachycardia diagnosis. The need is greatest in those with frequent atrial arrhythmia/SVT and VT with similar rates. Diagnostic algorithms vary by manufacturer, but share many of the same principles. Ventricular rates greater than atrial rates indicate ventricular arrhythmias. Detection of AF or SVT is based on algorithms that weigh relative rates and relationships of atrial and ventricular timing. . The two most difficult diagnostic situations, VT with 1:1 V-A conduction, and double tachycardias (e.g. AF in conjunction with VT) provide greater challenges, but are generally effectively dealt with by these devices. These algorithms, while designed primarily to inhibit inappropriate therapies, may occasionally serve to promote appropriate therapeutic interventions. For example, DDD-ICDs can be used in previously "unmanageable" patients with slower VTs, as a result of their ability to detect sinus tachycardia. Similarly, atrial EGMs, in conjunction with ventricular stability, can facilitate prompt recognition of "unstable VTs" unresponsive to ATP, thus, triggering immediate cardioversion.

Disadvantages and Costs

Progressive ease of implant has been a hallmark of ICD development over the past several years, and the introduction of the DDD-ICD reverses this trend. It has long been recognized that dual chamber pacemaker implantation is more complex, fraught with problems including prolonged implant time, increased risk of venous thrombosis, lead displacement and failure. Additionally, cross-chamber interactions may occur. All these issues are applicable to DDD-ICDs, only more so. The ventricular lead is larger in ICD systems, making lead placement more difficult and increasing the risk of venous thrombosis. Atrial far-field oversensing is particularly problematic in systems that utilize very high programmed sensitivity or automatic gain control settings, and can totally distort detection algorithms. Cross-talk may be promoted by the high outputs and sensitivities that typically follow an ICD discharge. Additionally, while not specific to DDD-ICDs, some post-defibrillation redetection algorithms deliver shocks in response to any non-sensed rhythms, and thus this is more likely to be an issue in patients with DDD-ICDs who have a greater prevalence of bradycardia. Needless to say, despite enhanced automaticity of features, programming and follow-up of these devices is far more complex and time consuming than that of single chamber ICDs. Furthermore, the likelihood for human error is undoubtedly greater.

Use of algorithms for increasing detection specificity raises the possibility of inappropriate inhibition of therapy. Ineffective atrial sensing may lead to incorrect conclusions about rhythm diagnoses. The benefit of older, single chamber based detection algorithms - e.g. stability criteria – may be lost if they are programmed off because of the perception that they are redundant or primitive.

The economic costs of shifting to a greater than 50% implant rate of DDD-ICDs, the current state of affairs in the US, are substantial. Dual chamber ICDs generally "list" at $4,000-$7,000 more than their single chamber counterparts. Finally, irrespective of the success in progressive downsizing of ICDs, battery longevity, output capacity, and pulse generator size must in some way be compromised to accommodate DDD-ICD capabilities.

Future potential uses of dual chamber defibrillation systems

Two additional uses of modified dual chamber ICD systems will be available in the near future. ICDs that provide antitachycardia therapy for both atrial and ventricular arrhythmias are likely to have a role, given the propensity for atrial arrhythmia occurrence in the ICD population. Though already in limited clinical use in Europe, the long term acceptability and tolerance of atrial defibrillation remains the major stumbling block for more widespread use of these devices. Still in its early investigative phase, modified dual chamber ICD systems are being developed to provide for dual site ventricular pacing, which may serve as primary CHF therapy in selected patients with intra-ventricular conduction defects. This combination of antiarrhythmic and hemodynamic therapy may hold out great promise, but clearly the current data does not justify its use out of the context of investigative trials.

Summary

This review has discussed the advantages and disadvantages of dual chamber versus single chamber ICD systems. Dual chamber ICDs represent a major advance in the management of ventricular arrhythmias, but at significant clinical and economic cost. Indiscriminate use of dual chamber ICDs for all patients with malignant ventricular arrhythmia appears unwarranted. Assessing where individual patients fit into the patient population spectrum is the key to cost-effective utilization of enhanced ICD technology. (See diagram below). On one extreme of the continuum are patients with chronic atrial fibrillation, or those with rare ventricular arrhythmia without concomitant conduction abnormalities or atrial arrhythmia. They represent a group of patients least likely to receive benefit from dual chamber ICDs, while still being subject to the risk of DDD-ICD associated complications. On the other end of the spectrum are ICD patients with clear clinical indications for bradyarrhythmia therapy. These patients ought to receive all the benefits of the state of the art pacing technology available to the general pacemaker population. Patients who sustain atrial arrhythmias with ventricular responses in the same range as their clinical VT, or those on pharmacological regimens likely to induce bradyarrhythmias, need to be seriously considered for dual chamber ICD therapy as well.

There is little room for debate that one of the central factors in device selection is cost. Health care systems with differing resources will clearly utilize different thresholds for use. Some health care systems may need to exclusively provide single chamber systems to all but a few select patients. Those receiving ICDs on a prophylactic basis might be targeted as candidates for limited forms of therapy in even "low threshold" environments. It should be noted that the constant evolution in ICD technology has been driven primarily by physician demands and patient need, but it has also surreptitiously served to prevent significant cost reduction in VT therapy. Thus, despite a huge explosion in the patient population, and significant competition within the medical device industry, no significant cost reduction in "top-of-the-line devices" has occurred. This undoubtedly will have to change if ICD therapy in general, and "enhanced technology" in particular, is to be provided to an ever expanding patient population.

The spectrum of patient population with variable utility of a dual chamber ICD

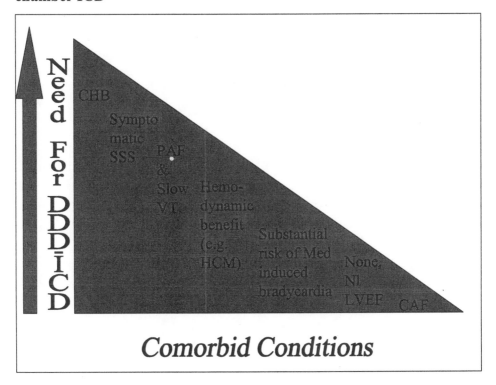

References

[1]Lamas GA, Orav EJ, Stambler BS et al.: Quality of life and clinical outcomes in elderly patients treated with ventricular pacing as compared

with dual-chamber pacing. Pacemaker Selection in the Elderly Investigators. N Engl J Med 1998; 338:1097

[2]Higgins SL, Williams SK, Pak JP et al.: Indications for implantation of a dual-chamber pacemaker combined with an implantable cardioverter-defibrillator. Am J Cardiol 1998; 81:1360

[3] Geelen P, Lorga Filho A, Chauvin M et al.: The value of DDD pacing in patients with an implantable cardioverter defibrillator. PACE 1997; 20:177

[4] Geiger MJ, O'Neill P, Sharma A et al.: Interactions between transvenous nonthoracotomy cardioverter defibrillator systems and permanent transvenous endocardial pacemakers. PACE 1997; 20:624

[5] A comparison of antiarrhythmic-drug therapy with implantable defibrillators in patients resuscitated from near-fatal ventricular arrhythmias. The Antiarrhythmics versus Implantable Defibrillators (AVID) Investigators. N Engl J Med 1997; 337:1576

[6] Kappenberger L, Linde C, Daubert C et al.: Pacing in hypertrophic obstructive cardiomyopathy. A randomized crossover study. PIC Study Group. Eur Heart J 1997; 18:1249

[7] Nishimura RA, Hayes DL, Holmes DR Jr et al.: Mechanism of hemodynamic improvement by dual-chamber pacing for severe left ventricular dysfunction: an acute Doppler and catheterization hemodynamic study. J Am Coll Cardiol 1995; 25:281

[8] Rosenqvist M, Beyer T, Block M, et al.: Adverse events with transvenous implantable cardioverter-defibrillators: a prospective multicenter study. European 7219 Jewel ICD investigators. Circ 1998; 98:663

28.
IMPLANTABLE CARDIOVERTER-DEFIBRILLATORS IN PEDIATRICS

Charles I. Berul, MD

Department of Cardiology, Children's Hospital • Boston
Harvard Medical School, Boston, Massachusetts, USA

Introduction

Implantable cardioverter defibrillator (ICD) placement in children involves specific issues related to patient size, growth, and congenital heart disease. Indications for pediatric ICD implantation include aborted sudden death and ventricular tachyarrhythmias. Children may have different implant techniques, medication dosing, anesthesia requirements, and psychosocial adaptation. There is not an ICD designed for children, as they comprise < 1% of implants. However, defibrillators have been shown to be valuable in children, especially with inheritable arrhythmia diseases and congenital heart disease.

Previous investigators have demonstrated that ICD use in pediatric patients is feasible and leads to a lower risk of sudden death in follow-up.[1] In a large series of pediatric ICD usage, 125 patients (age 1.9 – 19 years) were identified through manufacturer's records. In this group, the incidence of structural heart disease was high (74%) including hypertrophic and dilated cardiomyopathy. Indications for ICD in these children included aborted sudden death in 76%, refractory VT in 10%, syncope in congenital heart disease and a positive EP study in 10% of patients. Appropriate ICD shocks were seen in 68% of 125 patients and 20% received spurious shocks. The implant characteristics and incidence of ICD infections and lead revisions were not recorded. A smaller pediatric ICD series included 17 patients.[2] In this study, frequent ICD complications were seen, including erosion in 3 patients, lead dislodgment, and device infection. In another series of 11 children (age 4-16 yrs), implant indications included survivors of sudden cardiac death in 54%, refractory VT in 9%, syncope in congenital heart disease patients and a positive EP study in 18%, and high-risk familial disease in 18% of patients.[3] In this cohort, 55% had appropriate shocks and 55% also had inappropriate ICD discharges, while lead revisions for fractures or dislodgment were necessary in 3 of 11 (27%) patients.[3] A recent study evaluated ICD implantation in children compared with adults at the same institution over the same 5-year period, and found a notably higher frequency of complications in the pediatric group.[4] Infection and lead-related complications was higher in each of these studies on children with ICDs compared to adults[5,6], possibly

From Ovsyshcher IE. *Cardiac Arrythmias and Device Therapy: Results and Perspectives for the New Century.*
Armonk, NY: Futura Publishing Company, Inc., © 2000

because children are more active, resume daily activities and exercise, and may also be less vigilant with sterile wound care earlier than adults. Data between pediatric studies are consistent, and variability in shock frequency may be due to differences in patient selection, programming parameters, and disease severity.

ICD Leads in Children

Earlier pediatric ICD recipients were confined to epicardial systems, and even then only in older children.[7] The transvenous route has advantages of avoiding a thoracotomy, lower pacing thresholds and lower incidence of exit block and lead fractures. The epicardial route has advantages of not necessitating vascular continuity with the cardiac chambers, and avoiding venous thrombosis. The disadvantages of transvenous leads include a slightly higher dislodgment rate (particularly with passive fixation), venous occlusion, danger of embolic vascular events (especially in the presence of an intracardiac shunt), small risk of endocarditis, and subclavian crush syndrome. Leaving a generous amount of slack in the lead may decrease the likelihood of lead fracture or dislodgment with linear growth. There are vascular access challenges related to congenital heart diseases and surgical corrections.

Lead malfunctions requiring new leads are relatively common in pediatric patients. In the 1999 study by Link et al., 60% of lead problems were in epicardial systems, including 3 insulation breaks of the rate sensing lead and one high voltage lead fracture.[4] Undersensing of torsades de pointes or other low-amplitude ventricular signals may cause inappropriate inhibition of device therapy in both children and adults.[4,8,9] An increased incidence of lead failure in children may be due to the continued growth of the thorax and perhaps also due to the more dynamic activity in young patients. Many young patients are actively involved in sports and vigorous exercise programs and are not debilitated from heart failure, coronary artery disease or other issues present in older adults.

Congenital Heart Disease in ICD Recipients

The patient with structural heart disease presents many unique challenges in ICD placement. Transvenous lead placement in congenital heart patients often requires nonstandard positioning, due to variations in venous and intracardiac anatomy. The atrial appendage may be amputated during cardiac bypass. Use of active fixation leads, once uncommon in ICD lead systems but now available, allows for easier sampling of nonstandard pacing sites, and easier removal when necessary.[10] Future rhythm complications may arise in children who have undergone palliative repairs, and should be anticipated in advance of device implantation. For patients with repaired congenital heart disease, particularly tetralogy of Fallot, sudden death risk is estimated at 2 – 10%, varying among different studies and surgical era.[11] Patients with transposition of the great arteries, and aortic stenosis also are at risk of sudden death due to ventricular arrhythmias.[12] Ischemia is less common in pediatric ICD recipients compared with adults, yet conditions such as aberrant coronary arteries or coronary sequelae of Kawasaki disease, predispose to ventricular vulnerability from ischemic heart disease.

Children with myocarditis, ventricular dysfunction, or dilated cardiomyopathies and ventricular tachycardia may be better with an implantable defibrillator rather than risk exposure to antiarrhythmic medications, potentially causing further myocardial dysfunction or proarrhythmia.[13] The utility of ICD implantation for congenital long QT syndrome, hypertrophic cardiomyopathy, and other hereditary arrhythmia disorders has been assessed in children and studies have shown a greater frequency of arrhythmias and higher sudden death rate than adults.[14,15] A review of ICD therapy in children and adults with congenital long QT syndrome found that they were effective and life-saving in many cases.[16] Even the small infant with congenital long QT syndrome may necessitate ICD placement.[17] However, prominent U waves or T wave oversensing in long QT patients may promote inappropriate device therapy.[18] Additional concerns regarding electrical storms due to a catecholamine surge after receiving a defibrillation shock may be greater in patients with catecholamine-sensitive ventricular tachycardias and particularly patients with long QT syndrome.[19] Stored electrogram retrieval in modern ICD generators allows the review of inciting events and mechanism of sudden cardiac death,[20] which should be valuable in patients with congenital heart disease, primary electrical disease, and ventricular vulnerability.

Pediatric ICD Patient Follow-up

Implanting a device in a child necessitates the consideration of growth and development issues. Unlike adults, the pediatric patient is not fully mature, and these physical, hormonal, and emotional developmental changes need understanding. At the time of initial implantation, adequate slack should be left in the heart and vascular space to allow for future linear growth, yet avoiding the potential problem of redundant lead interfering with tricuspid valve function. Having multiple leads in the heart may promote electrical interactions, inappropriate oversensing, and thrombosis. Children will (hopefully) require multiple ICD system revisions, generator replacements, and lead extractions/abandonment. These "problems" of increased life expectancy are unique to the younger ICD recipient, and should be addressed at the initial implant to reduce future potential complications.

Summary

In conclusion, ICD use in pediatric patients is feasible and is associated with a high frequency of appropriate shocks. ICD use in this population may be associated with a higher incidence of infections and lead malfunctions. Future refinements in generator and lead designs may hopefully improve the long-term performance of these implanted devices in children. Differences in pediatric ICD implantation relate to clinical factors, including age, size, ventricular function, presence of congenital heart disease, and emotional maturity. The child has unique implant indications, unique considerations regarding device and lead choice, route of implantation, programmable parameters, and psychosocial aspects. The indications for ICD therapy in children are similar to adults, however, the data are less comprehensive, and therefore, risk-stratification criteria may have lower predictive value. Congenital heart disease patients have additional concerns relevant to ICD implantation and follow-up. The risk of sudden cardiac death is greater for patients with congenital heart disease. These patients necessitate individualized treatment, with overall generalizations applicable as guidelines.

References

1. Silka MJ, Kron J, Dunnigan A, et al.: Sudden cardiac death and the use of implantable cardioverter-defibrillators in pediatric patients. *Circulation* 1993; 87:800-807.

2. Kron J, Silka MJ, Ohm OJ, et al.: Preliminary experience with nonthoracotomy implantable cardioverter-defibrillators in young patients. *PACE* 1994; 17:26-30.

3. Hamilton RM, Dorian P, Gow RM, et al.: Five-year experience with implantable defibrillators in children. *Am J Cardiol* 1996; 77:524-526.

4. Link MS, Hill SL, Cliff DL, et al.: Comparison of frequency of complications of implantable cardioverter-defibrillators in children versus adults. *Am J Cardiol* 1999; 83:263-266.

5. Gallik DM, Ben-Zur UM, Gross JN, et al.: Lead fracture in cephalic versus subclavian approach with transvenous implantable defibrillator systems. *PACE* 1996; 19:1089-1094.

6. Molina JE. Undertreatment and overtreatment of patients with infected antiarrhythmic devices. *Ann Thorac Surg.* 1997; 63:504-509.

7. Kron J, Oliver RP, Norsted S, et al.: The automatic implantable cardioverter-defibrillator in young patients. *J Am Coll Cardiol.* 1990; 16:896-902.

8. Berul CI, Callans DJ, Schwartzman DS, et al.: Comparison of initial detection and redetection of ventricular fibrillation in a transvenous defibrillator system with automatic gain control. *J Am Coll Cardiol*. 1995; 25:431-436.

9. Natale A, Sra J, Axtell K, et al.: Undetected ventricular fibrillation in transvenous implantable cardioverter-defibrillators. *Circulation* 1996; 93:91-98.

10. Friedman RA, Moak JP, Garson A. Active fixation of endocardial pacing leads: the preferred method of pediatric pacing. *PACE* 1991; 14:1213-1216.

11. Berul, CI, Hill SL, Geggel RG, et al.: Electrocardiographic markers of late sudden death risk in postoperative tetralogy of Fallot children. *J Cardiovasc Electrophysiol* 1997; 8:1349-1356.

12. Keane JF, Driscoll DJ, Gersony WM. Second natural history study of congenital heart defects: results of treatment of patients with aortic valvular stenosis. *Circulation* 1993; 87:I16-27.

13. Kaminer SJ, Pickoff AS, Dunnigan A, et al.: Cardiomyopathy and the use of implanted cardioverter-defibrillators in children. *PACE* 1990; 13:593-597.

14. McKenna WJ, Franklin RC, Nihoyannopoulos P, et al.: Arrhythmia and prognosis in infants, children and adolescents with hypertrophic cardiomyopathy. *J Am Coll Cardiol* 1988; 11:147-153.

15. Fananapazir L, Epstein SE. Hemodynamic and electrophysiologic evaluation of patients with hypertrophic cardiomyopathy surviving cardiac arrest. *Am J Cardiol* 1991; 67:280-287.

16. Groh WJ, Silka MJ, Oliver RP, et al.: Use of implantable cardioverter-defibrillators in the congenital long QT syndrome. *Am J Cardiol* 1996; 78:703-706.

17. Tanel RE, Triedman JK, Walsh EP, et al.: High-rate atrial pacing as an innovative bridging therapy in a neonate with congenital long QT syndrome. *J Cardiovasc Electrophysiol*. 1997; 8:812-817.

18. Perry GY, Kosar EM. Problems in managing patients with long QT syndrome and implantable cardioverter defibrillators. *PACE* 1996; 19:863-867.

19. Credner SC, Klingenheben T, Mauss O, et al.: Electrical storm in patients with transvenous implantable cardioverter-defibrillators. *J Am Coll Cardiol*. 1998; 32:1909-1915.

20. Grubman EM, Pavri BB, Shipman T, et al.: Cardiac death and stored electrograms in patients with third-generation implantable cardioverter-defibrillators. *J Am Coll Cardiol*. 1998; 32:1056-1062.

29.

COST-EFFECTIVENESS OF IMPLANTABLE CARDIOVERTER-DEFIBRILLATOR THERAPY

Hindrik WJ Robbe, PhD, Fred W. Lindemans, PhD

Bakken Research Center, Maastricht, The Netherlands

Introduction

Since its clinical introduction in 1980, the implantable cardioverter-defibrillator (ICD) has been greatly improved with respect to its features, leads, longevity, volume, and, as a result, the required surgical procedure. Randomised studies have shown that ICD therapy provides better survival than antiarrhythmic drug therapy, both in secondary[1,2] and in primary[3] prevention of sudden cardiac death in high-risk populations. However, new technologies generally provide greater benefit only at higher costs and the economic impact of further proliferation of ICD therapy can be huge, particularly when considering prophylactic implantation. As resources are scarce, choices must be made, and cost-effectiveness of therapies will play an increasingly important role in the decision process.

Cost-effectiveness analysis

Cost-effectiveness analysis is the comparative analysis of alternative courses of action, both in terms of costs and in terms of results or outcome.[4] In designing cost-effectiveness studies, there are three different dimensions to consider: the type of costs and benefits, the viewpoint for the analysis, and the type of analysis.

Costs can be direct, indirect and intangible. Direct costs include both medical costs (e.g. cost of therapy and complications) and nonmedical costs (e.g. transportation and home help). Indirect costs include those that are borne by the patient or family because of the patient's impaired ability of daily living, and those borne by society as a whole because of the lost productivity of the patient and other family members involved in care. Intangible costs are the costs of pain, suffering, and grief, and are, like indirect costs, difficult to measure.

Besides actual costs, one may also use charges (fees for services) or reimbursements (e.g. from insurance programs). Charges typically include the provider's costs plus a mark-up for profits whereas insurance companies may reimburse only a percentage of charges billed.

The viewpoint one may take is that of the patient, the provider, the payer, or the society as a whole. For providers, for example, benefits from reductions

From Ovsyshcher IE. *Cardiac Arrythmias and Device Therapy: Results and Perspectives for the New Century.* Armonk, NY: Futura Publishing Company, Inc., © 2000

in hospital costs but not from reductions in lost productivity are important. The latter, however, do count for the society as a whole.

There are three types of analysis that compare the costs and outcomes of two treatment strategies according to the following equation:

$$\frac{Cost(A) - Cost(B)}{Outcomes(A) - Outcomes(B)}$$

where A and B are the treatments. The three analyses only differ in the way they measure outcomes.

Cost-effectiveness analysis measures outcomes in natural or physical units, such as "life expectancy." When no comparison is made to an alternative therapy, the calculation provides the therapy's average cost-effectiveness. If two treatments are compared, the calculation provides the incremental cost-effectiveness of one therapy over the other. For example, if ICD therapy is compared to antiarrhythmic drug therapy, the incremental cost of ICD therapy is divided by the incremental life expectancy, and the result is expressed as dollars per life year saved ($/LYS).

Cost-utility analysis takes also the value or utility of an outcome into account. For example, one could measure quality of life and express the score as a single number along a continuum from death (0) to good health (1), using this score to adjust life expectancy. The result of such an analysis is expressed as dollars per quality-adjusted life years (QALYs).

Cost-benefit analysis differs from cost-effectiveness analysis in that it measures not only costs but also the outcomes in financial terms. However, due to the difficulty to put a dollar value on medical benefits, cost-benefit analysis is only rarely used.

As uncertainties and bias may exist in the assumptions made, it is important to perform a "sensitivity analysis" to determine how critically dependent the final results are on given assumptions. For example, how sensitive are the results for changes in cost of therapy or longevity of the device.

Therapies that cost an additional $20,000 to $40,000/QALY are considered "cost-effective".[5] Less is considered "attractive"; greater than $60,000/QALY is considered "expensive". Thus treatment of patients with diastolic blood pressures of 90 to 105 mmHg is "attractive" in men and women aged 60 ($12,200 and $18,000/QALY), "cost-effective" in men and women aged 40 ($23,700 and $33,700/QALY), moderately "cost-effective" in men aged 20 ($42,600/QALY) and "expensive" in women aged 20 ($64,500/QALY).[6]

Cost-effectiveness of ICD therapy

A number of studies analysed the cost-effectiveness of ICD therapy. Kupperman et al.[7] used 1984 Medicare data and they were the first to address the issue of ICD cost-effectiveness in drug-refractory survivors of cardiac arrest. In their base-case scenario ICDs incur an additional $17,100/LYS, based on charges obtained from the Health Care Financing Administration over the life of the patient. Assuming a pectoral implant and a 5-yr device longevity, the additional cost of ICD therapy was reduced to $7,400/LYS.

Larsen et al.[8] used true costs from inpatient and outpatient care generated by a hospital's sophisticated cost-accounting system, and found an incremental cost-effectiveness ratio for ICD versus amiodarone therapy of $29,200/LYS in patients with recurrent sustained ventricular tachycardia (VT) and fibrillation (VF). Sensitivity analysis showed that with 3-yr and 8-yr longevity, the cost-effectiveness ratio would be $21,800/LYS and $13,800/LYS, respectively.

Kupersmith et al.[9] relied on Michigan Medicare discharge abstracts from 1989 to 1992 to calculate the incremental cost-effectiveness of ICD therapy compared with electrophysiologically guided therapy over a 6-yr time period in patients with sustained VT or VF. The base-case scenario resulted in a cost-effectiveness of $31,100/LYS. However, endocardial devices incurred an incremental cost of $25,700/LYS, and eliminating the pre-implant EP study dramatically reduced the incremental costs to $14,200/LYS.

Similar results have been observed in the UK by O'Brien et al.[10] who calculated ICD cost-effectiveness compared to amiodarone and reported ratios of £8,200 to £15,400 per life-year saved.

Owens et al.[11] used historical, clinical, economic and patient preference databases to construct a model comparing the cost-effectiveness of third-generation ICDs to amiodarone. Assuming a 20% mortality advantage for ICDs at year one and a perceived reduction of quality of life for both the ICD and amiodarone patients resulted in incremental costs of $74,400/QALY. If one assumed a 40% mortality advantage for ICDs in the first year and did not adjust for a perceived reduction in quality of life, the additional cost for ICD therapy was $27,300/LYS.

Two studies have been published that calculated cost-effectiveness from a prospective randomised study. The first was conducted over a 2-yr period in the Netherlands with 60 post-infarction sudden cardiac death survivors.[12] The study compared the incremental cost-effectiveness of initial ICD implantation with EP-guided treatment (antiarrhythmic drugs or ICD, if the arrhythmia could not be suppressed). In this study, early ICD implantation was a dominant strategy; i.e., it saved lives and costs.

The second prospective study was MADIT in which high-risk post-MI patients were randomised to prophylactic ICD therapy or conventional, primarily amiodarone, therapy. The base-case scenario resulted in a cost-effectiveness ratio of $27,000/LYS. Patients receiving a transvenous device incurred an additional $22,800/LYS; and assuming an 8-yr longevity reduced the incremental cost to $16,900/LYS.[13]

How to improve ICD cost-effectiveness

Although the above cost-effectiveness ratios are certainly not unfavourable, further dissemination of prophylactic ICD therapy will only happen with better cost-effectiveness ratios. This can be achieved either by lowering the costs or by improving the outcome of ICD therapy, or both.

The major cost drivers of ICD therapy are the cost of the ICD system and hospitalisation costs. Costs of ICD systems have gone down (both as a result of lower system prices and increased longevity) and hospitalisation costs have been decreased (simpler implant procedures, fewer complications, faster discharge).

The outcome of ICD therapy can be enhanced by increasing the gain in survival and quality-of-life, compared to alternative strategies. This can be achieved by better risk stratification so that only patients most likely to benefit from ICD therapy are implanted.

The result of optimal risk stratification is that a high percentage of patients selected for ICD therapy will indeed experience cardiac arrest; in other words, the positive predictive accuracy of risk stratification should be high. However, in patients who already experienced cardiac arrest, the probability of recurrence is so high that further risk stratification is only acceptable if most, if not all, patients who will experience recurrent cardiac arrest are selected. In short, in primary prevention, a high positive predictive accuracy is more important than a high sensitivity whereas in secondary prevention, a high sensitivity is more important.

Conclusion

Although ICD therapy is often viewed as expensive, cost-effectiveness analyses have shown favourable cost/benefit ratios and are well within the range of currently accepted life-saving technologies, particularly in secondary prevention. Several studies are now under way to test potential risk stratification procedures, particularly in primary prevention populations. Besides achievement of clinical benefit, improvements in quality of life and a favourable cost-effectiveness ratio will be important determinants for the further development and dissemination of this therapy.

References

1. The Antiarrhythmic Versus Implantable Defibrillators (AVID) Investigators. A comparison of antiarhythmic-drug therapy with implantable

defibrillators in patients resuscitated from near-fatal ventricular arrhythmias. N Engl J Med 1997;337:1576-1583.

2. Cappato R. Secondary prevention of sudden death: the Dutch study, the Antiarrhythmics Versus Implantable Defibrillator Trial, the Cardiac Arrest Study Hamburg, and the Canadian Implantable Defibrillator Study. Am J Cardiol 1999;83:68D-73D.

3. Moss AJ, Hall WJ, Cannom DS, et al. Improved survival with an implanted defibrillator in patients with coronary disease at high risk for ventricular arrhythmia. New Engl J Med 1996;335:1933-1940.

4. Kupersmith J, Holmes-Rovner M, Hogan A, et al. Cost-effectiveness analysis in heart disease – part I: general principles. Prog Cardiovasc Dis 1994;37:161-184.

5. Goldman L, Gordon DJ, Rifkind BM, et al. Cost and health implications of cholesterol lowering. Circulation 1992;85:1960-1968.

6. Littenberg B, Garber AM, Sox HC. Screening for hypertension. Ann Intern Med 1990;112:192-202.

7. Kupperman M, Luce BR, McGovern B, et al. An analysis of the cost effectiveness of the implantable defibrillator. Circulation 1990;81:91-100.

8. Larsen GC, Manolis AC, Sonnenberg FA, et al. Cost-effectiveness of the implantable cardioverter-defibrillator: effect of improved battery life and comparison with amiodarone therapy. J Am Coll Cardiol 1992;19:1323-1334.

9. Kupersmith J, Hogan A, Guerrero P, et al. Evaluating and improving the cost-effectiveness of the implantable cardioverter-defibrillator. Am Heart J 1995;130:507-515.

10. O'Brien B, Buxton MJ, Rushby JA. Cost effectiveness of the implantable cardioverter defibrillator: a preliminary analysis. Br Heart J 1992;68:241-245.

11. Owens DK, Sanders GD, Harris RA, et al. Cost-effectiveness of implantable cardioverter defibrillators relative to amiodarone for prevention of sudden cardiac death. Ann Intern Med 1997;126:1-12.

12. Wever EFD, Hauer RNW, Schrijvers G., et al. Cost-effectiveness of implantable defibrillator as first-choice therapy versus electro-physiologically guided, tiered strategy in postinfarct sudden death survivors. Circulation 1996;93:489-496.

13. Mushlin AI, Hall WJ, Zwanziger J, et al. The cost-effectiveness of automatic implantable cardiac defibrillators: results from MADIT. Circulation 1998;97:2129-2135.

30.
PREDICTORS OF LONG-TERM SURVIVAL IN PATIENTS WITH IMPLANTABLE CARDIOVERTER-DEFIBRILLATOR

Shimon Rosenheck, MD, FACC, FESC

Electrophysiology Laboratory, Cardiology Unit, Hadassah University Hospital, Mount Scopus, Jerusalem, Israel

Introduction

Recent studies have demonstrated better survival of patients with implantable cardioverter-defibrillator (ICD) when compared to the best medical antiarrhythmic treatment[1-17]. However the long-term survival after ICD implantation is determined and predicted by the left ventricular ejection fraction (LVEF) and the cardiac functional state[18-38], occurrence of shock therapy[19,225,26,36,38-46], high age and female sex. The prognostic importance of the background heart diseases, the presenting arrhythmia and coronary revascularization are still not definitely determined. The purpose of the present study was to evaluate the effect of left ventricular function, coronary revascularization, background heart disease, presenting arrhythmia, age, sex, and amount of residual brain damage on the prognosis in patients with ICD.

Methods

The study was conducted in 171 consecutive patients who had ICD implantation at our institution during the last 7 years and had regular follow-up in our clinic for at least 3 months. The mean age was 61±14 years, 133 were male and the mean LVEF was 0.36±0.16. The indication for ICD implantation was sudden cardiac death in 55 patients, ventricular tachycardia in 112 patients and prophylactic implantation in 5 patient. Coronary heart disease (CAD), was present in 117 patients, 16 patients had idiopathic dilated cardiomyopathy (IDC), 11 had hypertrophic cardiomyopathy (HCMO), 13 had valvular/congenital heart disease (VHD) and 9 had arrhythmogenic right ventricular dysplasia (ARVD).

The ICD was implanted using routine methods. Endocardial systems were implanted with active or passive generator can. In 21 patients ICD with dual chamber pacing and in two additional patients AV defibrillator (Jewel AF Model # 7258H, Medtronic, Minneapolis, MN) was implanted.

Kaplan Meier survival curves were compared using log-rank test. The relative risk was calculated using contingency table and the p value was

From Ovsyshcher IE. *Cardiac Arrythmias and Device Therapy: Results and Perspectives for the New Century.* Armonk, NY: Futura Publishing Company, Inc., © 2000

calculated using Fisher's exact test or the chi-square test. Analysis of variance was used to compare the groups. Confidence interval (95%CI) was calculated. A $p<0.05$ was considered significant. The data was recorded and evaluated using a statistical software package (GraphPad Prism version 2.0 for Macintosh, GraphPad Software, Inc., San Diego, CA).

Results

The population was divided into two groups, 81 patients with LVEF<0.35 (LEF) and 90 patients with LVEF≥0.35 (HEF). Patients with HEF had significantly better survival than those with LEF (Figure 1).

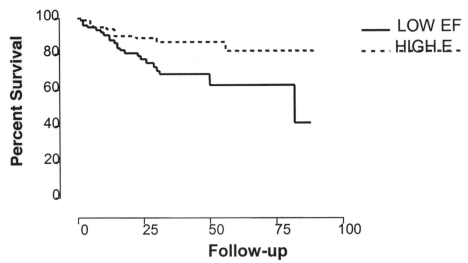

Figure 1. Survival curves in patients with LVEF<0.35 and LVEF≥0.35. (p=0.009, Hazard Ratio 2.51 with CI 95% from 1.25 to 4.99)

Patients without ICD treatment had significantly better survival than the users (Figure 2). There was no significant difference in the ejection fraction between the 78 non-users, 0.38±0.17, and the 93 users 0.35±0.15. After 7 years, in 105 patients without appropriate shock discharges, more than 90% long-term survival was observed and in patients with ICD discharges 52.4% survival was observed (p=0.0011, Hazard ratio 0.27 CI 95% from 0.13 to 0.60). The total mortality rate was only 7.6% in patients without ICD discharges and 31.8% in patients with discharges (p<0.0001, Relative Risk 0.74, CI 95% from 0.62 to 0.88). In the low LVEF group, the mortality rate was 13.9% in patients without discharges and 40.5% in patients with discharges (p=0.01, Relative Risk 0.69, CI 95% from 0.52 to 0.93). In the high LVEF group the mortality rate was 3.2% in patients without ICD discharges and 20.7% in patients with ICD discharges (p=0.01, Relative Risk 0.82, CI 95% from 0.68 to 0.99).

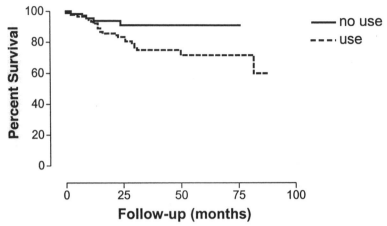

Figure 2. Survival curves in patients with and without appropriate ICD therapy (p=0.03, Hazard ratio 0.37 with CI 95% from 0.20 to 0.94).

Pacing treatment of ventricular tachycardia was effective in 88% of the episodes in 54 patients and in 12% of the episodes rescue shocks were needed. The mortality rate in patients with pacing therapy was 22.2% as compared to 15.8% in 117 patients without such treatment (p=0.1845). CAD was present in 68.4% of the patients and 18.4% of these patient died during the follow-up, surviving by 658.5±554.1 days the initial implantation (96% CI from 399 to 917.8). In the survivors with CAD the follow-up is for 1036±637 days (95%CI from 906.7 to 1166). From patients with IDC 6 died (37.5%). From 38 patients (22.2%) with HCMP, VHD, ARVD and normal heart, no one died during the follow-up. There was significant difference in the distribution of background heart disease between the LEF and HEF groups (Table 1).

Table 1. The background heart disease. (p<0.0001).

Heart Disease	Low LVEF	High LVEF	Total
CAD	63 (78.75%)	54 (59.34%)	117
IDC	14 (17.50%)	2 (2.20%)	16
Other			
HCMP	0	11	11
VHD	2	8	10
Cong.	1	2	3
None	0	5	5

Abbreviations: LVEF-left ventricular ejection fraction, CAD-coronary artery disease, IDC-idiopathic dilated cardiomyopathy, HCMP- hypertrophic cardiomyopathy, VHD-valvular heart disease, Cong.-congenital heart disease. Low LVEF- LVEF<0.35, High LVEF - LVEF≥0.35.

Patients with CAD and IDC were older than patients with OHD (Table 2). Patients with OHD had higher LVEF (p<0.0001), and had less ICD therapy (p=0.0198) and more of them were women (p=0.0001).

Table 2. Comparison between patients with coronary artery disease (CAD), idiopathic dilated cardiomyopathy (IDC) and other background pathologies.

	CAD	IDC	Other	p
Age	65±10	63±9	41±20	0.001
men/women	106/11	7/9	20/15	0.0001
VT/VF	84/33	10/6	19/16	0.1400
LVEF	0.32 (0.30 to 0.34)	0.24 (0.19 to 0.29)	0.55 (0.51 to 0.60)	0.0001
Use/no-use	67/50	12/4	14/24	0.0198
Follow-up	961 (844to 637)	775 (515 to 1037)	1079 (843 to 718)	0.2795

There was no difference in the presenting arrhythmia between the three groups. The cumulated survival during 7 years in patients with CAD and LEF was 44.66%, in patients with CAD and HEF was 84.18%, in patients with IDC was 57.29% and in patients with OHD was 100% (Figure 3).

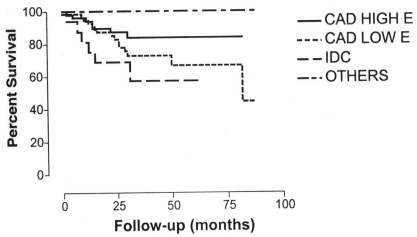

Figure 3. Survival curves in patients with CAD and LVEF<0.35, CAD and LVEF≥0.35, IDC and other heart diseases (p<0.001).

The difference between the users and non-users with CAD was not significant. Only 28.94% of the women had CAD versus 79.70% in men, 23.68% had IDC versus 5.26% and OHD in 47.37% versus 15.04% (p<0.0001). Women had higher LVEF than male patients, 0.34±0.15 versus 0.45±0.17 (p=0.0003) and were younger, 55.71±17.22 versus 61.95±12.95 (p=0.019). There was no difference in the presenting arrhythmia and percent of patients with ICD therapy. There was no difference between the survival in women and in men (Figure 4).

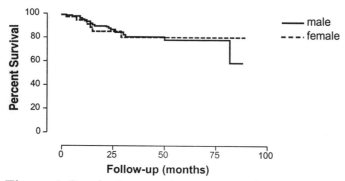

Figure 4. Survival curves in women and men.

Three patients had significant residual brain damage at the time of implantation, one after several previous episodes of aborted sudden cardiac death and 2 after one episode of sudden cardiac death. Two patients died during the first year after the implantation and one patient is alive 2 years after the implantation.

Discussion

Several predictors for favorable outcome in patients with implantable cardioverter defibrillator were suggested during the last 15 years. The left ventricular function was the strongest prognostic predictor for long-term survival[18-38]. However the low ejection fraction group includes mainly patients with CAD and IDC and they have limited survival[47]. Normal heart, arrhythmogenic right ventricular dysplasia, hypertrophic cardiomyopathy, valvular heart disease after surgical correction and certain congenital heart diseases, may be found only in the high ejection fraction group. They have an excellent prognosis[48,50], low rate of spontaneous arrhythmia and are younger than patients with CAD and IDC. If the burden of sudden cardiac death is eliminated there is no reason for limited survival in these patients. Therefore, the background heart disease may affect the survival curve even if the difference between the groups cannot reach statistical significance. A more adequate evaluation of the survival may be obtained in homogenous groups in regard to the background heart disease.

In our study the effect of ejection fraction in patients with coronary heart disease was evaluated and despite a trend towards better survival in those with higher ejection faction, the difference did not reach statistical significance. However, the ejection fraction still may be accepted as a strong prognostic predictor in patients with implantable cardioverter defibrillator and coronary artery disease. A similar analysis in the other patients was not feasible as most if not all the patients with idiopathic dilated cardiomyopathy had ejection fraction bellow 0.35 and patients with hypertrophic cardiomyopathy, arrhythmogenic right ventricular dysplasia and normal heart have normal or high LVEF. Patients with congenital heart disease and valvular heart disease, especially after successful surgical correction have normal left ventricular function.

Patients with non-coronary heart disease or idiopathic dilated cardiomyopathy had excellent prognosis. A large prospective study in patients with congenital and/or valvular heart disease without preserved left ventricular morphology and function has not been carried out.

Several studies evaluated the survival related to ICD discharges. The negative predictive value of ICD discharge was evident in certain studies[26,36,40,42,46], however other studies could not reconfirm this finding[25,38,39,41,43-45]. Multiple discharges for the same arrhythmia predicted a bed prognosis when single shocks had the same outcome as patients without ICD discharges[39]. However in this study the defibrillation threshold was high, except in a minority of patients enrolled in clinical studies. Most of the devices had no stored electrograms[39]. Electrical storm was not associated with bad prognosis[41].

In our study both total ICD treatment and appropriate ICD shock therapy were significantly correlated with a lower survival rate, independent of the ejection fraction. However the overdrive pacing therapy had no any prognostic value.

There is controversy about the worse prognosis in female patients. Women have more frequently idiopathic dilated cardiomyopathy and less often coronary artery disease. We could not reconfirm this finding.

The presenting arrhythmia has no prognostic value[51] and revascularization had a positive prognostic value[23,31,46,52].

Patients with residual brain damage had also a bed prognosis; however, their number was too low to come to any conclusion.

Independently, presence of extracardiac conditions which may limit the survival will significantly worsen the prognosis and the survival will depend on the progress of the extracardiac conditions.

Summary

The predictors of normal survival in patients with ICD are the preserved left ventricular function expressed by a high ejection fraction, normal functional state, no recurrence of rapid spontaneous ventricular tachyarrhythmias, adequate recovery from the anoxic brain damage and background heart disease different from CAD and IDC. Slow ventricular tachycardia terminated with overdrive pacing, age and female sex were not predictors of survival in our patients with ICD.

References

1. Anderson JJ, Hallstrom AP, Epstein AE, et al. Design and results of antiarrhythmics vs implantable defibrillators (AVID) registry. Circulation 1999;99:1692-1699.
2. Mittal S, Iwai S, Stein KM, et al. Long-term outcome of patients with unexplained syncope treated with electrophysiologic-guided approach in the implantable cardioverter-defibrillator era. JACC 1999;34:1082-1089.
3. Morris DC. Results from late-braking clinical trials sessions at ACCIS '99 and ACC '99. J Am Coll Cardiol 1999;34:1-11.
4. Nisam S. Can implantable defibrillators reduce non-arrhythmic mortality? J Interven Card Electrophysiol 1998;2:371-375.
5. Kuck KH, on behalf of CASH investigators. The CASH study: final results. Oral presentation at the Annual Session of the American College of Cardiology, Atlanta, March 29-April 1, 1998.
6. Connoly SJ, on behalf of CIDS investigators. The CIDS study: final results. Oral presentation at the Annual Session of the American College of Cardiology, Atlanta, March 29-April 1, 1998.
7. Pacifico A, Wheelan K, Nasir N, Wells PJ, Doyle TK, Johnson SA, Henry PD. Long-term follow-up of cardioverter-defibrillator implanted under conscious sedation in prepectoral subfacial position. Circulation 1997;95:946-950.
8. Nisam S, Breithardt G. Mortality trials with implantable defibrillators. Am J Cardiol 1997;79:468-471.
9. The Antiarrhythmics Versus Implantable Defibrillators (AVID) Investigators. A comparison of antiarrhythmic-drug therapy with

implantable defibrillators in patients resuscitated from near-fatal ventricular arrhythmias. N Engl J Med 1997;337:1576-1583.

10. Moss AJ, Hall J, Cannom DS, et al. Improved survival with an implanted defibrillator in patients with coronary artery disease at high risk for ventricular arrhythmia. N Engl J Med 1996;335:1933-1940.

11. Wever EFD, Hauer RNW, van Capelle FJI, et al. Randomized study of implantable defibrillator as first-choice therapy versus conventional strategy in post infarct sudden death survivors. Circulation 1995;91:2195-2203.

12. Bardy GH, Hofer B, Johnson G, et al. Implantable transvenous cardioverter-defibrillator. Circulation 1993;87:1152-1168.

13. Fogoros RN, Elson J, Bonnet CA, et al. Long-term Outcome of survivors of cardiac arrest whose therapy is guided by electrophysiologic testing. J Am Coll Cardiol 1992;19:780-788.

14. Wyndham CRC. Implantable cardioverter defibrillators: where do we go from here? J Am Coll Cardiol 1992;19:789-791.

15. Saksena, S, Poczobutt-Johanson M, Castle LW, et al. Long-term multicenter experience with a second-generation implantable pacemaker-defibrillator in patients with malignant ventricular tachyarrhythmias. J Am Coll Cardiol 1992;19:490-499.

16. Winkle RA, Mead RH, Ruder MA, et al. Long-term outcome with the automatic implantable cardioverter-defibrillator. J Am Coll Cardiol 1989;13:1353-1361.

17. Kelly PA, Cannom DS, Garan H, et al. The automatic implantable cardioverter-defibrillator: efficacy, complications ˋand survival in patients with malignant ventricular arrhythmias. J Am Coll Cardiol 1988;11:1278-1286.

18. Domanski MJ, Sakseena S, Epstein AE, et al. Relative effectiveness of the implantable cardioverter-defibrillator and antiarrhythmic drugs in patients with varying degree of left ventricular dysfunction who have survived malignant ventricular arrhythmias. J Am Coll Cardiol 1999;34:1090-1095.

19. Pacifico A, Ferlic LL, Cedillo-Salazar FR, et al. Shocks as predictors of survival in patients with implantable cardioverter-defibrillators. J Am Coll Cardiol 1999;34:204-210.

20. Anvari A, Gottsauner-Wolf M, Turel Z, et al. Predictors of outcome in patients with implantable cardioverter defibrillators. Cardiology 1998;90:180-186.

21. Bocker D, Bansch D, Heinecke A, et al. Potential benefit from cardioverter-defibrillator therapy in patients with and without heart failure. Circulation 1998;98:1636-1643.

22. Trappe HJ, Wezlaff P, Pfitzner P, Feiguth HG. Long-term follow-up of patients with implantable cardioverter-defibrillators and mild, moderate, or severe impairment of left ventricular function. PACE 1997;78:243-249.

23. Shahian DM, Williamson WA, Venditti FJ, et al. The role of coronary revascularization in recipients of an implantable cardioverter-defibrillator. J Thorac Cardiovasc Surg 1995;110:1013- 1022.

24. Schlepper M, Neuzner J, Pitschner HF. Implantable cardioverter defibrillator: effect on survival. PACE 1995;18:569-578.

25. Lessmeier TJ, Lehmann MH, Steinman RT, et al. Implantable cardioverter-defibrillator therapy in 300 patients with coronary artery disease presenting exclusively with ventricular fibrillation. Am Heart J 1994;128:211-218.

26. Tebbenjohanns J, Schumacher B, Jung W, et al. Predictors of outcome in patients with implantable transvenous cardioverter defibrillators. Am Heart J 1994;127:1086-1089.

27. Wood MA, Stambler BS, Damiano RJ, et al. Lessons learned from the data logging in a multicenter clinical trial using a late-generation implantable cardioverter-defibrillator. J Am Coll Cardiol 1994;24:1692-1699.

28. Kim SG, Maloney JD, Pinski LS, et al. Influence of left ventricular function on survival and mode of death after implantable defibrillator therapy (Cleveland Clinic Foundation and Montefiore Medical Center Experience). Am J Cardiol 1993;72:1263-1267.

29. Leissmeier TJ, Lehmann MH, Stenman R, et al. Outcome with implantable cardioverter-defibrillator therapy for survivors of ventricular fibrillation secondary to idiopathic dilated cardiomyopathy or coronary artery disease without myocardial infarction. Am J Cardiol 1993;72:911-915.

30. Grimm W, Flores BT, Marchlinski FE. Shock occurrence and survival in 241 patients with implantable cardioverter-defibrillator therapy. Circulation 1993;87:1880-1888.

31. Nath S, DeLacey WA, Haines DE, et al. Use of regional wall motion score to enhance risk stratification of patients receiving an implantable cardioverter-defibrillator. J Am Coll Cardiol 1993;22:1093-1099.

32. Bocker D, Block M, Isbruch F, et al. Do patients with implantable defibrillator live longer? J Am Coll Cardiol 1993;21:1638-1644.

33. Crandall BG, Morris CD, Cutler JE, Kudenchuk PJ, Peterson JL, Liem LB, Bruody DR, Greene HL, Halperin BD, et al. Implantable cardioverter-defibrillator therapy in survivors of out-of-hospital sudden cardiac death without inducible arrhythmias. J Am Coll Cardiol 1993;21:1186-92.

34. Mehta D, Saksena S, Krol RB, et al. Survival of implantable cardioverter defibrillator recipients: Role of left ventricular function and its relationship to device use. Am Heart J 1992;124:1608-1614.

35. Kim S, Fisher J, Choue CW, et al. Influence of left ventricular function on outcome of patients treated with implantable defibrillators. Circulation 1992;85:1304-1310.

36. Levine JH, Mellits D, Baumgardner RA, et al. Predictors of first discharge and subsequent survival in patients with automatic implantable cardioverter-defibrillators. Circulation 1991;84:558-566.

37. Fogoros RN, Elson JJ, Bommet CA, et al. Efficacy of the automatic implantable cardioverter defibrillator in prolonging the survival in patients with severe underlying cardiac disease. J Am Coll Cardiol 1990;16:381-386.

38. Myerburg RJ, Luceri RM, Thurer R, et al. Time to first shock and clinical outcome in patients receiving an automatic implantable cardioverter-defibrillator. J Am Coll Cardiol 1989;14:508-514.

39. Villacastin J, Almedral J, Arenal A, et al. Incidence and Clinical significance of multiple consecutive, appropriate, high-energy discharges in patients with implanted cardioverter-defibrillators. Circulation 1999;93:753-762.

40. Endoh Y, Ohnishi S, Kasanuki H. Clinical significance of consecutive shocks in patients with left ventricular dysfunction treated with implantable cardioverter defibrillators. PACE 1999;22:187-191.

41. Credner SC, Klingenheben T, Mauss O, et al. Electrical storm in patients with transvenous implantable cardioverter-defibrillators. Incidence, management and prognostic implications. J Am Coll Cardiol 1998;32:1909-1915.

42. Reiter MJ, Fain ES, Senelly KM, et al. Predictors of device activity for ventricular arrhythmias and survival in patients with implantable pacemaker/defibrillators. PACE 1994;17:1487-1498.

43. Tchou P, Axtell K, Keim S, et al. Does reception of appropriate shocks from the implantable cardioverter defibrillator affect survival ? PACE 1991;14:1929-1934.

44. Gross JN, Song SL, Buckingham T, et al. Influence of clinical characteristics and shock occurrence on ICD patient outcome: a multicenter report. PACE 1991;14:1881-1886.

45. Fogoros RN, Elson JJ, Bonnet CA. Survival of patients who have received appropriate shocks from their implantable defibrillators. PACE 1991;14:1842-1845.

46. Zilo P, Gross JN, Benedek M, et al. Occurrence of ICD shock and patient survival. PACE 1991;14:273-279.

47. Knight BP, Goyal R, Pelosi F, et al. Outcome of patients with nonischemic dilated cardiomyopathy and unexplained syncope treated with an implantable defibrillator. J Am Coll Cardiol 1999;33:1964-1970.

48. Elliott PM, Sharma S, Varnava A, Poloniecki J, Rowland E, McKenna WJ. Survival after cardiac arrest or sustained ventricular tachycardia in patients with hypertrophic cardiomyopathy. J Am Coll Cardiol 1999;33:1596-1601.

49. Geelen P, Primo J, Wellens F, Brugada P. Coronary artery bypass grafting and defibrillator implantation in patients with ventricular tachyarrhythmias and ischemic heart disease. PACE 1999;22;1132-1139.

50. Meissner MC, Lehmann MH, Steinman RT, et al. Ventricular fibrillation in patients without significant heart disease: a multicenter experience with

implantable cardioverter-defibrillator therapy. J Am Coll Cardiol 1993;21:1406-1412.

51. Menz V, Schwartzman D, Nallamothu N, Grimm W, Hoffmann J, Callans DJ, Gottlieb CD, Marchlinski FE. Does the initial presentation of patients with implantable defibrillator influence the outcome? PACE 1997;20:173-176.

52. Nath S, Haines D, DeLacey WA, et al. Comparison of the usefulness of the implantable cardioverter-defibrillator and subendocardial resection in patients with sustained ventricular arrhythmias and poor regional wall motion associated with coronary artery disease. Am J Cardiol 1993;72:652-657.

31.
PACEMAKER – ICD INTERACTIONS – ARE THEY STILL RELEVANT? PAST, PRESENT AND FUTURE

Michael Glikson, MD, *Paul Friedman, MD

Sheba Medical Center and Tel Aviv University, Israel
*Cardiovascular Division, Mayo Clinic, Rochester, MN, USA

Introduction

Pacemaker – ICD interactions were the subject of numerous studies and publications over the last fifteen years. Patients with concomitant pacemaker and ICD were studied thoroughly according to various protocols to prevent hazardous interactions between the devices. Multiple publications in that field demonstrate the diversity and complexity of the problem [1].

Over the past three years, ICDs with dual chamber rate adaptive pacing capabilities have become readily available, making the implantation of concomitant pacing systems unnecessary and even obsolete. The need for de-novo implantation of concomitant systems has dropped to nearly zero.

However, although new implants of dual systems are only rarely performed nowadays, the subject is still pertinent, as there are still many patients being followed with concomitant pacemaker – ICD systems, and many new patients with old pacemaker systems present with a need for new ICD implantation. Moreover, understanding of pacemaker – ICD interactions may have implications on the development of future systems, some of which will incorporate dual chamber defibrillation with atrial – biventricular pacing for the treatment of patients with both atrial and ventricular arrhythmias and congestive heart failure.

In this paper we will review the past, present and future of pacemaker – ICD interactions.

The Past

In the past, concomitant pacemakers were necessary in almost 20% of patients with first generation ICDs, which lacked any antibradycardia pacing capability. This need decreased dramatically subsequent to the introduction in the late 1980s of ICDs capable of bradycardia pacing. However, for nearly a decade, ICDs had only basic VVI pacing ability, which was sufficient for most ICD patients who were not pacemaker dependent and needed the bradycardia pacing only for backup purposes. Nevertheless, some patients still required pacemakers in addition to ICDs, particularly those in need of dual chamber pacing, rate adaptive pacing,

From Ovsyshcher IE. *Cardiac Arrythmias and Device Therapy: Results and Perspectives for the New Century.* Armonk, NY: Futura Publishing Company, Inc., © 2000

and or a high frequency of pacing (in order to avoid premature ICD battery depletion). The requirement of two separate arrhythmia devices added significant implant complexity and the introduced the possibility of potentially dangerous interdevice interactions.

A host of interactions between pacemakers and ICDs have been described, and numerous testing protocols have been developed to detect them, which became more and more sophisticated over time, especially since the development of telemetered EGMs. When tested rigorously during implantation, up to 50% of patients may demonstrate significant pacemaker – ICD interactions that can be avoided if properly identified. The most important interactions included the following:

The most hazardous interaction was inhibition of ventricular fibrillation (VF) detection by the pacemaker pacing artifacts. This problem is caused by the combination of the large amplitude of pacemaker artifacts, the small amplitude of ventricular fibrillation and the auto adjusting sensing mechanism that exists in all modern ICD systems. By adjusting to the amplitude of the pacemaker artifacts, the sensing mechanism may become blinded to the underlying small amplitude ventricular fibrillation, resulting in nondetection or delayed detection of the arrhythmia. All Protocols of pacemaker – ICD interactions call for rigorous testing of this potential interaction under worst case conditions of maximal output, rapid rate asynchronous pacing by the pacemaker in the presence of induced ventricular fibrillation. Electrode repositioning is required when such interactions cannot absolutely be avoided.

Asynchronous pacemaker activity is necessary for inhibition of VF detection by that mechanism. The two main reasons for asynchronous pacing in VF are undersensing of the VT or noise reversion mechanisms, which exist in most pacemakers. Understanding of that mechanism and its difference from undersensing enables the operator to minimize asynchronous pacing in VF [2].

Another mechanism of interaction is inappropriate detection of tachycardia due to detection of pacemaker stimulus artifacts in addition to subsequent QRS, resulting in double or (in some cases of low atrial pacing) triple counting of the rate, which may trigger inappropriate therapies.

Various post-shock phenomena have been described, including loss of pacemaker capture while pacing artifacts still inhibit pacing by the ICD, resetting of the pacemaker by the delivered ICD shock, inhibition of redetection by pacemaker artifacts, and others.

Our approach to screening for ICD-pacemaker interactions has been published [1] and is beyond the scope of this review. In addition to testing, several measures to avoid inadvertent pacemaker – ICD interactions were used during implantation. They included the use of bipolar pacing leads, implanting ventricular leads of the pacemaker and ICD as far as possible and perpendicular to each other, and the use of pacemakers with no potential for resetting to unipolar configuration.   It is critical to note that most of the interactions can be avoided with utilization of meticulous testing protocols during implantation and follow-up [3-6].

The Present

Despite the decrease in implantation of concomitant systems, the issue of pacemaker – ICD interactions is still pertinent in several situations:

Many patients with previously implanted concomitant pacemakers - ICD systems are still being followed. The problems of pacemaker – ICD interactions have to be dealt with in these patients, as delineated in the previous section. Upon replacement, most will undergo ICD upgrading to a dual chamber ICD, and the pacemaker will be removed. The pacemaker atrial lead will be tunneled, if possible, to the ICD pocket and will serve as the atrial lead of the ICD, while the ventricular lead will either be abandoned or removed.

ICDs often have to be implanted in patients who already have old but well functioning pacemaker systems. This situation raises the dilemma of whether the old pacing system should be removed or abandoned prior to ICD implantation, or whether a new ICD system should be combined with the preexisting pacing system, and programmed so as to avoid interactions between them. This dilemma is probably most important in the presence of a very old (but well functioning) pacing system, the removal of which may impose significant difficulties and risks, as discussed below.

Patients with recently implanted "simple " ICDs (capable of VVI pacing only) which have several years of battery life remaining may develop AV block or sinus node dysfunction, requiring dual chamber or rate responsive pacing. In these cases, there may be a significant economic advantage to separate pacemaker implantation, as this may be much less expensive than upgrading the relatively new, preexisting ICD to a dual chamber ICD.

When facing a patient with a well functioning pacing system, who needs an ICD implantation, three options are available. The first is to implant an additional single chamber ICD system with continued use of the existing pacemaker while testing for interactions. The second option is to extract the preexisting pacemaker system and to implant a new dual chamber ICD system with complete pacing functionality. The third is to remove the old pulse generator, but abandon extant leads, and insert the new ICD.

Despite our experience with pacemaker – ICD interactions we tend to favor new dual chamber ICD systems over pacemaker – ICD combinations. This is especially true when the old atrial lead can be used for the atrial channel of the ICD and the old ventricular lead can be removed. However, removal of old leads may be technically difficult and associated with significant procedural risk, particularly with very mature systems.   However, recent advances in lead extraction are reducing procedural morbidity[7,8].

Abandonment of the old pacing leads is another option, which is usually feasible. However, the problem of leaving redundant leads with subsequent potential venous complications, as well as possible interference with the location and function of the new ICD leads should be weighed against the complexity and risks of lead extraction. Notably, when lead extraction is being considered, it should be carried out to completion, as partially removed leads may subsequently interfere with ICD function. We have seen a case of intractable electrical noise created by pacemaker lead that was severed and consequently irretrievable during attempted extraction in anticipation of an ICD implantation. The noise created by the damaged lead caused inappropriate tachycardia detection as well as inhibition of pacing, and an ICD could not be implanted. Others observed similar phenomena [9].

Therefore, when a patient with a pacemaker needs an ICD, we usually prefer to use the old atrial lead for the ICD if possible, extract or abandon the old ventricular lead, and implant a new dual chamber ICD. The choice between extraction and abandonment of old leads depends upon the estimated chances of successful complete removal, which depend on their implant duration as well as on local expertise and available tools. Only rarely will we choose to combine the old pacing system with a new ICD, and perform extensive testing during implantation to avoid interactions.

The patient with an existing recently implanted single chamber ICD system, who becomes pacemaker dependent and needs physiological pacing, presents another dilemma. The ideal approach is to upgrade such a patient to a dual chamber ICD system. However, given the costs of upgrading vs. pacemaker implantation and potential lack of reimbursement for yet another ICD, one may be forced to implant a concomitant pacemaker system to provide physiological pacing. Some manufacturers now provide financial credit for the preexisting system if a newer system with greater functionality from the same manufacturer is employed, diminishing the financial burden associated with this approach.

The Future

With recent advances in technology, we will see progressively fewer patients with concomitant pacemaker and ICD systems, and more patients with combined systems of dual chamber ICDs, sometimes with biventricular pacing capabilities. These systems present a new aspect of interactions – those between pacing/sensing and antiarrhythmia features in the same device. The understanding of pacemaker – ICD interactions gives us better insight into the function of complex future devices.

New Dual chamber ICDs, when used in patients who are pacemaker dependent or who have supraventricular arrhythmias, present a whole spectrum of actual and potential interactions between pacing and ICD mechanisms incorporated in the same device. The same applies to new systems with biventricular pacing capabilities. Following are some examples out of the many potential interactions:

The high sensitivity of the ventricular channel is sometimes the cause of pacing inhibition due to various noises, such as diaphragmatic myopotential sensing, which is not uncommon with certain ICD leads. Notably, the ventricular channel in an ICD may be ten times as sensitive as the similar channel in a regular pacemaker. This problem is especially pertinent in patients who have received their DDD® ICDs due to their pacemaker dependency. Whereas detection duration may prevent inappropriate therapy delivery with short-lasting noises, pacing inhibition of a few seconds may occur, which may result in symptomatic asystole, or may sometimes trigger ventricular arrhythmias.

Far field sensing of ventricular activity by the atrial channel is not uncommon. While this is usually a benign phenomenon in simple dual chamber pacemakers, it may have ominous consequences in dual chamber ICDs. These may include inhibition of ventricular VT therapies by false detection of simultaneous atrial tachyarrhythmias which is actually far field sensing, and, in cases of ICDs with atrial therapy capabilities, triggering of atrial therapies by the far field sensing superimposed on normal atrial electrical activity.

In cases of ICDs with biventricular pacing, there is a potential for double sensing of normal sinus beats. Sensing in these cases involves the two ventricular leads, which are positioned as far as possible from each other. Given the wide QRS of regular sinus beats, which is a prerequisite for most cases of biventricular pacing, double sensing may occur in sinus rhythm, which may cause inappropriate detection of VT, especially during sinus tachycardia. Oversensing may also occur if capture is lost on the left ventricular electrode, resulting in a very wide paced QRS complex, originating from the right ventricular electrode, then sensed by the left ventricular electrode.

The fact that the left ventricular lead is positioned in the coronary sinus, in the vicinity of the left atrium, creates a tendency for oversensing of atrial activity. This mechanism may result in inhibition of ventricular pacing by atrial activity, which may endanger dependent patients and in oversensing, leading to inappropriate ventricular arrhythmia detection.

Summary

Pacemaker – ICD interactions were very important when ICDs had no physiological pacing functions. Since the appearance of full feature DDD ICD system, the relevance of pacemaker – ICD interactions is limited to patients previously implanted with dual systems, as well as to patients with old pacemakers who need new ICD or vice versa. New devices are currently available with complex dual chamber and biventricular pacing – sensing algorithms. They present a whole new spectrum of interactions between their pacing/ sensing and their anti-arrhythmia functions.

REFERENCES

1. Glikson M, Trusty JM, Grice SK, et al. A stepwise testing protocol for modern implantable cardioverter-defibrillator systems to prevent pacemaker-implantable cardioverter- defibrillator interactions. *Am J Cardiol*. 1999;83:360-6.
2. Glikson M, Trusty JM, Grice SK, et al. Importance of pacemaker noise reversion as a potential mechanism of pacemaker-ICD interactions. *PACE* 1998;21:1111-21.
3. Brooks R, Garan H, McGovern BA, et al. Implantation of transvenous nonthoracotomy cardioverter-defibrillator systems in patients with permanent endocardial pacemakers. *Am Heart J* 1995;129:45-53.
4. Clemo HF, Ellenbogen KA, Belz MK, et al. Safety of pacemaker implantation in patients with transvenous (nonthoracotomy) implantable cardioverter defibrillators. *PACE* 1994;17:2285-91.
5. Geiger MJ, O'Neill P, Sharma A, et al. Interactions between transvenous nonthoracotomy cardioverter defibrillator systems and permanent transvenous endocardial pacemakers. *PACE*1997;20:624-30.
6. Epstein AE, Wilkoff BL. Pacemaker - defibrillator interactions. In: Ellenbogen KA, Kay GN, Wilkoff BL, eds. *Clinical cardiac pacing*. Philadelphia: W.B. Saunders; 1995:757-769.
7. Wilkoff BL, Byrd CL, Love CJ, et al. Pacemaker lead extraction with the laser sheath: results of the Pacing Lead Extraction with the Excimer Laser sheath (PLEXES) trial. *JACC*1999;33:1671-6.
8. Smith HJ, Fearnot NE, Byrd CL, et al. Five year experience with intravascular lead extraction. *PACE* 1994;17:2016-20.
9. Lickfett L, Wolpert C, Jung W, et al. Inappropriate implantable defibrillator discharge caused by a retained pacemaker lead fragment [In Process Citation]. *J Interv Card Electrophysiol*. 1999;3:163-7.

Part VI.

Sudden Death

32.
THE GENETICS OF SUDDEN DEATH

Dan M. Roden, M.D.

Professor of Medicine and Pharmacology, Vanderbilt University, Nashville, Tennessee, USA

Sudden death is a common problem, affecting 300,000-500,000 Americans each year. In most patients, underlying heart disease (usually coronary atherosclerosis) is present. Nevertheless, occasional patients with structurally normal hearts and sudden death have been identified, and recent molecular studies have begun to identify mutations in ion channel or structural cardiac genes that appear to account for sudden death in some of these cases. As this work has progressed, patients with such mutations but lacking any electrocardiographic or phenotype have been identified; whether such individuals are at increased risk for sudden death at baseline or during certain forms of stress (such as myocardial ischemia or drug challenge) is an area of active investigation. In addition, while specific mutations that predispose subjects to sudden death can be identified, common genetic polymorphisms may also eventually be added to traditional "risk factors" in evaluation of sudden death risk in large populations.

The Long QT Syndromes

Clinical Characteristics:
The typical features in the congenital long QT syndrome (LQTS) include QT prolongation, labile and morphologically bizarre TU complexes, syncope and sudden death - in the proband and in family members - due to Torsades de Pointes and ventricular fibrillation. Most cases are autosomal dominant or arise de novo (the Romano-Ward Syndrome). Occasional cases are transmitted in an apparently autosomal recessive fashion (the Jervell-Lange-Nielson Syndrome [JLN]); patients with JLN have congenital deafness, and a high incidence of syncope and sudden death in childhood. Although the disease is autosomal, events such as syncope and sudden death are commoner among women, particularly after puberty, and the period at the end of pregnancy and immediately post-partum is one of especially high risk for events. Spectacular advances have been made in the last five years in understanding the molecular genetic basis of the LQTS, and it is now

From Ovsyshcher IE. *Cardiac Arrythmias and Device Therapy: Results and Perspectives for the New Century.* Armonk, NY: Futura Publishing Company, Inc., © 2000

apparent that the "typical" clinical case probably represents a minority of individuals with LQTS mutations, and that the clinical presentation may be determined at least in part by the specific mutation present in a given patient.

Molecular Genetics:

The technique of genetic linkage has been used to identify loci in the genome at which mutations are associated with the disease. At least six such loci have been reported, and specific disease genes have been identified at five of these. All five LQTS disease genes encode proteins involved in the structure and normal function of ion channels, the protein complexes whose function underlie the ion currents that make up the cardiac action potential.

The commonest forms of LQTS are LQT1 and LQT2, caused by mutations in *KvLQT1* and *HERG*, respectively. *KvLQT1* encodes the major structural ion channel protein (the -subunit) responsible for the slowly-activating potassium current I_{Ks}, while *HERG* encodes the -subunit for the rapidly-activating potassium current I_{Kr}. LQT5 is caused by mutations in *minK*, an ancillary protein (-subunit) that co-assembles with *KvLQT1* (and possibly *HERG*) to modify function of I_{Ks} (and possibly I_{Kr}). LQT6 is caused by mutations in *MiRP1*; *MiRP1* co-assembles with *HERG* to modify I_{Kr} function. When the functional effects of mutations in any of these four genes are studied *in vitro*, a decrease in the encoded potassium currents (I_{Ks} and/or I_{Kr}) is observed. Since K^+ currents are outward (repolarizing), an increase in action potential duration results. Interpreting the effects of these mutations is complicated by the fact that potassium channel complexes are tetrameric; that is, they are composed of at least 4 -subunits (such as *KvLQT1* or *HERG*) as well as an unknown number of ancillary subunits, such as *minK* or *MiRP1*. In some cases, mutations can be shown not only to decrease current through homotetrameric channels (i.e. those composed entirely of mutant proteins), but also to disproportionately decrease current through heterotetrameric channels, composed of mutant and wild type proteins. This situation likely occurs *in vivo*, since most cases of LQTS are autosomal dominant, i.e. the patient inherits one set of abnormal alleles from an affected parent and another set of wild type (normal) of alleles from an unaffected parent. Regardless of whether such a "dominant negative" suppression of potassium current is present or not, multiple defects in potassium channel physiology, such as alterations in trafficking protein complexes to the cell surface or altered gating of protein complexes that arrive at the cell surface, have now been reported in various forms of potassium channel-associated LQTS.

The LQT3 variant is caused by mutations in *SCN5A*, the cardiac sodium channel gene. Here, unlike the situation with the potassium channel gene mutations (which decrease outward repolarizing currents), *SCN5A* mutations actually increase inward current through sodium channels during the plateau of the action potential. The result is similar to that with potassium channel mutations: an increase in net inward current during the plateau, and hence action potential prolongation. Another difference is that the sodium channel protein is approximately four times larger than individual potassium channel proteins, and expression of a single sodium channel gene gives rise to the sodium channel; thus, no dominant negative effects are postulated in LQT3.

The typical clinical features of LQTS are now being reinterpreted in a contemporary molecular genetic context. These analyses have focused on LQT1, LQT2, and LQT3, as they constitute the vast majority of cases, and only a handful of cases of LQT4 (where no disease gene has yet been found), LQT5, and LQT6, have been identified. Patients with LQT1 mutations tend to have broad -based TU complexes, and do not shorten their QT interval with exercise. Syncopal events occur with emotional or physical stress. In LQT2, the typical ECG morphology is a flat or bifid TU complex. QT intervals shorten near-normally with exercise. Syncope in LQT2 occurs either with stress or at rest, and syncope with an auditory stimulus (e.g. an alarm clock going off) is highly suggestive of LQT2. Patients with LQT3 have a long isoelectric ST segment with peaked T waves. QT intervals shorten supra-normally with exercise, and syncopal events and/or sudden death occur almost exclusively at rest or at night. In one study from the large International Long QT Registry, 68% of patients with *KvLQT1* mutations had "events" (syncope or sudden death) by age 40, compared to 54% of those with *HERG* mutations, and only 22% of those with *SCN5A* mutations.

JLN arises when a child inherits an abnormal *KvLQT1* or *minK* allele from each parent. The "double-dose" of abnormal I_{Ks} genes explains why these subjects have marked QT prolongation. Expression of *KvLQT1* and *minK* is also important for normal endolymph homeostasis in the inner ear, and thus absence of functional I_{Ks} channels likely underlies the deafness observed in these patients. Importantly, although JLN parents have been described as normal, they do in fact have mutations in LQTS disease genes.

One of the most intriguing findings to emerge from evaluation of the molecular genetics of LQTS is the identification of subjects who carry the mutations and yet who appear to have normal electrocardiograms. Parents of children with JLN are one example, as described above, and sudden death occurring under emotional stress in a JLN parent has now been reported. A second example are asymptomatic and phenotypically normal relatives of patients with manifest LQTS who nevertheless carry mutations, i.e. the phenomenon of "incomplete penetrance" of the phenotype. A third example are some patients with drug-associated Torsades de Pointes. The apparently unpredictable nature of the drug-associated arrhythmia has lead some to speculate that some patients may be susceptible because of sub-clinical mutations in LQTS disease genes. Indeed, occasional examples of this phenomenon have now been reported. For example, a mutation of the arginine at position 555 in the C-terminus of *KvLQT1* to cysteine appears to confer little QT prolongation but a susceptibility to drug-associated LQTS. Similarly, a common polymorphism in the *minK* gene, which results in an asparagine instead of aspartate at position 85 in the C-terminus, appears over-represented among patients with drug-associated LQTS, and may therefore be a risk factor. Finally, *MiRP1* mutations have been proposed as risk factors for the drug-associated form of a syndrome. Overall, mutations such as these have been identified in only a small minority of patients with LQTS, and the state-of-the-art is not yet advanced sufficiently to allow routine genetic screening to identify susceptible patients prior to drug exposure.

Arrhythmia Mechanisms in LQTS:

While the molecular lesions outlined above are sufficient to explain QT prolongation, they cannot, themselves, explain the development of arrhythmias. Rather, a consensus view is that action potential prolongation sets in motion other alterations in cellular homeostasis that are themselves directly arrhythmogenic. These alterations, occurring through genetically-normal and drug-unmodified mechanisms, may include increased inward current through L-type calcium channels and/or sodium-calcium exchange, as well as intracellular calcium overload. These mechanisms, in turn, cause two important changes that underlie Torsades de Pointes. The first is the development of early (and conceivably in some cases delayed) afterdepolarizations, the proximate triggers for Torsades de Pointes. The second is increased dispersion of action potential durations, which forms the substrate for intramural re-entry, which is thought to be the mechanism whereby Torsades de Pointes is sustained. It is conceivable that similar mechanisms underlie arrhythmias in other situations in which intracellular calcium homeostasis is impaired, such as congestive heart failure.

Implications of a Modern Understanding of LQTS for Therapy:

The "standard" therapy for LQTS is anti-adrenergic interventions, usually beta-blockade. One current explanation for this efficacy is that the commonest mutations are in *KvLQT1*, and that a contributor in this situations is increased inward current through L-type calcium channels. It seems likely that beta-blockers and similar interventions are so effective because L-type calcium channels can be activated by -stimulation (and suppressed by -blockade). On the other hand, whether anti-adrenergic interventions will be as effective in rarer forms of LQTS is not so clear. One argument is that increased inward current through L-type calcium channels is a common underlying mechanism (regardless of the mutation) and therefore beta-blockade will be effective. On the other hand, *in vitro* and clinical studies both suggest that sodium channel blockade with drugs such as mexiletine or flecainide maybe especially effective in reducing inward current through mutant sodium channels in LQT3; whether this is more desirable than beta-blockade is not known. In patients in whom bradycardia, or bradycardia-dependent onset of arrhythmias is known or strongly suspected, pacing can be useful in conjunction with beta-blockade. The role of the ICD in LQTS is evolving. One view is that patients with LQTS in whom syncope or cardiac arrest recurs are candidates for ICDs, while another view is that, because while a first event may be a cardiac arrest in some patients (the proportion is not yet known), ICDs should evolve to first line therapy in this disease. Finally, both in LQTS as well as in the other syndromes described below, increasing availability of genetic testing has identified asymptomatic individuals who nevertheless carry these or other mutations. Whether such individuals should be treated, and how, is not known, although a consensus in favor in at least beta-blockade is emerging.

The Brugada Syndrome

In the late 1980's and early 1990's, rare individuals with distinctive J-point elevation in the right precordial leads, a right bundle branch block-like appearance on ECG, and idiopathic ventricular fibrillation (VF) were recognized by Brugada and Brugada, and others. This entity appears to underlie a relatively high incidence of sudden death (often occurring at night) in young men in the Far East. In other populations, the gender distribution is more balanced. Some patients display the abnormal electrocardiogram at all times, whereas in others it is intermittent, and can be provoked by administration of sodium channel blocking drugs or beta-blockers.

Since sodium channel block exacerbates the syndrome, the cardiac channel gene *SCN5A* became a "candidate" for the Brugada syndrome. Indeed, *SCN5A* mutations in patients with the Brugada syndrome have now been identified. The mechanisms whereby the mutations actually cause the electrocardiographic pattern, and ventricular fibrillation, are not yet well understood. The mutations probably result in decreased I_{Na}, unlike those causing LQTS. At least one large kindred in which the Brugada phenotype is not linked to the sodium channel gene has now been described (i.e., as in LQTS, mutations in multiple genes will likely be found to cause the Brugada phenotype). *In vitro* studies suggest that sodium channel block results in loss of the typical "spike and dome" configuration of the epicardial action potential, resulting in a markedly abbreviated action potential duration. The endocardium seems relatively immune to these changes, so the presence of sodium channel block can set up marked heterogeneity of repolarization times in the right ventricular epicardium, likely leading to re-entrant excitation that underlies VF. Interestingly, similar changes are observed with myocardial ischemia, raising the possibility that the combination of sodium channel block plus ischemia might lead to a very high incidence of ventricular fibrillation (perhaps accounting for the result of the Cardiac Arrhythmia Suppression Trial).

No effective therapies to prevent VF in patients with the Brugada syndrome have yet been identified. In patients with the manifest syndrome, the ICD has been used. As in LQTS, the management of asymptomatic family members identified by molecular genetic testing to have mutations remains uncertain.

Genetically Determined Cardiomyopathies Associated With Sudden Death

The best studied disease in this group of these is hypertrophic cardiomyopathy (HCM). The clinical characteristics of HCM vary widely among subjects, and increasingly are recognized to arise in part from the fact that mutations arise in different genes. Just as LQTS is a disease of the action potential, HCM is a disease of the contractile apparatus, with mutations in the -myosin heavy chain being the commonest. Mutations with particularly "malignant" clinical courses have been described. The most widely-recognized of these is the -myosin heavy chain R403G mutation, in which 50% of individuals have died suddenly by age 50. Another is troponin T mutations, which appear to be associated with an especially high incidence of sudden death prior to age 30 in men. A disturbing feature of the troponin T mutations is that hypertrophy may be relatively mild, so the echocardiogram may be near-normal.

The mechanisms whereby disruption of the contractile apparatus causes hypertrophy are unknown, as are the mechanisms whereby patients with HCM are especially susceptible to VF. One possibility is that the hypertrophic ventricle is susceptible to myocardial ischemia, particularly during rapid supraventricular tachycardias to which these patients are subject. Another possibility is that the myocardial fibrillar disarray typically seen on histopathological examination forms the substrate for re-entrant excitation.

In addition to HCM, many other inherited cardiac diseases associated with myocardial dysfunction and various forms of conduction system disease and/or death due to ventricular arrhythmias are now being reported. Examples include dilated cardiomyopathies including those associated with muscular dystrophy and (increasingly recognized to be attributable to mutations in the cytoskeleton), mitochondrial cardiomyopathies. It seems likely that as our understanding of these genetic basis of these syndromes, and how mutations directly or indirectly alter the electrophysiology of the heart in these situations, rational forms of risk stratification and therapy may evolve.

Summary

The last five years has seen dramatic advances in our understanding of the molecular genetics of cardiovascular disease. One important consequence of this new understanding is the identification of specific syndromes that appear to confer a high risk for sudden death, often in the absence of other manifestations of heart disease. Examples include troponin T mutations, patients with the Brugada syndrome, and certain patients with the long QT syndromes. Whereas mutations are defined as rare, function-altering genetic changes, it is also increasingly appreciated that DNA polymorphisms are relatively common and may contribute to interindividual variability in physiology and its response to external stimuli. Interestingly, analysis of the large Seattle out-of-hospital resuscitation experience has identified a family member with an out-of-hospital cardiac arrest as a risk factor. Whether the Seattle data represent the sorts of mutations described above, mutations in other genes regulating cardiac electrophysiology, or a cumulative effect of multiple common polymorphisms, remains to be determined. The imminent availability of the first draft of the human genome will therefore represent a crucial starting point for further work to identify the way in which variations in the genome influence risk for sudden death.

33.

PATHOLOGY OF THE CONDUCTION SYSTEM IN SUDDEN DEATH IN THE YOUNG, ATHLETES AND HEALTHY

Saroja Bharati, M. D.

Maurice Lev Congenital Heart and Conduction System Center, The Heart Institute for Children, Hope Children's Hospital, Christ Hospital and Medical Center, Oak Lawn, IL, University of Illinois at Chicago and Rush Medical College, Chicago, IL

Introduction

Sudden death does occur in the young, athletes and healthy with or without a previous history of arrhythmias.[1-8] In order to understand the pathologic findings in the conduction system, it is understood that a thorough examination of the heart, both at the gross and light microscopy level, including toxicological examinations, have ruled out the possible causes of sudden death. Despite a very careful analysis of the heart, if the cause of death could not be determined, it is then assumed that the sudden death is due to arrhythmias.[1-8] It is our opinion that the conduction system in the above hearts may shed some light as to the possible cause for arrhythmias. The study of the conduction system is therefore mandatory in these individuals. However, it is to be noted that the method of study of the conduction system is equally important in order to derive useful information.

Method of Study of the Conduction System–Light Microscopy–

Since the conduction system in a broad sense comprises the entire heart, it is important that one examines at least every 20th or 30th section by serial section examination from the beginning to the end and compare the findings with a similar age matched controlled conduction system. Furthermore, the specialized myocardial fibers of the conduction system is located in strategic parts of the heart in the form of an arc or a curve. The various parts of the specialized myocardium cannot be identified by random single sections. Therefore, a meaningful semi quantitative examination of the conduction system may be obtained by the above described manner.[5, 7]

Findings in the Conduction System

An examination of the conduction system studied in the above described manner, in more than 150 young, healthy, people, including athletes, revealed varying types of congenital anomalies as well as acquired pathology.[1-8] The congenital abnormalities included abnormally formed sinoatrial (SA) node, atrioventricular (AV) node (fig 1) and AV bundle. In addition, there were

From Ovsyshcher IE. *Cardiac Arrythmias and Device Therapy: Results and Perspectives for the New Century.* Armonk, NY: Futura Publishing Company, Inc., © 2000

abnormalities in the formation of the central fibrous body, the atrioventricular part of the membranous septum, the coronary sinus, the tricuspid, and the mitral valves. The acquired changes included frequent association of mononuclear cell infiltration in the SA node and its approaches, fibrosis and fat to a varying extent in all parts of the conduction system, and focal fibrotic scars in the ventricular septum (fig 2) with or without fat and occasional mononuclear cells.[1-8]

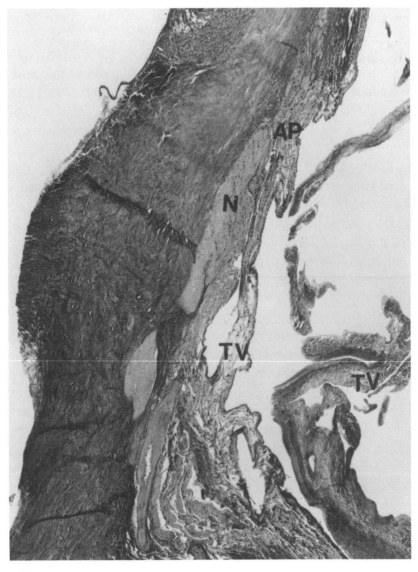

Figure 1
Photomicrograph of AV node (N) and its approaches (A) demonstrates the AV node within the tricuspid valve (TV) anulus in a 34 year old athletically

trained bicyclist who collapsed suddenly while bicycling in preparation for races. Paramedics found him in coarse ventricular fibrillation. Weigert van Geison stain X17.

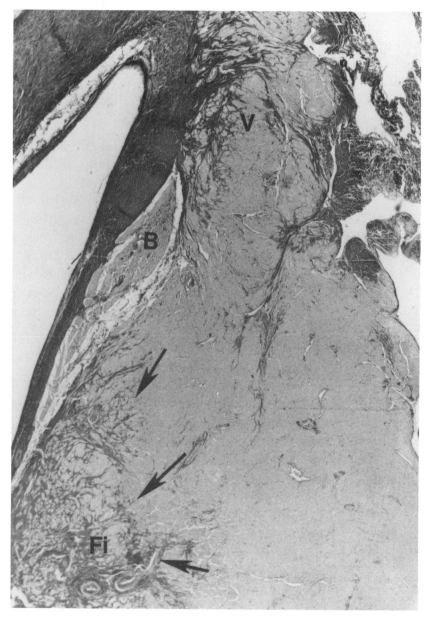

Figure 2
Photomicrograph of a left sided branching bundle (B) with marked fibrosis (Fi) in the left side of the ventricular septum (V) in a 14 year old athletic boy who complained of chest pain while playing soccer, then collapsed and died suddenly. Weigert van Geison stain x 22.5

(Fig 1 and 2 with permission from Bharati, S, Lev, M. The Cardiac Conduction System in unexplained sudden death. Futura Publishing Co., Mt. Kisco, NY 1990, 1-416.)

Is There A Difference in the Pathological Findings Between the Athletes and the Otherwise Healthy Youngsters?

The examination of the conduction system in sudden death in more than 150 hearts suggests that there are no significant differences in the findings of the conduction system between the otherwise healthy and/or an athlete or an athletically trained individuals.[1-8]

Athletes, Athletically Trained Individuals and the Young, Healthy With Known Arrhythmias or Other Known Diseases

Is there a difference in pathology in athletically trained individuals, athletes and other healthy non athletes with known arrhythmias and/or diseases? In order to answer this question, we compared the findings of the conduction system of athletes, athletically trained individuals and other youngsters with a history of known arrhythmias and/or other diseases with those without arrhythmias who died suddenly. There were significant pathologic changes in the conduction system and the surrounding myocardium in the group with known arrhythmias than in the group without a history of known diseases and or arrhythmias.[1-8]

Sudden death in Alaskan Sled Dogs

Sudden death also occurs in Alaskan sled dogs during the Iditarod Race or during the training period. We studied the conduction system of these animals and compared the findings with the findings in the human athletes who died suddenly to see if the findings were similar and if there were differences, what part of the conduction system was vulnerable in both.[1-10]

The Conduction System in Sudden Death in Alaskan Sled Dogs During the Iditarod Race and/or During Training

The conduction system in sled dogs revealed considerable amount of fibrosis in the SA node and/or its approaches, narrowing of the SA nodal artery, marked fatty infiltration and fibrosis in and around the AV node in all, with almost isolation of the AV node from its surrounding approaches in some, fat and fibrosis in the AV bundle and bundle branches to a varying degree, with focal fibrotic scars in the left ventricle with fat and some myocardial disarray.[9]

Is There A Difference Between The Pathological Findings in Sudden Death in Human Athletes versus Sudden Death in Alaskan Sled Dogs

The acquired pathological findings in both the human and the sled dog appear to be more or less similar, but not identical. The fatty infiltration in the AV junction including the AV node and its approaches seem to be more affected in the sled dog than the human. However, the Alaskan sled dogs did not reveal any congenital anomalies of the conduction system.[1-10]

The Acquired Changes in the Heart of Athletes and Their Significance

The frequent association of mononuclear cell infiltration in and around the SA node and elsewhere in the myocardium and focal fibrosis in the myocardium especially in the ventricular septum, and the fibro fatty changes in the conduction system. might have played a role in sudden death of the athletes. However, the mononuclear cell infiltration is not sufficient to call it a myocarditis. Although the findings are not significant enough to call it a myocarditis, they cannot be ignored and will require further research. Could this, however, represent a peculiar type of a myocarditis and/or an auto-immune reaction to some foreign material? The fibrotic scars in the ventricular septum, fat and focal myocardial disarray may be related in part to the aging process and/or to hypertrophy of the ventricular mass. Or, the above acquired pathologic changes may indeed be related to chronic ischemic episodes of a hypertrophied left ventricle. Or is it conceivable that the arrhythmias might have been present and the athletes were "asymptomatic" and were not able to appreciate the arrhythmias and that the arrhythmias might have produced the focal scars in the ventricular myocardium? The significance of long term effects of silent arrhythmias on the myocardium is not known today. At the moment it is not clear how these acquired pathological changes occurred in the athletes' heart.[1-10]

Assumed Patho–Physiology of Sudden Death in the Young, Athletes and Healthy

It is obvious that the findings in the conduction system were present in the young, athletes and healthy. for a considerable period of time. The question then arises is, why then does death occur <u>suddenly</u> in these young people. We hypothesize that the congenital and/or acquired pathological changes in and around the conduction system may remain silent during one's life and indeed may permit a "normal life" for a long period of time. However, during an altered physiologic state, the acquired pathological findings in and around the conduction system and/or the congenitally abnormally formed conduction system may become vulnerable and promote or stimulate a re-entry mechanism or an abnormal automaticity or fractionization of an impulse or some other unknown mechanism to induce an arrhythmic event. For example: slowing of impulse conduction may occur in the congenitally abnormally formed conduction system and/or the acquired pathological sites with the healthy myocardium that may trigger a ventricular premature contraction during an altered physiological state. The ventricular premature contractions may degenerate into ventricular tachycardia, fibrillation and sudden death. Further, there may be a tendency for sudden death to occur in a genetically, abnormally formed conduction system.[1-8]

It is emphasized that this is a very brief discussion of the findings in the conduction system and the surrounding myocardium in cases of sudden death in the young, athletes and healthy and the interested reader is therefore encouraged to read the original works described in this chapter for further details.

References

1. Bharati S, Lev M, Bauernfeind R, et al.: Sudden death in three teenagers: Conduction system studies. J Am Coll Cardiol 1983; 1:879-886.
2. Bharati S, Lev M: Congenital abnormalities of the conduction system in sudden death in young adults. J Am Coll Cardiol 1986; 8:1096-1104.
3. Bharati S, Lev M, Dreifus LS, et al.: Conduction system in a trained jogger with sudden death. Chest 1988; 93:348-351,.
4. Brookfield L, Bharati S, Denes P, et al: Familial Sudden Death: Report of a Case and Review of the Literature. Chest 1988; 94:989-993.
5. Bharati S and Lev M: The cardiac conduction system in unexplained sudden death. Armonk, NY, Futura Publishing Co, 1990; 1:416.
6. Bharati S, Lev M: The conduction system findings in sudden cardiac death. J of Cardiovasc Electrophysiology 1994; 5:356-366.
7. Bharati S, Lev M: Sudden death in athletes - conduction system: practical approach to dissection and pertinent pathology. Cardiovascular Pathology 1994; 3:117-127.
8. Bharati S, Lev M: Role of Specialized Conduction System Abnormalities in Sudden Cardiac Death. Akhtar, M, Myerberg, J., Ruskin, JN (ed): In Sudden Cardiac Death, Andover Medical Publishers, Inc.,1994; pp. 274-289.
9. Bharati S, Cantor GH, Leach JB III, et al.: The conduction system in sudden death in Alaskan sled dogs during the Iditarod race and/or during training. PACE, 1997; 20:654-663.
10. Bharati S: The Cardiac Conduction System in Sudden Death in Athletes NAM Estes III, Salem, DN, Wang, PJ.(ed): In Sudden Cardiac Death in the Athlete, Armonk, NY, Futura Publishing Co, 1998; pp. 483-514.

34.
SUDDEN CARDIAC DEATH IN THE YOUNG: GENETIC ASPECTS
Melvin M. Scheinman, M.D.

Cardiac Electrophysiology Service, Cardiology Division, University of California, San Francisco, San Francisco, CA

It is estimated that approximately 300,000 Americans die suddenly. Of these deaths, approximately 10% occur in patients without significant structural cardiac disease. The bulk of these patients would appear to be those with the long QT syndrome, Brugada's syndrome or, more rarely, catecholeminergic polymorphic ventricular tachycardia or short-coupled torsade. This is emerging evidence that most of these conditions are related to genetic abnormalities. Other genetically linked causes of sudden death associatedwith structural disease include those with hypertrophic myopathy, right ventricular dysplasia and familial cardiomyopathy. The purpose of this essay to review the various genetically determined cardiac abnormalities associated with cardiac death. The long QT syndrome has been discussed separately.

Arrhythmogenic Right Ventricular Dysplasia (ARVD)
ARVD is a disease entity first described by Dr. Fontaine,[1,2] as an entity comprising malignant ventricular arrhythmias appearing to arise from the right ventricle. In a study from Northern Italy, 20% of 60 patients with sudden death under age 35 had ARVD[3]. The anatomic features of this disease have been reported by Lobo et al [4] and Boffa et al[5]. The findings include fatty tissue replacement of the right ventricular myocardium or marked thinning of the myocardium. The locations of the abnormalities appear to be restricted to the free wall of the right ventricle which has been coined the "triangle of the dysplasia"[2]. Other features include dilation of the right ventricle, focal right ventricular aneurysm, and/or areas of mononuclear infiltrates.

Patients with ARVD present with palpitations due to either ventricular ectopics or sustained left bundle branch block type ventricular tachycardia. The symptoms are often exercise-induced and there is a 4:1 male predominance. The ECG may be very helpful in diagnosis, usually showing a pattern of inverted T waves in V_1-V_3, additional findings include an epsilon wave (a slight defection following the QRS) or a right

From Ovsyshcher IE. *Cardiac Arrythmias and Device Therapy: Results and Perspectives for the New Century.* Armonk, NY: Futura Publishing Company, Inc., © 2000

bundle branch block pattern. In addition, abnormal signal averaged ECG may be recorded[6] but the specificity of this finding is not known.

The diagnosis rests on finding evidence for structural right ventricular disease. Unfortunately, apart from the postmortem examination, no gold standard is available for firm diagnosis. It is oftentimes difficult to discern minor abnormalities in the normally heavily trabeculated right ventricle. Similarly, there are no generally agreed standards for right ventricular enlargement by echocardiography. Suggested criteria include a right ventricular/left ventricular end-diastolic diameter >0.5 or using radioscintigraphy, a right ventricular/left ventricular end-diastolic volume ration 71.8 or right ventricular exercise ejection fraction of <50%7. Other non-invasive tests include magnetic resonance imaging (MRI). Since epicardial fat is a normal finding, the cardiac MRI cannot be interpreted as being abnormal except if there are areas of full thickness fat or areas of marked thinning of the right ventricular wall. An invasive electrophysiology study is only of value if inducible sustained ventricular tachycardia is initiated.

Genetics

Sporadic reports of familial right ventricular dysplasia have been reported in the past[2,8]. In an extended study by Nava et al[9], who studied 72 members of 9 families and found that the disorder was inherited as an autosomal dominant with variable penetrance. This group described twins with this disorder and were the first to localize the abnormal gene on chromosome 14q23-24. Subsequently, a number of abnormal genes have been located on 5 different chromosomes (see Table 1)[10,11].

Treatment

A recent report by Wichter et al[12] suggests that sotalol may be effective but recurrences of 10% were reported over a 34 month follow-up. Others prefer use of amiodarone alone or in combination with other drugs have been reported. Multiple groups have reported success with catheter ablation of the right ventricular focus but, unfortunately, other ventricular tachycardia foci may appear with time[13]. Patients with recurrent ventricular tachycardia (or ventricular fibrillation) refractory to drug therapy should be treated with a defibrillator.

Brugada's Syndrome
Diagnosis
The hallmark of diagnosis is the typical ECG changes seen in the early precordial leads. These are characterized in V_1-V_5 with an elevated terminal QRS deflection (or J wave) followed by a downsloping ST segment with negative T wave[14]. The ECG abnormality is not entirely specific and may be mimicked by ischemia, drugs (tricyclic agents), electrolyte or metabolic disorder[15,16], Table 2. It may be very difficult or impossible to distinguish Brugada's syndrome from right ventricular dysplasia[17] since these ECG abnormalities have been described in patients with fibrofatty replacement of the right ventricular musculature. Hence, imagining techniques are often required to differentiate the two entities.

Presentation
Patients with Brugada's syndrome usually present with palpitations, syncope, seizures, or sudden cardiac death. The prevalence appears to be especially high among Asian males. Nademanee et al[18] found this ECG pattern in 17 of 27 victims of either aborted sudden death or syncope. All were young males with a history of sudden cardiac death.

Genetics and Pathogenesis of Brugada's Syndrome
The first gene to be linked to the Brugada's syndrome was described by Chen et al[19] and was found to be the sodium channel gene SCN5A which is also the gene responsible for one form of the long QT syndrome. The SCN5A mutation differs from that described in LQT3 and are associated with either an accelerated recovery of the Na^+ channel or non-functional Na^+ channels.

ST segmental elevation akin to that observed for patients is a normal characteristic of some of the rodents. This finding is due to outward gradients owing to strong I_{to} currents in the epicardial cells. Normally, the action potential plateau is due to strong inward Ca^{++} currents. If these currents are overwhelmed by I_{to}, then the epicardial cells will show loss of the dome and show an abbreviated action potential duration. Potential differences between mid-myocardial and epicardial lead to an unbalanced current explaining the ST elevation while marked differences in cellular action potential can lead to propagated responses (phase 2 reentry) and ultimately to ventricular fibrillation[20].

Diagnostic Considerations

It has been amply documented that the characteristic ECG pattern may wax and wane. Drugs that tend to accentuate the abnormal pattern include potent Na^+ channel blockers (i.e., flecainide, Ajmaline), alpha agonists or beta blockers. Drugs that tend to abolish the pattern include quinidine, disopyramide and beta agonists. Use of these drugs may be helpful in diagnosing difficult case[21]. In addition, imaging is required to exclude structural cardiac disease and electrophysiologic studies may show prolongation of the H-V interval or inducible ventricular arrhythmias.

Treatment

No prospective treatment studies are available but available data suggest efficacy of the internal defibrillator[22]. Since drugs which also block Ito current tend to normalize the ECG, it is conceivable that such drugs may be effective for long-term chronic therapy. Treatment of asymptomatic individuals remain a problem. In such individuals, inducibility of malignant arrhythmias would suggest need for a defibrillator.

Catecholeminergic Polymorphic Ventricular Tachycardia and Short Coupled Torsade

Coumel and colleagues described patients with recurrent episodes of polymorphous ventricular tachycardia associated with either enhanced sympathetic tone or in those with short coupled PVCs[23]. These patients may have a familial history but to date, the precise chromosomal abnormality has not been defined.

Hypertrophic Cardiomyopathy

A full explanation of the genetic basis of hypertrophic cardiomyopathy is beyond the scope of the present effort and the reader is referred to several excellent recent reviews[24,25]. In brief, hypertrophic cardiomyopathy is characterized by inappropriately large left ventricular mass, predominantly in the septum. The overall prevalence of this disease appears to be 1:1,000. Recent studies suggest an annual mortality due to sudden cardiac death of approximately 1%/year and appears to be higher in younger patients. Reports from the United States have identified hypertrophic cardiomyopathy as the most common cause of sudden death in athletes, accounting for almost 50% of sudden death in competitive athletes <35 years of age[26].

Predictors of Sudden Cardiac Death

Left ventricular mass as a predictor of sudden death remains controversial while symptoms of chest pain, magnitude of left ventricular outflow gradient or left ventricular and diastolic pressure are not reliable predictors of sudden death[25,26]. More reliable predictors of sudden death appear to be a positive family history, history of syncope, younger age, history of non-sustained ventricular tachycardia on Holter or history of prior sudden cardiac death[27,28].

Molecular Basic for Hypertrophic Cardiomyopathy

Clark et al[29] and van Dorp et al[30] using echocardiography found that hypertrophic cardiomyopathy was inherited in an autosomal dominant pattern with high penetrance. In more recent years, a large variety of abnormal genes responsible for mutations in the sarcomeric proteins have been found. The most common disorder being in the encoding of beta myosin heavy chain (BM4HC), cardiac troponin T (cTnT or I, and tropomysin, myosin binding protein C and myosin light chain. Genotype-phenotype interactive studies have shown a strong influence on specific genetic abnormalities and the potential for malignant events, Table 3. While the described genetic abnormalities help explain the structural changes noted, no clear-cut linkage between sarcomeric protein abnormalities and sudden death has emerged.

References

1.   Fontaine G, Guiraudon G, Frank R, et al: Stimulation studies and epicardial mapping in VT: Study of mechanisms and selction for surgery. In HE Kulbertus (ed): Reentrant Arrhythmias. Lancaster, PA, MTP Publishers, 1977, pp 334-350.
2.   Marcus FI, Fontaine G, Guiraudon G, et al: Right ventricular dysplasia: A report of 24 cases. Circulation 1982;65:384-399.
3.   Thiene G, Nava A, Corrado D, et al: Right ventricular cardiomyopathy and sudden death in young people. N Engl J Med 1988;318:129-133.
4.   Lobo FV, Heggtveit HA, Butany J, et al: Right ventriculardysplasia: Morphological findings in 13 cases. Can J Cardiol 1992;8:261-268.

5.   Boffa GM, Thiene G. Nava A, et al: Cardiomyopathy: A necessary revision of the WHO classification. Int J Cardiol1991;30:1-7.

6.   Blomstrom-LundqvistC,HirschI, Olsson SB: Quantitative analysis of thesignal-averaged QRSin patients with arrhythmogenic right ventricular dysplasia. Euro Heart J 1988;9:301-312.

7.   Manyari DE, Duff HJ, Kostuk WJ, et al: Usefulness of noninvasive studies for diagnosis of right ventricular dysplasia. Am J Cardiol 1986;57:1147-1153.

8.   KirschLR, Weinstock DJ, Magid MS, et al: Treatment of presumed arrhythmogenic right ventricular dysplasiainan adolescent. Chest 1993;104:298-300.

9.   Nava A, Thiene G., Canciani B, et al: Familial occurrence of right ventricular dysplasia: A study involving nine families. J Am Coll Cardiol 1988;12:1222-1228.

10.   Ahmad F, Li D, Karibe A, et al: Localization of a gene responsible for arrhythmogenicright ventricular dysplasia to chromosome 3p23. Circulation 1998:98:2791-2795.

11.   Rampazzo A, Nava A, Danieli GA, et al: The gene for arrhythmogenic right ventricular cardiomyopathy maps to chromosone 14q 23-q24. Hum Mol Genet 1994;3:959-962.

12.   Wichter T, BorggrefeM, Haverkamp W, et al: Efficacy of antiarrhythmic drugs in patients with arrhythmogenic right ventricular disease. Results in patients with inducible and noninducibleventricular tachycardia. Circulation 1992;86:29-37.

13.   Shoda M, Kasanuki H, Ohnishi S, et al: Recurrence of new ventricular tachycardia after successful catheter ablation in patients with arrhythmogenic right ventricular dysplasia. (abstract) Circulation 1992;86:(Suppl 1):580.

14.   Brugada P, Brugada J: A distinct clinical and electrocardiographic syndrome: right bundle-branch block, persistent ST segment elevation with normal QT interval and sudden cardiac death (abstract)PACE 1991;4:746.

15.   Scheinman MM. Is Brugada syndrome a distinct clinical entity? JCardiovasc Electrophysiol 1997;8:332336.

16.   Gussack I, Antzelevitch C, Bjerregaard P, et al: The Brugada syndrome: clinical, electrophysiologic and genetic aspects. J Am Coll Cardiol 1999;33:5-15.

17.   Martini B, Nava A, Cancinani B, Thiene G: Right bundle branch block, persistent ST segment elevation and sudden cardiac death (letter). J Am Coll Cardiol 1993;22:633.

18.   Nademanee K, Veerakul G, Nimmannit S, et al: Arrhythmogenic marker for the sudden unexplained death syndrome in Thai men. Circulation 1997;96:2595-2600.

19. Chen Q, Kirsch GE, Zhang D, et al. Genetic basis and molecular mechanisms for idiopathic ventricular fibrillation. Nature 1998;392:293-345.

20. Lukas A, Antzelevitch C: Phase 2 reentry as a mechanism of iinitiation of circus movement reentry in canine epicardium exposed to simulated ischemia. The antiarrhythmic effects of 4-aminopyridine. Cardiovasc Res 1996;32:593-603.

21. Antzelevitch C. The Brugada syndrome. J Cardiovasc Electrophysiol 1998;9:513-516.

22. Brugada J, Brugada R, Brugada P: Right bundle-branch block and ST segment elevation in leads V_1 through V_3. A marker for sudden death in patients without demonstrable structural heart disease. Circulation 1998;97:457-460.

23. CoumelP, Leclercq JF, Lucet V: Possible mechanisms of the arrhythmias in the long QT syndrome. Eur Heart J 1985;6(suppl D):115-129.

24. Marian AJ, Roberts R: Molecular genetic basis of hypertrophic cardiomyopathy: Genetic markers for sudden cardiac death. J Cardiovasc Electrophysiol1998;9:88-99.

25. Marian AJ: Sudden cardiac death in patients with hypertrophic cardiomyopathy: from bench to bedside with an emphasis of genetic markers. Clin Cardiol 1995;18(4):189-198.

26. Maron BJ, Epstein SE, Roberts WC: Causesof sudden death in competitive athletes. J Am Coll Cardiol 1986;7:204-214.

27. Maron BJ, Roberts WC, Edwards JE, et al: Sudden death in patients with hypertrophic cardiomyopathy: Characterization of 26 patients without functional limitation. Am J Cardiol 1978;41:803-810.

28. McKenna W, Deanfield J,Farugui A, et al: Prognosisin hypertrophic cardiomyopathyP: Role of age and clinical electrocardiographic and hemodynamic features. Am J Cardiol1981;47:532-538.

29. Clark CE, Henry WL, Epstein SE: Familial prevalence and genetic transmission of idiopathic hypertrophic subaortic stenosis. N Engl J Med 1973;289:709-714.

30. van Dorp WG,Ten Cate FJ, Vletter WB, et al: Familial prevalence of asymmetric septal hypertrophy. Eur J Cardiol 1976;4:349-357.

Table 1.   Abnormal Chromosomes Identified for Arrhythmogenic Right Ventricular Dysplasia

1q42
1q12
14a23
2q32
3p23

Table 2.   Abnormalities That Can Lead to ST Segment Elevation in the Right Precordial Leads

Right or left bundle branch block, left ventricular hypertrophy (66,108)
Acute myocardial infarction (109
Left ventricular aneurysm (109)
Exercise test-induced (110)
Acute myocarditis (111)
Right ventricular infarction (112)
Dissecting aortic aneurysm (113)
Acute pulmonary thromboemboli (114)
Various central and autonomic nervous system abnormalities (115,116)
Heterocyclic antidepressant overdose (117)
Duchenne muscular dystrophy (118)
Friedreich ataxia (119)
Thiamine deficiency(120)
Hypercalcemia (121)
Hyperkalemia (108,122)
Cocaine intoxication (124
Compression of the right ventricular outflow tract by metastatic tumor (123)

Modified from Gussak et al, JACC 1999; 33:8[16].

Table 3. Cardiomyopathy Mutations

Gene	Mutation		
	Benign	Intermediary	Malignant
βHC	Leu^{908}Val	Arg^{249}Gln	Arg^{403}Gln
	Val^{606}Met	Glu^{930}Lys	Arg^{719}Trp
	Gly^{256}Glu	--	Arg^{453}Cys
cTnT	--	--	Arg^{92}Gln
			Arg^{92}Trp
MyBP-C	All	--	--
α-Tropomyosin	Asp1^{75}Asn	--	--

Marian AJ et al, J Cardiovasc Electrophysiol 1998;

35.
THE NEED FOR POWERFUL RISK STRATIFICATION OF SUDDEN CARDIAC DEATH IN THE ERA OF PROPHYLACTIC ICD

Nabil El-Sherif, MD, Gioia Turitto, MD

Cardiology Division, Department of Medicine, State University of New York Health Science Center and Veterans Affairs Medical Center, Brooklyn, NY, USA

Introduction

In spite of recent improvement in overall cardiovascular mortality, post-hospital mortality remains high in survivors of acute myocardial infarction (AMI). Approximately one third of late deaths in survivors of AMI are sudden and unexpected and the risk of sudden death persists for years after the AMI [1,2]. Prevention of sudden cardiac death (SCD), which, in the majority of cases is due to malignant ventricular tachyarrhythmias (VT – defined as hypotensive ventricular tachycardia/ventricular fibrillation) in survivors of AMI remains a formidable clinical challenge. Management strategy of this major health care problem has centered over the years on two closely related aspects: one, how to identify those at risk of SCD, and two, what are the best management modalities, vis-à-vis pharmacotherapy or the implantable cardioverter-defibrillator (ICD). Following recent publications of the results of several multicenter studies, pharmacotherapy, mainly antiarrhythmic drugs, has not proven, so far, to be an effective management modality for those at risk of SCD. This cleared the way for more widespread use of the ICD as the sole, or main, management modality. Primarily because of the high cost of the ICD, and the invasive nature of this therapeutic modality, the prophylactic use of the device for primary prevention of SCD did not gain momentum until recently. This aspect of management strategy for SCD is still in the clinical research domain with several primary ICD prevention trials currently underway. However, this trend has highlighted the urgent need for more powerful risk stratification algorithms for SCD in this population.

The most recent results of the MADIT [3] and AVID [4] trials on one hand and the CABG-PATCH trial [5] on the other hand, underscored the point that the ICD works only when implanted in patients at high risk of arrhythmic death. Besides the invasive electrophysiologic study (EPS), commonly utilized non invasive risk stratifiers include: left ventricular

From Ovsyshcher IE. *Cardiac Arrythmias and Device Therapy: Results and Perspectives for the New Century.* Armonk, NY: Futura Publishing Company, Inc., © 2000

ejection fraction (LVEF), ventricular arrhythmias on ambulatory Holter recording, signal averaged electrocardiography (SAECG), heart rate variability (HRV), baroreflex sensitivity (BRS), QT dispersion, and T wave alternans (TWA). In addition, there is a number of other less commonly utilized markers of arrhythmic death. However, with the exception of LVEF, none of the other tests, at present, has proven to be solely adequate as a powerful risk stratifier. An optimal algorithm that combines more than one index of high risk has not yet been identified or agreed upon.

LVEF – LV function is one of the best predictors of cardiac mortality and morbidity in patients with coronary artery disease (CAD), especially after AMI. For example, in the Multicenter Postinfarction Study, patients with LVEF <20% had an approximately 45% 1-year mortality rate, compared to a 4% rate in patients with LVEF >40% [6]. However, LV systolic dysfunction is not a very sensitive marker of sudden or arrhythmic death [7]. The combination of severely depressed LVEF and NYHA class IV seems to identify patients who will die from pump failure or electromechanical dissociation rather than from malignant VT. On the other hand, in patients with moderate-to-severe LV dysfunction, approximately one third die suddenly, relatively independent of the severity of LV dysfunction [7]. It is important to remember that the extent of LV dysfunction can influence significantly the predictive power of other risk stratifiers, such as the SAECG and EPS.

Ambulatory Holter recording – The finding of complex ventricular arrhythmias on a Holter recording is not specific enough to identify individual patients at high risk of SCD. Spontaneous variation from day to day in the incidence of complex ventricular arrhythmias makes interpretation of the results of therapy guided by Holter recording subject to large errors. A more difficult question that remains unanswered at present is the relationship of asymptomatic complex ventricular arrhythmias to symptomatic VT. It is not clear whether these rhythm disorders are related mechanistically, and therefore whether alterations in spontaneous ectopy by antiarrhythmic therapy will impact on the prognosis.

SAECG – The SAECG appears useful in risk stratification of post-MI patients. Late potentials have been shown to predict future arrhythmic events [8,9]. However, a recent NIH study has shown that time-domain (TD) SAECG indices of late potentials do not provide the best prediction criteria for serious arrhythmic events in the first year post-MI, but rather the filtered QRS duration at 40 Hz [10]. The SAECG has some limitations; although it appears to have an excellent negative predictive value, both its sensitivity and positive predictive value are low. Recently, combined time- and frequency-domain analysis of the SAECG was shown to improve its overall predictive accuracy [11,12]. The rationale for combined time- and frequency-domain analysis of the SAECG is the observation that TD analysis has a high incidence of false positive results in patients with inferior wall MI, while spectral turbulence analysis (STA) has high incidence of false positive results in anterior MI. In a recent study of 602 post-MI patients, receiver operated characteristics curves were utilized to optimize cutoff values for each SAECG parameter separately, and also for the combined TD+STA model [12]. The negative predictive accuracy of all three analysis was high (98%). On the other hand, the positive predictive accuracy of TD (19.6%) or STA (18.3%) was quite low, and significantly improved to 35.8% by combined TD+STA analysis. The best results were obtained in patients with LVEF<40%, where the positive predictive accuracy of combined TD+STA analysis was 51.2%. The study concluded that combined TD+STA analysis of the SAECG significantly improves risk stratification power for VT in post-MI patients compared to TD and STA separately.

HRV and BRS – Many studies have revealed an association between the autonomic nervous system and SCD [13]. Both HRV and BRS are measures of the sympathovagal balance. Methods to analyze HRV employ both time- and frequency-domain measurements that quantify periodicities in the data. Prognostic information to risk stratify patients for future VT or other cardiac events leading to premature death may be possible by quantifying HRV [14,15]. Baroreflex sensitivity assessed with phenylephrine injection is an alternative non invasive test to evaluate sympathovagal balance [16]. Two major questions concerning HRV remain to be clarified. First, many methods to measure HRV have been reported, and it is very difficult to conclude which one is most appropriate for establishing normal values and for particular patient subgroups. There is a need to standardize the measurement of HRV and to quantify normal values under various circumstances, including patient age and gender. A recent effort in this regard is the report of the Task Force of the European Society of Cardiology and the North American Society of Pacing and Electrophysiology [17]. Low HRV is associated with increased all-cause mortality in middle aged and elderly men [18]. HRV did not add independent prognostic value to LV function and ventricular arrhythmias on predischarge Holter recording [19]. On the other hand, in the ATRAMI study, low values of BRS and HRV were significantly associated with an increased mortality risk in a multivariate model in which LVEF and premature ventricular complexes were included[16].

QT interval and QT dispersion – Previous studies have shown that prolongation of the QT interval is a risk factor for VT and SCD in patients with previous MI [20], but there has been some controversy as to the predictive accuracy of the prolonged QT interval. QT dispersion may be a more powerful predictor of susceptibility to VT, suggesting that inhomogeneity of repolarization is more closely associated with arrhythmic risk than is prolongation of repolarization itself [21]. Spatial dispersion of recovery times may be a fundamental electrophysiologic substrate for the genesis of reentrant VT. Day et al first proposed that interlead variability of QT interval in 12-lead electrocardiograms, QT dispersion, reflects dispersion of ventricular recovery time, thus providing a convenient tool for clinical studies[22]. However, the role of QT dispersion for risk stratification of SCD remains controversial which, in large measure, may be due to methodologic discrepancies. Some studies suggest that increased QT dispersion is related to susceptibility to VT, independent of the degree of LV dysfunction or clinical characteristics of the patients [21]. Other studies have shown that determination of QT dispersion from the surface ECG, even when performed with the best available methodology, failed to predict subsequent risk in post-MI patients [23]. Some investigators have found an association between measures of dispersion of ventricular repolarization and susceptibility to ventricular fibrillation [24]. However, because of considerable overlap between groups, these measures failed to provide a useful marker for the risk of SCD.

TWA – Alternation of the configuration and/or duration of the repolarization wave of the ECG, usually referred to as TWA, is seen under diverse experimental and clinical conditions [25]. Interest in repolarization alternans is attributed to the hypothesis that it may reflect underlying dispersion of repolarization in the ventricle, a well recognized electrophysiologic substrate for reentrant VT. Although overt TWA in the ECG is not common, in recent years digital signal-processing techniques capable of detecting subtle degrees of TWA have suggested that the phenomenon may be more prevalent than previously recognized and could represent an important marker of vulnerability to VT[26]. The electrophysiological basis of arrhythmogenicity of QT/T alternans in long QT syndrome has been recently investigated in an experimental surrogate model of long QT syndrome [27]. The arrhythmogenicity of QT/T alternans was primarily due to the greater degree of spatial dispersion of repolarization during alternans than during slower rates not associated with alternans. The dispersion of repolarization was most marked between midmyocardial and epicardial zones in the LV free wall. In the presence of a critical degree of dispersion of repolarization, propagation of the activation wavefront could be blocked between these zones to initiate reentrant excitation and polymorphic VT. An important observation was that marked repolarization alternans could be present in local electrograms without manifest alternation of the QT/T segment in the surface ECG. The latter was seen at critically short cycle lengths associated with reversal of the gradient of repolarization between epicardial and midmyocardial sites, with a consequent reversal of polarity of the intramyocardial QT wave in alternate cycles. These observations provide a strong impetus for studies that explore the use of microvolt TWA as a strong predictor for SCD.

Recent technical improvements allow the detection of microvolt TWA during sinus rhythm with the heart rate moderately elevated using bicycle exercise test. Several studies have shown that microvolt TWA detected with heart rate elevation with bicycle exercise is a strong predictor of arrhythmia inducibility at EPS [28,29]. In a prospective multicenter study of 148 patients, the relationship between TWA and the induction of VT on EPS was assessed. TWA was a moderately sensitive but specific predictor of the results of EPS. However, TWA more accurately predicted future arrhythmic events compared to EPS [29]. TWA compared favorably with EPS and other non invasive risk markers in predicting recurrence of VT in ICD recipients[30]. The heart rate at the onset of TWA in normals and in patients with VT was also investigated[31]. False positive TWA developed in 7% of age-matched normal subjects at higher heart rate compared to patients with VT. A target heart rate of 110 beats/min was found to be highly sensitive and specific. However, because of their lower symptom-limited heart rate, many patients may not be able to achieve the target heart rate associated with TWA resulting in an indeterminate tests. In these patients, non invasive or pharmacologic means to increase heart rate may be considered.

EPS – The role of EPS in risk stratification of post-MI patients for arrhythmic events remains controversial. Inducible VT were reported in 9-20% of survivors of recent MI by EPS and after a follow-up period of one to two years, serious arrhythmic events occurred in 14-36% of patients with inducible sustained VT [32-34]. In the MADIT study, patients with one or more prior MI, LVEF ≤35%, non-sustained VT and inducible nonsuppressible VT had significantly improved survival with the ICD compared to conventional medical therapy [3]. The MUSTT study investigated a very similar population (the only difference was an LVEF ≤40%) and found that in patients with inducible VT, EP-guided antiarrhythmic therapy improved survival primarily due to therapy with the ICD rather than "effective" antiarrhythmic drugs [35]. In this study, the 5-year arrhythmic death or cardiac arrest in patients who had no inducible

VT was 26% compared to 32% in patients with inducible VT who were followed on no antiarrhythmic therapy. However, the 5-year total mortality was similar (48%). Both MADIT and MUSTT trials failed to shed light on the one crucial question regarding the future role of EPS in risk stratification, namely, whether non inducibility of VT in post-MI patients is a strong marker of low risk independent of other variables, such as the degree of LV dysfunction, TWA, etc.

In search for other risk stratifiers for SCD

In addition to the more commonly investigated techniques for risk stratification of SCD, several other risk indices have been reported. For instance, QT dispersion detected by magnetocardiograph [36] or by precordial mapping techniques [37] was reported to be a sensitive marker of the susceptibility to malignant VT. However, the prohibitive cost of a magnetocardiography laboratory and the technical demands of precordial mapping techniques are obvious deterrents to their wide application in a clinical setting. Beat-to-beat repolarization lability was found in one study to be a better identifier of SCD than other indicators of abnormal repolarization, including spatial QT dispersion and TWA[38]. Low variability of cycle lengths of non-sustained VT was also suggested as an independent predictor of mortality after AMI [39]. Increased heart rate, assessed from a 24-hour Holter recording, or even from a standard ECG tracing, was found to be a strong predictor of mortality after AMI [23,40]. On the other hand, "non electrophysiologic" indices may also be associated with increased risk for SCD, for instance, LV mass and hypertrophy [41].

The practical value of many of the risk stratifiers of SCD remains largely unanswered. Although risk stratification for SCD may be improved by using several variables in combination, one problem that has been alluded to is that dichotomous limits derived from univariate analysis may be different when used in the multivariate setting [42].

Review of ongoing ICD studies of primary prevention of SCD

The MADIT study was the first to examine the role of ICD in primary prevention of SCD in high-risk coronary patients with LVEF $\leq$35%, asymptomatic non-sustained ventricular tachycardia, and inducible nonsuppressible sustained VT[3]. The significant protection afforded patients who received the ICD provided the impetus for a number of ICD studies of primary prevention of SCD. Unfortunately, these studies utilize different risk stratification indices as well as different management strategies. Table I provides a brief outline of those studies currently ongoing or recently initiated.

Table I – Current ICD primary prevention trials

Study	Patients	Randomization
MADIT II (Multicenter Automatic Defibrillator Implantation Trial)	Late post-MI, LVEF <30%	ICD vs conventional □
SCD-HeFT (Sudden Cardiac Death in Heart Failure Trial)	NYHA Class II/III LVEF <35%	ICD vs amiodarone vs placebo
CAT (German Dilated Cardiomyopathy Trial)	NICM, LVEF ≤30%, NYHA Class II/III	ICD vs conventional □
AMIOVIRT (Amiodarone Vs ICD Randomized Trial)	NICM, LVEF ≤35%, NSVT	ICD vs amiodarone
BEST+ICD (Beta-blocker Strategy Plus ICD Trial)	Recent MI, LVEF ≤35%, HRV or NSVT or +SAECG	EP-guided (including ICD in EP+ pts vs conventional □)
DINAMIT (Defibrillator In Acute Myocardial Infarction Trial)	Recent MI, LVEF ≤35%,HRV or mean RR≤750 ms	ICD vs no ICD
DEFINITE (DEFibrillators in Non Ischemic Cardiomyopathy Treatment Evaluation)	NICM, LVEF <35%, NSVT or >10 VPC/ hour, symptomatic heart failure	Heart failure drugs+ beta-blockers vs ICD
SEDET (South European Defibrillator trial)	AMI ineligible for thrombolysis, LVEF, 15-40%,≥ 10 VPC/ hour or ≥ 1 NSVT	ICD vs conventional □

EP= electrophysiology; HRV= heart rate variability; MI = myocardial infarction; NICM = non-ischemic cardiomyopathy; NSVT= non-sustained ventricular tachycardia; SAECG = signal averaged electrocardiogram, □=therapy

A review of Table I reveals that, besides a low LVEF, different indices of increased arrhythmic risk are utilized for patient selection. These include: non-sustained ventricular tachycardia (AMIOVIRT, BEST+ICD, DEFINITE); inducible sustained VT (BEST+ICD); and abnormal heart rate variability (DINAMIT). Two of the studies compare the ICD versus amiodarone versus conventional therapy (SCD-HeFT, AMIOVIRT).

Critique of current ICD trials of primary prevention of SCD

LVEF is one of the best predictors of cardiac morbidity and mortality. However, LV systolic dysfunction is not a very sensitive marker of sudden or arrhythmic death[7]. Fifty percent of cardiac mortality in patients with low LVEF is nonsudden and is attributed to progressive deterioration of myocardial function[46]. Those patients are not expected to benefit from the ICD. Thus, the major critique of ICD primary prevention trial of SCD is their **redundancy**, that is to say, many patients who may not benefit from the ICD will still receive it, based only on their low LVEF. An obvious strategy is to restrict the use of the ICD to those patients with low LVEF who have a high risk for arrhythmic, not nonarrhythmic, cardiac death. The problem with this strategy is that, so far, there is no available index of increased arrhythmic risk with sufficiently high predictive accuracy that would justify its inclusion in the selection algorithm for eligible candidates for the ICD. Some of the arrhythmic risk stratifiers utilized in the studies listed in Table I have limited predictive accuracy (non-sustained ventricular tachycardia in AMIOVIRT, BEST+ICD, DEFINITE, SEDET; inducible sustained VT on electrophysiology study in BEST+ICD; and heart rate variability in DINAMIT). An additional critique of some of the studies in Table I, specifically SCD-HeFT and AMIOVIRT, is the use of amiodarone as one of the management strategies. Several trials have evaluated the role of amiodarone in decreasing mortality in patients at high risk of SCD. However, current evidence does not support the prophylactic use of amiodarone or, for that matter, the use of other antiarrhythmic agents, for patients at high arrhythmic risk[47].

Conclusions

At present it remains uncertain how to manage patients at high risk for arrhythmic death. Although combinatorial algorithms that utilize several non invasive and invasive tests may provide better risk stratification, there is still no consensus as to what is the best way to characterize the patient's arrhythmic risk and whether antiischemic measures, antiarrhythmic pharmacologic therapy, the ICD, or a combination of measures represent the best management strategy. The current impression in the field is that, other than low LVEF, no other "electrophysiologic" marker is powerful enough to be included in the risk stratification strategy for primary prevention of SCD. The validity of this approach remains to be defined.

References

1. Rouleau JL, Talajic M, Sussex B, et al.: Myocardial infarction patients in the 1980s – their risk factors, stratification and survival in Canada: The Canadian Assessment of Myocardial Infarction (CAMI) Study. J Am Coll Cardiol 1996;27:1119-1127.
2. De Vreede-Swagemakers JJM, Gorgels APM, Dubois-Arbouw WI, et al.: Out-of-hospital cardiac arrest in the 1990s: A population-based study in the Maastricht area on incidence, characteristics and survival. J Am Coll Cardiol 1997;30:1500-1505.
3. Moss AJ, Hall WJ, Cannom DS, et al.: Improved survival with an implanted defibrillator in patients with coronary artery disease at high risk for ventricular arrhythmias. N Engl J Med 1996;35:1933-1940.
4. The Antiarrhythmics Versus Implantable Defibrillators (AVID) Investigators: A comparison of antiarrhythmic drug therapy with implantable defibrillators in patients resuscitated from non-fatal ventricular arrhythmias. N Engl J Med 1997;337:1576-1583.
5. Bigger JT, for the Coronary Artery Bypass Graft (CABG) Patch Trial Investigators: Prophylactic use of implanted cardiac defibrillators in patients at high risk for ventricular arrhythmias after coronary-artery bypass graft surgery. N Engl J Med 1997;337:1569-1575.
6. The Multicenter Post-Infarction Research Group: Risk stratification and survival after myocardial infarction. N Engl J Med 1983;309:331-336.
7. Kober L, Torp-Pedersen C, Elming H, Burchardt H, on behalf of the TRACE Study Group: Use of left ventricular ejection fraction or wall-motion score index in predicting arrhythmic death in patients following an acute myocardial infarction. PACE 1997;20:2553-2559.
8. Kuchar DL, Thornburn CW, Sammel NL: Prediction of serious arrhythmic events after myocardial infarction: signal averaged electrocardiogram, Holter monitoring and radionuclide ventriculography. J Am Coll Cardiol 1987;9:531-538.
9. El-Sherif N, Ursell SN, Bekheit S, et al.: Prognostic value of the signal averaged ECG depends on the time of recording in the postinfarction period. Am Heart J 1989;118:256-264.
10. El-Sherif N, Denes P, Katz R, et al.: Definition of the best criteria of the time-domain signal-averaged electrocardiogram for serious

arrhythmic events in the post-infarction period. J Am Coll Cardiol 1995;25:908-914.

11. Ahuja RK, Turitto G, Ibrahim B, Caref EB, El-Sherif N: Combined time-domain and spectral turbulence analysis of the signal-averaged electrocardiogram improve its predictive accuracy in post-infarction patients. J Electrocardiol 1994;27(Suppl):202-206.

12. Vazquez R, Caref EB, Torres F, Reina M, Espina A, El-Sherif N: Improved diagnostic value of the combined time- and frequency-domain analysis of the signal-averaged electrocardiogram after myocardial infarction. J Am Coll Cardiol 1999;33:385-394.

13. Baron HV, Lesh MD: Autonomic nervous system and sudden cardiac death. J Am Coll Cardiol 1996;27:1053-1060.

14. Kleiger RE, Miller JP, Bigger JT Jr, Moss AJ, and the Multicenter Post-Infarction Research Group: Decreased heart rate variability and its association with increased mortality after acute myocardial infarction. Am J Cardiol 1987;59:256-262.

15. Bigger JT, Steinman RC, Rolnitzky LM, Fleiss JL, Albrecht P, Cohen RJ: Power law behavior of RR-interval variability in healthy middle-aged persons, patients with recent acute myocardial infarction, and patients with heart transplants. Circulation 1996;93:2142-2151.

16. La Rovere MT, Bigger JT Jr, Marcus FI, Mortara A, Schwartz PJ, for the ATRAMI (Autonomic Tone and Reflexes After Myocardial Infarction) Investigators: Baroreflex sensitivity and heart-rate variability in prediction of total cardiac mortality after myocardial infarction. Lancet 1998;351:478-484.

17. Task Force of the European Society of Cardiology and the North American Society of Pacing and Electrophysiology: Heart rate variability. Standards of measurement, physiological interpretation, and clinical use. Circulation 1996;93:1143-1165.

18. Dekker JM, Schouten EG, Klootwijk P, Pool J, Swenne CA, Kromhout D: Heart rate variability from short electrocardiographic recordings predict mortality from all causes in middle-aged and elderly men. Am J Epidemiol 1997;145:899-908.

19. Lanza GA, Guido V, Galeazzi N, et al: Prognostic role of heart rate variability in patients with a recent acute myocardial infarction. Am J Cardiol 1998;82:1323-1328.

20. Ahnve S, Gilpin E, Madsen EB, Frolicher V, Henning H, Ross J: Prognostic importance of QT interval at discharge after acute myocardial infarction: a multicenter study of 865 patients. Am Heart J 1984;108:395-400.

21. Higham PD, Campbell RFW: QT dispersion. Br Heart J 1994;71:508-510.

22. Day CP, McComb JM, Campbell RFW: QT dispersion: An indication of arrhythmia risk in patients with long QT intervals. Br Heart J 1990;63:342-344.

23. Zabel M, Klingenheben T, Franz MR, Hohnloser SH: Assessment of QT dispersion for prediction of mortality or arrhythmic events after myocardial infarction. Results of a prospective, long-term follow-up study. Circulation 1998;97:2543-2550.

24. Oikarinen L, Toivonen L, Viitasalo M: Electrocardiographic measures of ventricular repolarization: dispersion in patients with coronary artery disease susceptible to ventricular fibrillation. Heart 1998;79:554-559.

25. El-Sherif N: T-wave alternans. A marker of vulnerability to ventricular tachyarrhythmias. In: Raviele A (ed) Cardiac Arrhythmias 1995. Springer, Milan, 1996;pp 12-16.

26. Rosenbaum DS, Jackson LE, Smith JM, et al.: Electrical alternans and vulnerability to ventricular arrhythmias. N Engl J Med 1994;330:235-241.

27. Chinushi M, Restivo M, Caref EB, El-Sherif N: Electrophysiological basis of the arrhythmogenicity of QT/T alternans in the long QT syndrome. Tridimensional analysis of the kinetics of cardiac repolarization. Circ Res 1998;83:614-628.

28. Estes NAM, Michaud G, Zipes DP, et al.: Electrical alternans during rest and exercise as a predictor of vulnerability to ventricular arrhythmias. Am J Cardiol 1997;80:1314-1318.

29. Gold MR, Bloomfield DM, Anderson KP, et al.: T wave alternans predicts arrhythmia vulnerability in patients undergoing electrophysiology study (abstr). Circulation 1998;98 (Suppl I):647.

30. Hohnloser SH, Klingenheben T, Li Y G, Zabel M, Peetermans J, Cohen RJ: T-wave alternans as a predictor of recurrent ventricular tachyarrhythmias in ICD recipients: prospective comparison with conventional risk markers. J Cardiovasc Electrophysiol 1998;9:1258-1268.

31. Turitto G, Caref EB, Pedalino R, et al.: Comparison of heart rate at onset of T-wave alternans in normals and patients with malignant ventricular tachyarrhythmias (abstr). Circulation 1998;98 (Suppl I):647.

32. Roy D, Marchand E, Theroux P, Waters DD, Pelletier GB, Bourassa MG: Programmed ventricular stimulation in survivors of an acute myocardial infarction. Circulation 1985;72:487-494.

33. Iesaka Y, Nogami A, Aonuma K, et al.: Prognostic significance of sustained monomorphic VT induced by programmed ventricular stimulation using up to triple extrastimuli in survivors of acute myocardial infarction. Am J Cardiol 1990;65:1057-1063.

34. Bourke JP, Richards ADB, Ross DL, Wallace EM, McGuire MA, Uther JB: Routine programmed electrical stimulation in survivors of acute myocardial infarction for prediction of spontaneous ventricular tachyarrhythmias during follow-up: results, optimal stimulation protocol and cost-effective screening. J Am Coll Cardiol 1991;18:780-788.

35. Buxton AL: MUSTT results. 1999, Personal communication.

36. Oikarinen L, Paavola M, Montonen J, Viitasalo M, et al.: Magnetocardiographic QT interval dispersion in postmyocardial infarction patients with sustained ventricular tachycardia: validation of automated QT measurements. PACE 1998;21:1934-1942.

37. Hubley-Kozey CL, Mitchell LB, Gardner MJ, et al.: Spatial features in body-surface potential maps can identify patients with a history of sustained ventricular tachycardia. Circulation 1995;92:1825-1838.

38. Atiga Wl, Calkins H, Lawrence JH, et al.: Beat-to-beat repolarization lability identifies patients at risk for sudden cardiac death. J Cardiovasc Electrophysiol 1998;9:899-908.

39. Dabrovski A, Kramarz E, Piotrowicz R: Low variability of cycle lengths in nonsustained ventricular tachycardia as an independent predictor of mortality after myocardial infarction. Am J Cardiol 1997;80:1347-1350.

40. Copie X, Hnatkova K, Staunton A, Fei L, Camm AJ, Malik M: Predictive power of increased heart rate versus depressed left ventricular ejection fraction and heart rate variability for risk stratification after myocardial infarction: results of a two-year follow-up study. J Am Coll Cardiol 1996;27:270-276.

41. Haider AW, Larson MG, Benjamin EJ, Levy D: Increased left ventricular mass and hypertrophy are associated with increased risk for sudden death. J Am Coll Cardiol 1998;32:1454-1459.

42. Redwood SR, Odemuyiwa O, Hnatkova K, et al.: Selection of dichotomy limits for multifactorial prediction of arrhythmic events and mortality in survivors of acute myocardial infarction. Eur Heart J 1997;18:1278-1287.

43. Moss AJ, Cannom DS, Daubert JP, et al, for the MADIT-II Investigators: Multicenter Automatic Defibrillator Implantation Trial II (MADIT-II): design and clinical protocol. Ann Noninvasive Electrocardiol 1999;4:83-91.

44. Bardy GH, Lee KL, Mark DB, and the SCD-HeFT Pilot Investigators: The Sudden Cardiac Death in Heart Failure Trial: pilot study (abstr). PACE 1997;20:1148.

45. Raviele A, Bongiorni MG, Brignole M, et al.: Which strategy is "best" after myocardial infarction? The beta-blocker strategy plus implantable cardioverter defibrillator trial: Rationale and study design. Am J Cardiol 1999;83(5B):104D-111D.

46. Narang R, Cleland JGF, Erhardt L, et al: Mode of death in chronic heart fail: a request for more accurate classification. Eur Heart J 1996;17:1390-1403.

47. Farre J, Romero J, Robio JM, et al: Amiodarone and "primary" prevention of sudden death: critical review of a decade of clinical trials, Am J Cardiol 1998;83:55D-63D.

36

MADIT AND THE PRIMARY PREVENTION OF SUDDEN CARDIAC DEATH

Arthur J. Moss, M.D.

Cardiology Unit, Department of Medicine, University of Rochester Medical Center, Rochester, New York, USA

Introduction

The Multicenter Automatic Defibrillator Implantation Trial (MADIT) had its origin in the 1980s with the publications of the risks posed by left ventricular dysfunction and ventricular ectopic beats in the setting of subacute coronary heart disease.[1] Other relevant background for MADIT included the findings from the Cardiac Arrhythmia Suppression Trial (CAST)[2] and the publication by Wilber, et al. in 1990 on the value of electrophysiologic testing for risk stratification in patients with non-sustained ventricular tachycardia, coronary heart disease, and ejection fraction <0.40.[3] In December 1990, the MADIT investigators initiated a prophylactic trial in which high-risk patients with coronary heart disease and asymptomatic NSVT were randomly assigned to receive an implanted cardioverter-defibrillator (ICD) or conventional medical management. To ensure a population at high risk for malignant ventricular arrhythmias, eligible patients had to have an ejection fraction ≤0.35, NSVT unrelated to an acute coronary event, and an inducible, sustained, nonsuppressible ventricular tachyarrhythmia on electrophysiologic testing. The end point of the trial was overall mortality during long-term follow-up. The primary hypothesis of MADIT was that prophylactic ICD therapy in high-risk coronary patients with ejection fraction ≤0.35, NSVT, and inducible-nonsuppressible ventricular tachyarrhythmia would be associated with improved survival when compared to patients managed with conventional treatment not involving ICD therapy. The finding from MADIT were published in 1996.[4]

Study Population

The eligibility and exclusion criteria for MADIT are presented in Table 1. Eligibility included patients of either sex age 25 to 80 years with a documented Q-wave or enzyme-positive myocardial infarction three weeks or more before entry, an episode of asymptomatic NSVT unrelated to an acute myocardial infarction, an ejection fraction ≤0.35, NYHA Class I-III, and no indication for coronary revascularization. Patients were excluded from enrollment if they had a previous cardiac arrest,

From Ovsyshcher IE. *Cardiac Arrythmias and Device Therapy: Results and Perspectives for the New Century.* Armonk, NY: Futura Publishing Company, Inc., © 2000

documented sustained ventricular tachycardia, coronary artery bypass graft surgery within the past two months, coronary angioplasty within the past three months, NYHA Class IV, or major non-cardiac comorbidity. Patients were referred to MADIT investigators at the discretion of their primary attending physician. Eligible, non-excluded patients underwent electrophysiologic testing according to a prespecified protocol[5] and qualified for enrollment if sustained monomorphic ventricular tachycardia (with 2 or 3 extrastimuli) or polymorphic ventricular tachycardia/ventricular fibrillation (with 2 extrastimuli) were reproducibly induced and not suppressed after intravenous procainamide.

Table 1. MADIT Eligibility and Exclusion Criteria

ELIGIBILITY CRITERIA
1. Male or female age 25 to 80 years of age
2. One or more prior myocardial infarctions
3. Documented episode of nonsustained ventricular tachycardia (run of 3 to 30 VEBs at a rate >120 bpm) within the three months before enrollment
4. Ejection fraction ≤ 0.35
5. NYHA Class I – III
6. Inducible, nonsuppressible ventricular tachycardia at electrophysiologic study

EXCLUSION CRITERIA
1. Aborted cardiac arrest at any time in the past
2. History of sustained ventricular tachycardia unrelated to an acute myocardial infarction
3. Enzyme positive myocardial infarction in the past 3 weeks
4. Coronary artery bypass graft surgery within the past 8 weeks or coronary angioplasty within the past 12 weeks
5. Indication for coronary revascularization in the foreseeable future
6. Major comorbidity with a reduced likelihood of survival for the duration of the trial
7. Cardiogenic shock, symptomatic hypotension, or NYHA Class IV
8. Participation in other clinical trials
9. Patients unwilling to sign a consent form for participation in MADIT

Findings

The clinical characteristics of the 196 patients enrolled in MADIT by treatment group are presented in Table 2. The baseline characteristics

Table 2. Baseline Characteristics of 196 Patients Randomized to Conventional or Defibrillator Therapy

	Treatment Group	
	Conventional (n = 101)	Defibrillator (n = 95)
Mean age (yr)	64±9	62±9
Sex (M/F)	92/8	92/8
Cardiac history		
Two or more prior MIs	29	34
Treatment for ventricular arrhythmias	35	42
NYHA Class II-III	67	63
Treatment for congestive heart failure	51	52
Treatment for hypertension	35	48
Insulin-dependent diabetes	5	7
Coronary bypass surgery	44	46
Implanted pacemaker	7	2
Cardiac findings at enrollment		
Blood urea nitrogen >25 mg/dl	21	22
Left bundle branch block	8	7
Mean ejection fraction	0.25±0.07	0.27±0.07
Qualifying nonsustained ventricular tachycardia		
Number of consecutive beats	9±10	10±9

*Figures are percentages unless otherwise indicated; plus-minus values are mean ± SD. Modified from N Engl J Med 1996;335:1933-1940,[4] with permission.

of the two treatment groups were clinically similar. The MADIT-defined patient was predominantly male, average age 63 years, with an ejection fraction of 0.26. More than half the patients had been treated previously for heart failure and almost half the patients had prior coronary artery bypass graft surgery. Of special note, the average number of repetitive beats in the qualifying run of NSVT was 9-10 beats. At electrophysiologic study, monomorphic ventricular tachycardia was induced by double or triple extrastimuli in about 90% of the patients, with the remaining 10% induced into either polymorphous ventricular tachycardia or ventricular fibrillation by double extrastimuli. At the time of enrollment, more than one-half of the patients were receiving angiotensin converting enzyme inhibitors and diuretics, and more than one-third were receiving a digitalis preparation.

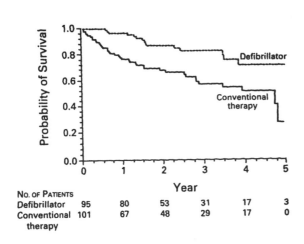

Fig. 1. Probability of survival by treatment assignment.
From N Engl J Med 1996;335;1933-1940,[4] with permission.

During an average follow-up of 27 months per patient, there were 15 deaths in the defibrillator group and 39 deaths in the patients receiving conventional-therapy. The hazard ratio (ICD:No-ICD) by Cox analyses for overall mortality was 0.46 (95% CI =0.26-0.82 P=0.009). The Kaplan Meier survival curves by assigned treatment are presented in Fig.1. The two mortality curves separate early and remain well separated throughout the five-year trial, with a significantly higher survival rate for patients randomized to ICD than to conventional therapy. Of note, there were no operative deaths due to implantation of the ICD. Further analyses revealed that the major beneficial effect from ICD therapy occurred in the subset with ejection fraction <0.26. The cumulative time to the first shock in the ICD group was analyzed, and 40% of the ICD patients had a shock discharge within 1 year after device implantation, 60% within 2 years, and 90% within 5 years.

A MADIT cost-effectiveness analysis was carried out.[6] The costs of all healthcare services during the trial were determined, including hospitalizations, physician visits, medications, laboratory tests, and procedures, in patients randomized to ICD and non-ICD therapy. Incremental cost-effectiveness ratios were calculated by relating these costs to the increased survival associated with the use of the defibrillator. The average survival for the ICD group over a 4-year period was 3.66 years compared with 2.80 years in the non-ICD group. Accumulated net costs were $97,560 for the ICD group compared with $75,980 for individuals randomized to conventional therapy. The resulting incremental cost-effectiveness ratio of $27,000 per life-year saved compares favorably with other cardiac interventions like coronary artery bypass graft surgery.

Comments

MADIT was the first randomized device trial to evaluate the safety and efficacy of prophylactic ICD therapy in high-risk patients with coronary heart disease. The implanted cardioverter-defibrillator was associated with a 54% reduction in all-cause mortality in this patient population when compared to conventional, non-ICD therapy. MADIT was a primary prevention trial in that the patients did not have a malignant arrhythmia, arrhythmogenic syncope, or aborted cardiac arrest before implantation of the defibrillator. Following the MADIT publication, the Antiarrhythmics Versus Implantable Defibrillator (AVID) trial showed that ICD was also effective in secondary prevention with improved survival among survivors of ventricular fibrillation or sustained tachycardias causing severe symptoms,[7] but especially in those with ejection fractions <0.35.[8] Recently, the Multicenter Unsustained Tachycardia Trial (MUSTT), a primary prevention trial using a somewhat different design from that of MADIT, found that ICD therapy was superior to selected antiarrhythmic drug therapy based on electrophysiologic testing, with the ICD results in excellent alignment with those of MADIT.

The ICD has also been used effectively as primary and secondary prevention of sudden cardiac death in high-risk patients with inherited cardiac disorders such as the long QT syndrome (LQTS), hypertrophic cardiomyopathy (HCM), and the Brugada syndrome. Although no randomized clinical trials have been carried out with ICDs in subjects with these conditions, individual case reports with interrogated data from implanted defibrillators have clearly shown the life-saving value of ICD therapy in selected patients with these arrhythmogenic conditions. In patients with LQTS, the presence of overt T-wave alternans, recurrent syncope unresponsive to beta-blockers, a documented episode of torsades de pointes, or an aborted cardiac arrest are reasonable indications for ICD therapy unless specific contraindications exist. In the International LQTS Registry, 88 high-risk LQTS patients have had an ICD implanted because of the presence of life-threatening arrhythmogenic risk potential. During an average follow-up of over 2 years, numerous life-saving defibrillations have been documented by interrogation, and no deaths have occurred in this group of patients. In a recent study involving over 100 patients with HCM and extreme septal hypertrophy, an ICD was implanted for primary prevention of sudden cardiac death. During an average follow-up of over 1 year, device interrogation revealed appropriate ventricular tachycardia termination or life-saving defibrillation in 15% of the study group.[9] The Brugada syndrome presents a particularly difficult problem since sudden death may be the first symptomatic manifestation of this disorder. Experts in the field are now recommending prophylactic ICDs once the diagnosis of the condition has been established by electrocardiogram, appropriate testing, and family history.

Conclusion

As a result of the MADIT experience, the overall improved survival documented with ICD therapy in the aforementioned clinical trials, and the favorable experience with defibrillators in patients with rare genetic arrhythmogenic disorders, the U.S. Health Care Financing Administration (HCFA) recently liberalized their reimbursement guidelines for ICD therapy.[10] The implantation of an automatic defibrillator is a covered service for patients with the following conditions: 1) A documented episode of cardiac arrest due to ventricular fibrillation not due to a transient or reversible cause; 2) Ventricular tachyarrhythmia, either spontaneous or induce, not due to a transient or reversible cause; or 3) Familial or inherited conditions with a high risk of life-threatening ventricular tachyarrhythmias such as long QT syndrome or hypertrophic cardiomyopathy.

References

1. The Multicenter Postinfarction Research Group. Risk stratification and survival after myocardial infarction. N Engl J Med 1983;309:331-6.
2. Echt DS, Liebson PR, Mitchell LB, et al., and the CAST Investigators. Mortality and morbidity in patients randomized to receive encainide, flecainide, or placebo in the Cardiac Arrhythmia Suppression Trial. N Engl J Med 1991;324:781-8.
3. Wilber DJ, Olshansky B, Moran JF, et al. Electrophysiologic testing and nonsustained ventricular tachycardia: use and limitation in patients with coronary artery disease and impaired ventricular function. Circulation 1990;82:350-8.
4. Moss AJ, Hall WJ, Cannom DS, et al. Improved survival with an implanted defibrillator in patients with coronary disease at high risk for ventricular arrhythmia. N Engl J Med 1996;335:1933-40.
5. MADIT Executive Committee. Multicenter automatic defibrillator implantation trial (MADIT): Design and Clinical Protocol. PACE 1991(II):14:920-7.

6. Mushlin AI, Hall WJ, Zwanziger J, et al. The cost-effectiveness of automatic implantable cardiac defibrillators: results from MADIT. Circulation 1998;97:2129-2135.
7. The Antiarrhythmics Versus Implantable Defibrillators (AVID) Investigators. A comparison of antiarrhythmic-drug therapy with implantable defibrillators in patients resuscitated from near-fatal ventricular arrhythmias. N Engl J Med 1997;337:1576-83.
8. Domanski MJ, Sakseena S, Epstein AE, et al. Relative effectiveness of the implantable cardioverter-defibrillator and antiarrhythmic drugs in patients with varying degrees of left ventricular dysfunction who have survived malignant ventricular arrhythmias. J Am Coll Cardiol 1999;34:1090-1095.
9. Maron B. Minneapolis, MN. Personal communication.
10. Medicare Coverage Issues Manual 35.85 Implantation of Automatic Defibrillators. July 1, 1999.

Part VII.

Cardiac Pacing

37.
THE HISTORY OF THE COMPREHENSION OF AV CONDUCTION, HEART BLOCK AND STOKES-ADAMS SYNDROME

Seymour Furman, MD, FACC, FACS

Montefiore Medical Center, Albert Einstein College of Medicine, Bronx, New York, United States of America; Member of NASPE

Galen, the compiler of Roman medical knowledge had written that the ears (auricles, atria) beat prior to the heart (as the ventricles were then named), and that there was a pause between the beating of the upper chambers (ears, auricles, atria) and the lower. That was the state of knowledge and belief based on acceptance of this physiology until the nineteenth century. The case reports, now believed to be precursors of the description of heart block and ventricular standstill (asystole) did not appreciate the dissociation of the sequential auricular and ventricular contractions. The history of heart block and the syncopal episodes that have been called Stokes-Adams disease (syndrome) runs through the past three hundred years of medical and cardiologic history, though only Stokes (1846) described syncope associated with "*a very remarkable pulsation in the right jugular vein ...more than double the number of the manifest ventricular contractions...*" In addition to his describing seven cases which he considered similar and of cardiac origin, an association not clearly recognized by earlier workers, he added the dissociation of auricular and ventricular function. Initially and to the end of the nineteenth century, the syncopal episodes, which are part of the syndrome, were considered by some to be a category of epilepsy. It was only at the beginning of the eighteenth century that the first distinction of "epilepsy" associated with a slow pulse was made. Before Stokes described seven cases, eleven other case descriptions had been made, one by Adams.[1]

The earliest recorded description of what can now be regarded as bradycardia with syncope was by the Slovene Marko Gerbec (1658-1718) (in Latin, Marcus Gerbezius) who wrote, "*I noticed something even more unusual about the pulse of two patients, one of whom, a melancholic, a hypochondriac, otherwise basically healthy, had such a slow pulse that the pulse of a healthy person would beat three times before his pulse would beat for a second time: Otherwise the man had been robust, precise in his movements, but very sluggish, frequently dizzy, and from time to time subject to mild epileptic seizures...*"[2]

From Ovsyshcher IE. *Cardiac Arrythmias and Device Therapy: Results and Perspectives for the New Century.* Armonk, NY: Futura Publishing Company, Inc., © 2000

Further descriptions of slow pulse with syncope, all categorized as epilepsy variants, were provided by Morgagni[3] in 1769, *"He was in his sixty-eighth year, of a habit moderately fat, and of a florid complexion, when he was first seized with the epilepsy, which left behind it the greatest slowness of pulse, and in like manner a coldness of the body."* Other descriptions were by Spens[4] in 1793, Burnett[5] in 1824 and that of Adams[6] in 1826, *"An officer in the revenue, aged 68 years, ...was just then recovering from the effects of an apoplectic attack. ...What most attracted my attention was, the irregularity of his breathing, and remarkable slowness of pulse, which generally ranged at the rate of 30 in a minute....November 4, 1819, he was suddenly seized with an apoplectic attack, which in two hours carried him off..."* and that of his later contemporary William Stokes[7] who in 1846 added seven cases including *Case I-Repeated pseudo-apoplectic attacks, not followed by paralysis: slow pulse, with valvular murmur.* His further case descriptions associated syncope with slow cardiac rate and cardiac standstill as the cause of syncope.

Harvey[8] (De Motu Cordis-1628) observed that, *"There are as it were at one time two motions, one of the ears, and another of the ventricles themselves, for they are not just at one instant, but the motion of the ears goes before and the motion of the heart follows; and the motion seems to begin at the ears, and to pass forward to the ventricles; when all things are already in a languishing condition, ..."* and added that before agonal asystole, differential beating of the ears and ventricles could be observed, that the right ear beat last of all and that, *"So the heart first leaves beating before the ears, so that the ears are said to out-live it: the left ventricle leaves beating first of all, then its ear, then the right ventricle, last of all (which Galen observes) all the rest giving off and dying, the right ear beats still: so that life seems to remain last of all in the right. And whilst by little and little the heart is dying, you may see after two or three beatings of the ear, the heart will, being as it were rowsed, answer... Knowledge that the cardiac appendages and ventricles beat in succession with a pause, separated by about a fifth a second, between. ...."* He noted that the dying heart had a prolonged interval between auricular and ventricular contractions and might have multiple auricular beats for each ventricular.

Purkinje[9], an anatomist working in Prague in the 1840s described the existence of a muscular bundle between the auricles and the ventricles but did not assign it any function. It remained mysterious as the burgeoning electrophysiology of the middle of the nineteenth century developed the two competing theories of cardiac contraction and its sequence. One explanation was that the heart, like striated muscle beat in response to nervous stimulation and the other that cardiac muscle, unlike striated muscle had intrinsic rhythmicity though its action could be affected by those nerves which reached the heart.

During the mid nineteenth century cardiac physiology, Haller postulated that the heart beat because of the direct action of the blood passing through the chambers of the heart. Soon it was repeatedly demonstrated that in vertebrates such as the frog and tortoise when the heart was removed from the body and from the flow of blood it continued to beat and was therefore independent of transiting blood flow and was a cardiac characteristic. The heart possessed automatic rhythmic capability. In 1848 Remak discovered ganglion cells in the sinus venosus of the frog's heart, Bidder two large masses of ganglion cells at the junction of the auricles and ventricles and Ludwig ganglion cells in the interauricular septum. The rhythmic contraction of the invertebrate heart was rapidly attributed to the presence of these nerve ganglia and gave impetus to the neurogenic theory of cardiac contraction. This hypothesis was further supported by rudimentary experimental work of Stannius (1852) in which both an incision and a fully constricting ligature at the junction of the sinus and the auricle caused cardiac standstill presumably because it obstructed impulses from Remak's ganglia.[10]

At the beginning of the second half of the nineteenth century, the concept of the origin and propagation of the heart beat was of a continually active nervous motor center in the sinus, which resembled the control of respiration, and which stimulated auricles and ventricles. It was suggested that there was a less excitable center in the auriculo-ventricular groove which was usually inactive, providing a slower rate and less excitability but could be activated in unusual situations. It was soon demonstrated that electricity could cause denervated cardiac muscle to contract continuously if it was bathed in artificial nutrient solution and that intact ventricles would beat readily and rhythmically at a rate which varied directly with fluid pressure within its cavity. Further, it was recalled and reemphasized that the dying heart beat irregularly in response to auricular contraction so that a continuous muscular connection, driven at the auricular level was not possible.

Beginning work in 1881 and writing in 1882[11]-1883[12] Gaskell attempted to resolve the issues at least as far as the cold-blooded vertebrate heart was concerned. He invented a suspension device in which threads were attached to the apex of the ventricle and the auricle and to levers which recorded their motion on a smoked drum. A precision clamp occupied the auriculo-ventricular groove and was progressively tightened, so that he was able to produce increase in block in the frog and tortoise while recording auricular and ventricular contractions. The progressive increase in block while maintaining a consistent numerical relationship between the number of auricular and ventricular beats and its reversibility with release of clamp pressure was convincing evidence of a conductive mechanism that might imply that the auricles and ventricles were a continuous sheet of muscle. By placing a clamp or a ligature at different levels, e.g. between sinus and auricle, along the auricle or the ventricle, more rapid beating from above was interrupted and it became rapidly obvious that after a period of asystole the excluded section assumed spontaneous, though slower, beating. A portion of frog cardiac muscle cut from the ventricle and properly nourished in a solution of sodium, calcium and potassium ions can continue to beat spontaneously for as long as 100 hours. So that *"...the part in connection with the sinus continues its regular beat; the part separated from it remains still for a variable time, and then, according to its inherent rhythmical power, develops a rhythmical beat of its own, the rate of that rhythm when developed, and the length of time the standstill lasts, being correlated with the rhythmicity of the tissue. Further, the same experiment can be applied to every part of the heart,...* [13] Finally, gradual thinning of any strip of muscle between auricle and ventricle allowed continuation of the muscular contraction as a peristaltic wave from the auricle to the apex of the ventricle. Only thinning of a muscular bridge eventually produced 2:1, then greater degrees of block.

By 1893 Kent could write, *"...inasmuch as it is well known that the muscular tissue constituting the various chambers of the heart is in these (cold-blooded) animals –perfectly continuous from the sinus venosus through the auricles into the ventricle, and the explanation of the passage of a wave of contraction of the various chambers is upon exactly the same footing as the explanation of the passage of a wave of contraction along any other continuous stretch of muscular tissue. With the mammal, however, the case has up to the present appeared to be different, inasmuch as no such continuity has been known to exist, but on the contrary a distinct break has always been described as existing between the muscular fibres of auricle and ventricle."* Further he wrote, *"Instead of complete muscular continuity throughout the heart, there occurs in the mammalian heart a distinct break—a distinct interval—between the muscle of the auricles and the muscle of the ventricles. The auricular fibres and the ventricular fibres belong to systems of their own, and are separated by a considerable amount of connective tissue at the auriculo-ventricular junction."* [14]

Kent added, *"In the case of the Mammalian heart almost precisely similar results may be obtained by the use of a suitably constructed clamp, and using such an instrument I have been able to verify for the Mammal almost all the effects described by Gaskell as obtained in the frog."* And later, *"For whereas in the past it has been supposed that the mammalian heart differs from the heart of cold-blooded animals in having a complete break of muscular continuity between auricles and ventricles, it has now been shown that no such break exists, but that the auricles are connected with the ventricles both by strands of altered muscular tissue...and by a more complex system of branching and anastomosing fibers which penetrate the fibrous tissue between the two chambers..."* With these and many other supporting publications it had been established that the synchronous rhythmic contraction of the auricle and ventricle was based on the beginning of the contraction at a collection of cells adjacent to the enlargement in the embryologic sinus venosus which became the auricle. Thereafter the contraction wave spread across the auricle to the auriculo-ventricular groove and then, after a pause (which remained unexplained), via a larger or smaller muscular bridge, to the ventricle. Still the general physiology community remained unconvinced.

In spite of Gaskell's work which demonstrated muscular continuity between the two chambers in lower vertebrates, i.e. the tortoise, uncertainty had remained concerning the myogenic hypothesis in mammals where a clear and distinct break existed between the muscle of the auricles and the muscle of the ventricles. Kent in 1893, ten years after Gaskell's publications demonstrated that a muscular connection did exist in the mammalian heart. He found that in young rats well defined continuity of auricular and ventricular muscle existed at birth. While connective tissue separation within the auriculo-ventricular groove developed with maturity, still in adults, well demarcated bands of muscular tissue persisted between the two chambers over a substantial area of the auriculo-ventricular groove, especially at the junction of the septum. The degree of this muscular connection varied in different animals he studied but was found in each.

In the same year (1893) Wilhelm His, Jr independently published his major contribution which more exactly defined and described the auriculo-ventricular bundle and gave its precise location.[15,16] In the embryologic study he demonstrated continuity of the auricular and ventricular musculature and that coordinated contraction existed in the absence of neurons or ganglion cells and that the heart, in all classes of vertebrates beat in the adult, coordinated, sequential manner before it contained cerebrospinal nerves or ganglia.[17,18] He demonstrated further that the assumption of complete separation of the muscles of the two chambers was not accurate. A single site of muscular union did exist as a strand of muscle fibers of the right auricular posterior wall which penetrated the upper portion of the ventricular septum, and forked into right and left branches.

His then had the occasion to examine a patient who had had the Adams-Stokes syndrome, which had not been known by that name in Germany[19] (His Jr. worked in Leipzig). Huchard[20] had given the syndrome that name only in 1889 but the elements which constituted that syndrome had not yet been fully defined. Previous careful studies by contemporary writings had also not clearly defined the components of the syndrome. Charcot, for example, had described episodic syncope associated with a permanently slow pulse in a patient who, on autopsy, had changes in the medulla oblongata and therefore referred to the syndrome as *"pouls lent permanent"* (permanent slow pulse) and considered it a primarily neurologic condition. His Jr's patient had suffered from episodic unconsciousness with respiratory disturbances but without interruption of the slow radial pulse. Arterial and venous pulse recordings had shown the independent contractions of auricular and ventricular beats and the continued auricular beating during the ventricular bradycardia. No ECG was possible in 1893. He considered that the block resulted from damage or destruction of the auriculo-ventricular bundle and hoped that pathology of the bundle could be demonstrated in addition to the anatomy and physiology he had already demonstrated. The patient, however, died without an autopsy and His awaited a second case which, he later wrote, never appeared during his entire clinical career. Still, the coupling, by the discoverer of the muscular conduction system which bears his name, of dissociation of auricular and ventricular activity and the bradycardia and syncope of the Adams-Stokes syndrome gave great impetus to the establishment of the pathophysiology of the diagnosis. In the same year Wenckebach too published a case of Adams-Stokes syndrome and both he and His Jr. suggested a lesion of the auriculo-ventricular bundle (bundle of His) as the cause[21]. In 1903 the syndrome had received sufficient attention that Osler attempted to collect many related conditions into a report of twelve of his cases, without any graphic documentation. 'ON THE SO CALLED STOKES-ADAMS DISEASE (SLOW PULSE WITH SYNCOPAL ATTACKS, &c) and included multiple conditions including presumed bradycardia-asystole caused by carotid sinus massage. Of his twelve cases, one was a young man with bradycardia following a streptococcal infection who recovered; five others he considered severe, four died. A senile group of four, of whom three died during syncopal episodes and a group of two younger healthy men with bradycardia and syncope who survived. In one the bradycardia eventually reversed to a normal cardiac rate and the other who became accustomed to the bradycardia and syncope and also survived at the time of the writing of the manuscript.[22]

Nevertheless, it remained to be demonstrated, that in the mammal, destruction of the atrioventricular pathway would produce partial or complete auriculo-ventricular block as Gaskell had demonstrated in the tortoise. Several years after his 1893 description of the auriculo-ventricular bundle His Jr. verbally described experiments in rabbits which he stated had shown that destruction of the area of the bundle produced block, but he never published this data.[23] In 1904 Humblet[24] reported having cut the auriculo-ventricular bundle of the perfused heart of the dog and produced partial and complete heart block in a way that suggested that, indeed, the anatomic bundle did conduct the impulse. Within a year Hering[25] and Erlanger[26] repeated and improved upon these demonstrations. Erlanger modified Gaskell's twenty year old technique of clamping the auriculo-ventricular groove and applied it to mammals. He placed one blade of the clamp within the left ventricle, so that with increasing compression, and while maintaining continuity of the cardiac tissue, i.e. without cutting or otherwise separating the tissue, progressively greater degrees of block could be produced and then reversed with release of the pressure. Erlanger concluded:

1- Slight increase of pressure will increase the duration of the intersystolic pause;
2- An occasional ventricular beat will be lost;
3- Regularly recurring ventricular asystole will occur, e.g. 9:1, 8:1, etc;
4- Two auricular beats to each ventricular beat (2:1 block);
5- Three auricular beats to each ventricular beat (3:1 block);
6- Complete dissociation, ie complete heart block.

A major impetus to the understanding of the anatomy of the conduction system was the publication in 1906 of Tawara's monograph *"The Conduction System of the Mammalian Heart"*.[27] This beautifully researched and illustrated work described the auriculo-ventricular node, its connection to the previously described His bundle and the Purkinje fibers and tied the entire conduction system from auricle to ventricle into a consistent network. There were four major findings in Tawara's contribution:

1- In all mammals he investigated, including man, the Purkinje fibers formed a spreading and branching network uniting the auricular and ventricular musculature;
2- The muscular system had a similar and uniform appearance in all mammals. It runs from the auricular wall through the fibrous septum between auricle and ventricle and eventually spreads and branches throughout the ventricular wall.

3- This conduction system is an embryologic development and continues to grow with the increase in size of the heart but otherwise does not change.

4- The anatomic and histologic properties of the system suggest that its function is not that of a muscular pump, rather the fibers have different characteristics.

Treatment of the Stokes-Adams syndrome remained elusive and it was rapidly recognized that if that diagnosis were made, early death usually occurred. Following the anatomic descriptions of the normal conduction system came clinical and autopsy descriptions of cases of Stokes-Adams syndrome, each demonstrated degrees of dissociation of auricular and ventricular contractions and more general acceptance of the term "heart block" by which this dissociation was also named. The clinical syndrome was accepted and associated with heart block by most investigators. During a symposium *A Discussion on Some Aspects of Heart-Block* published in the British Medical Journal in 1906, Mackenzie[28] could write: *"The term "heart-block is applied to that condition where the stimulus for contraction passing from auricle to ventricle by the muscular fibres joining the auricle and ventricle, is stopped or "blocked" on account of some defect in those muscle fibres. The main function of the a-v fibres is to convey the stimulus for contraction from auricle to ventricle."* The effect of this dissociation was clearly demonstrated in multiple auricular and ventricular pulse tracings which were commonly used at that time, though the ECG, which had already been described by Waller[29] and Einthoven[30] was not yet used in establishing the diagnosis. In the same symposium Erlanger[31] described that *"...the contraction wave which normally originates in the venous end of the heart is transmitted rapidly through the bulged portions of the heart wall, but suffers an appreciable delay in crossing the auriculo ventricular junction. This normal block to the excitation wave has in man a duration of about one-fifth of a second. By the term "heart-block" as applied to mammals, is understood a state in which the passage of this wave through the auriculo-ventricular junction is interfered with".* By 1908 Lewis had collected 27 additional reported cases of Adams-Stokes syndrome in which lesions were described at the bundle.[32] The lesions included gumma, tumor, infection, sclerosis and deterioration of the bundle. He was then able to conclude, *"Surveying the evidence as a whole, we may say that, knowing that heart block can occur in man, and that it may be associated with lesions of a bundle which has been shown to be essential to conduction in the lower animals, we are justified in concluding that heart block in man may arise as the result of such a lesion."*

By 1910 the major anatomic determinants of auriculo-ventricular conduction in the mammalian heart and specifically in the human had been determined. The function of the Purkinje fibers, which had been described sixty years earlier, had been ascertained and their connection with the conduction bundle described by Kent and His in 1893 established. The auriculo ventricular node at the auricular termination of the His bundle had been described by Tawara working in Aschoff's laboratory and the effect of partial or complete interruption of the bundle had been demonstrated. The clinical complex of bradycardia, syncope and sudden death had been named the Stokes-Adams syndrome by Huchard after those who had described it in earlier years and several series of published cases had begun with descriptions by His and Wenckebach followed by many others who provided pathologic descriptions of destruction of the conduction pathway by infection, sclerosis, gumma and tumor. The anatomic substrate, physiology, pathophysiology, pathology and clinical syndrome were all in place, awaiting significant therapeutic intervention which would not appear for another forty years.

Note: To be consistent, the archaic term auricle has been used throughout instead of atrium.

References

[1] Lewis JK. Stokes-Adams disease. An account of important historical discoveries. Arch Int Med 1958; 101:130-142.

[2] Music D, Rakovec P, Jagodic A, Cibic B. The first description of syncopal attacks in heart block. PACE 1984; 7:301-303.

[3] Morgagni G. Letter the Ninth, Which Treats Epilepsy. In De Sedibus et Causis Morborium, 1761. (The Seats and Causes of Diseases, trans by Benj Alexander). London, Millar & Cadell; 1762:92.

[4] Spens T. History of a case in which there took place a remarkable slowness of the pulse. Medical Commentaries, Edinburgh 1793; 7:463.

[5] Burnett, W. Case of epilepsy, attended with remarkable slowness of the pulse. Med Chir Trans 1827; 13:202.

[6] Adams R. Cases of diseases of the heart accompanied with pathological observations. Dublin Hosp Rep 1827; 4:396.

[7] Stokes R. Observations on some cases of permanently low pulse. Dublin Quart J Med Sci 1846; 2:73-85.

[8] Harvey W.. Exercitatio Anatomica de Motu Cordis et Sanguinis et Animalibus Frankfurt 1628.

[9] Purkinje JE. Mikroskopisch-neurologische Beobachtungen; Arch Anat Physiol Wiss Med 1845; 2/3:281-295.

[10] Gaskell WH. The Contraction of Cardiac Muscle. In Schafer EA. Text-Book fo Physiology, Volume Second. Edinburgh & London, Young J Pentland, 1900, pp 169-180.

[11] Gaskell WH. On the Rhythm of the Heart of the Frog and the Nature of the Action of the Vagus Nerve. Phil Trans 1882; p.993.

[12] Gaskell WH. On the innervation of the heart, with especial reference to the heart of the tortoise. J Physiol 1883; 4:43-127.

[13] Gaskell WH. The Contraction of Cardiac Muscle-The Meaning of the Heart-Beat. In Schafter EA. Text-Book of Physiology. Volume Second. Edinburgh & London, Young J Pentland, 1900, p. 176.

[14] Kent AFS. Researches on the structure and function of the mammalian heart. J Physiol 1893; 14:233-254.

[15] His W, Jr. Die Thetigkeit des embryonalen Herzens und deren Bedeutung fur die Lehre von der Herzbewegung beim Erwacsenen. Arch Med Klin Leipzig 1893; 14:14-49.

[16] His W, Jr. The activity of the embryonic human heart and its significance for the understanding of the heart movement in the adult. Reprinted in English: J Hist Med Allied Sci 1949;4:289-318.

[17] His W, Jr. Zur geschichte des atrioventricul-bundels nebst bemerkungen uber die embryonale Herztetigkeit. Klin Wchnschr 1933; 12:569-574.

[18] His W, Jr. The Story of the Atrioventricular Bundle with Remarks Concerning Embryonic Heart Activity. J Hist Med Allied Sci 1949;4:319-333.

[19] His W, Jr. Ein Fall von Adams-Stokes'scher Krankheit mit ungleighzeitigem Schlagen der Vorhof und Herzkammern (Herzblock). Deutsches Arch fur Klin Med 1899; 64:316-331.

[20] Huchard H. Le maladie de Stokes-Adams. Bull med, Paris 1890; 4:937

[21] Wenckebach KF. Zur Analyse des unregelmessigen Pulses. III. Ueber einige Formen von Allorhythmie und Bradycardie. Zeitschr f klin Med 1900; 39:293-304.

[22] Osler W. On the so-called Stokes-Adams disease (slow pulse with syncopal attacks, etc.). Lancet 1903; 2:516-524.

[23] His W, Jr. Report given at 3rd internation physiological congress in Bern. Zentrallbl Physiol 1895; 9:469.

[24] Humblet M. Allorythmie cardiaque par section du Faisceau de His. Arch Internat de Physiol 1905-1906; 3:330-337.

[25] Hering HE. Uber die Erregungsleitung zwischen Vorkammer und Kammer des Saugethier herzens. Arch ges Physiol 1905; 107:97.

[26] Erlanger J. On the physiology of heart-block in mammals, with especial reference to causation of Stokes-Adams disease. Part I. Observations on an instance of heart block in man. J Exp Med 1905; 7:676-724.

27 Tawara S. Das Reizleitungsystem des Saugetierherzens. Jena, 1906.

28 Mackenzie J. Definition of the term, heart block. Brit Med J 1906; 2:1107-1111.

29 Waller AD. Introductory address on the electromotive properties of the human heart. Brit Med J 1888; 2:751-754.

30 Einthoven W. Ueber die Form des menschlichen Electrocardiogramms. Pfluger's Arch 1895; 60:101-123.

31 Erlanger J. A review of the physiology of heart block in mammals. Brit Med J 1906; 2:1111.

32 Lewis T. A lecture on the occurrence of heart block in man and its causation. Brit Med J 1908; 2:1798-1802.

38.
THE 1998 ACC/AHA GUIDELINES FOR PACEMAKER IMPLANTATION SHOULD BE REVISED

S. Serge Barold, Helen S. Barold, Robert S. Fishel.

Boca Raton and Palm Beach, Florida, USA.

Authoritative guidelines concerning the indications for permanent pacing were originally published in 1984 by a joint committee established by the American College of Cardiology (ACC) and the American Heart Association (AHA). These guidelines were revised in 1991 and 1998[1]. The documents recognize that indications for permanent pacing in an individual patient may not always be clear-cut; however they have been classified into three well known groups. This chapter focuses on a number of shortcomings in the 1998 ACC/AHA guidelines. Some of the problems stem from inherent inconsistencies, lack of detail and imprecise definitions whereas others reflect the rapid evolution of pacing technology and practice in the last few years.

Complete AV Block

The guidelines designate *asymptomatic* complete AV block with ventricular escape rates >40 bpm as a class II indication for pacing. The rate criterion of >40 bpm is arbitrary and unnecessary. It is not the escape rate that is critical to stability, but rather the site of origin of the escape rhythm (junctional or ventricular). Rate instability may not be predictable or obvious. Irreversible acquired complete AV block should be a class I indication for pacing[2].

Neuromuscular Disease. The 1998 guidelines advocate pacing in asymptomatic patients with neuromuscular disease only in complete AV block (class I). Pacing should be considered much earlier in the course of the disease and offered to the asymptomatic patient once any conduction abnormality is noted and subsequent follow-up shows progression[2]. Waiting to satisfy the guidelines may expose patients to a significant risk of syncope or even sudden death.

Second-Degree AV Block

The 1998 guidelines state that second-degree AV block is classified as type I, type II and advanced AV block. The current and past guidelines fail to discuss 2:1 AV block. Although 2:1 AV block can occur either in the AV node or the His-Purkinje system, it cannot be classified as type I or type II, an important concept clearly explained in the 1985 and 1995 ACC/AHA guidelines for clinical intracardiac electrophysiologic studies[3,4].

From Ovsyshcher IE. *Cardiac Arrythmias and Device Therapy: Results and Perspectives for the New Century.* Armonk, NY: Futura Publishing Company, Inc., © 2000

2:1 AV block is best considered as advanced second-degree AV block as are higher degrees of block such as 3:1, 4:1, etc. , according to the definitions promulgated by the World Health Organization and the ACC[5,6]. Confusion arises when the term "advanced AV block" (defined in the guidelines as block of 2 or more P waves) is used in the current guidelines to describe both second- and third-degree AV block (in the section on acute myocardial infarction).

Type I Second-Degree AV Block. Most authorities recommend an electrophysiologic study in *asymptomatic* patients with type I block and bundle branch block (BBB) to determine the site of block (AV node or His-Purkinje system)[7].The 1998 guidelines do not fully endorse this concept because they state that "type I second-degree AV block at intra- or infra-His levels found *incidentally* at electrophysiologic study performed for *other indications*" is a class IIa indication for pacing. Yet it is widely believed that the prognosis of type I and type II infranodal block is similar. Type I second-degree AV block in the His-Purkinje system represents diffuse conduction system disease and should be a class I indication for pacing in the asymptomatic patient.

His bundle recordings are unnecessary in an asymptomatic patient with narrow QRS type I block. However if an electrophysiologic study (performed for other reasons) in such a patient reveals infranodal block, a pacemaker should be recommended as a class I indication because diffuse conduction system disease is likely to be present.

Type II second-degree AV block. The definition of type II second-degree AV block remains problematic even 31 years after the introduction of invasive cardiac electrophysiology[8,9]. The definition in the 1998 guidelines is incomplete and likely to be misinterpreted (…no progressive prolongation of the PR intervals before a blocked beat). The guidelines do not mention the importance of a stable sinus rate in the diagnosis of type II block[8,10-12]. Stability of the sinus rate is an important diagnostic criterion of type II block because a vagal surge can cause simultaneous sinus slowing and AV nodal block, generally a benign condition that can superficially resemble type II block. The literature is replete with diagnostic errors because the requirements of rate stability and an unchanged PR interval after the single blocked impulse are often ignored for the diagnosis of type II block. Furthermore when the PR interval after a blocked impulse is shorter or the P wave is missing (if preempted by an escape complex), the diagnosis of type II block cannot be made regardless of the constancy of *all* the PR intervals before the single nonconducted P wave. Such an arrangement should be considered as unclassifiable in terms of type II block.

With regard to acquired AV block "asymptomatic type II second-degree

AV block" is a class IIa indication and the duration of the QRS complex is not stated. In the section on intraventricular block the guidelines state that bifascicular and trifascicular block with type II block (symptoms not specified) constitutes a class I indication for pacing. This discrepancy is strange considering that 65-80 % of type II blocks are associated with a wide QRS complex[14,15]. Type II block should be a class I indication regardless of QRS duration, symptoms or whether it is paroxysmal or chronic.

First-Degree AV Block

The guidelines now advocate pacing in first-degree AV block (PR >0.30 sec) as a class IIa indication provided there is "documented alleviation of symptoms with temporary pacing"[15]. This subject is discussed in detail in the chapter "Cardiac pacing in patients with marked first-degree AV block" (IE. Ovsyshcher and SS. Barold). Most of the symptomatic patients with symptoms of AV dyssynchrony do not have substantial depression of left ventricular function. The necessity and appropriateness of an acute hemodynamic study are questionable. During a resting AV pacing study, it may not be possible to demonstrate symptomatic improvement and exercise data with a temporary pacemaker are difficult to perform. Therefore it is justifiable to implant a pacemaker without a prior study in selected symptomatic patients whose very long PR interval does not shorten on exercise thereby avoiding additional risk and cost[2].

Intraventricular Conduction Blocks

The guidelines use the term "trifascicular" rather loosely. Electrocardiographic documentation of trifascicular block during 1:1 AV conduction is rare and manifested by right BBB alternating with left BBB or fixed right BBB with alternating left anterior hemiblock and left posterior hemiblock[16]. The guidelines do not mention these conditions that are generally recognized as class I indications for pacing in view of their poor prognosis[17,18]. Like 2:1 AV block the guidelines totally ignore right BBB. Is it because it is neither bifascicular nor trifascicular block? This is an important omission because all the recommendations for pacing in bifascicular block also apply to right BBB itself.

Provocable AV Block

The 1998 guidelines do not address clearly certain types of AV block that require provocative maneuvers for diagnosis[19]. Many workers believe that most of these situations should provide class I indications for pacing. 1) Second- or third-degree His-Purkinje block induced by a "stress test" that involves gradually increasing the rate of atrial pacing[20]. 2) "Fatigue" phenomenon in the His-Purkinje system induced only after cessation of rapid ventricular pacing, a challenge usually performed after the response to an atrial pacing "stress test" is normal[19]. 3) Bradycardia-dependent (phase 4) block (not bradycardia-associated as in vagally-induced AV block) is always *infranodal* and can be evaluated with His bundle recordings by producing bradycardia and pauses by the electrical induction of atrial or ventricular premature beats. 4)Positive response to pharmacological challenge with drugs such as procainamide according to published criteria[21]. 5) Permanent pacing is recommended as a class I indication in symptomatic or asymptomatic patients with exercise-induced AV block (absent at rest) because the vast majority are due to tachycardia-dependent block in the His-Purkinje system and carry a poor prognosis[19,22]. Exercise-induced AV block secondary to myocardial ischemia is rare and does not require pacing unless ischemia cannot be alleviated. The current guidelines also fail to mention that exercise-induced AV block could conceivably be a manifestation of malignant vasovagal syncope a condition treatable pharmacologically.

Reversible AV Block

The guidelines do not address AV block in sleep apnea and related disorders, an important omission because treament of the sleep disorder may eliminate the need for pacing[23].

Acute Myocardial Infarction

The 1998 guidelines and the 1999 ACC/AHA guidelines for the treatment of acute myocardial infarction (MI) introduced "persistent and symptomatic AV block" as a new class I indication for pacing[24]. This statement is vague, and ignores the simple fact that any form of AV block in acute MI can be symptomatic before it resolves completely as in inferior MI. The 1998 ACC/AHA guidelines recommend that in transient second- or third-degree AV block with BBB, an electrophysiologic study should be considered in uncertain cases to assess the site and extent of heart block. Missing from these new guidelines is how to interpret the data from an EPS in the decision process to implant a permanent pacemaker[2].

The 1998 ACC/AHA guidelines classify persistent AV nodal block as a class II indication without defining what "persistent" means, a limitation that also appears in the 1999 ACC/AHA guidelines for the treatment of acute MI. It is therefore possible that pacemakers may be implanted unnecessarily considering the wide latitude of the ACC/AHA recommendation[25]. The guidelines should state categorically that permanent pacing is almost never needed in patients with inferior MI and narrow QRS AV block. Even relatively uncommon intra-Hisian block in inferior MI is almost always reversible, and rarely requires permanent pacing[26]. The term "persistent" has been interpreted by some workers to mean 14-16 days, a cut-off point that seems satisfactory[25]. More conservative workers have indicated that pacemaker implantation should not be considered unless second- or third-degree AV block is present 3 weeks after MI. On the basis of the 14-16 day criterion the need for permanent pacing in survivors who develop second- and/or third-degree AV block should not exceed 1-2% of the entire AV block group whether or not they are treated with thrombolytics[25].

Rarely, a patient with preexistent right BBB block and left anterior hemiblock presents with an acute inferior MI complicated by left posterior hemiblock and the development of complete heart block in the His-Purkinje system. A permanent pacemaker seems justified in this situation.

Other Types of Bradycardia

Many authorities agree that spontaneous sinus pauses are abnormal if they exceed 3 sec without intervening escape. However, the role of permanent pacing in these patients has not been established. Nevertheless some feel that such a pause justifies a permanent pacemaker even in an asymptomatic patient. Does a pause >3 sec or rate < 30bpm during sleep (in the absence of sleep apnea) constitute a class II indication? The guidelines should discuss these difficult issues and provide a practical approach to these common problems.

Technology of Antibradycardia Pacing in Specific Situations

Clear recommendations for the optimal use of pacing technology are required for patients with associated conditions such as coronary artery disease, paroxysmal supraventricular tachyarrhythmias, cardiac transplantation, vasovagal syncope and implanted defibrillators.

Hypertrophic Obstructive Cardiomyopathy

The guidelines are vague about what a "significant" resting or provoked left ventricular outflow tract gradient should be in patients with hypertrophic obstructive cardiomyopathy. No firm consensus exists, but a resting gradient >30mm Hg or a provoked gradient >50 mmHg (or both) are generally considered as significant to consider pacing in drug-refractory patients[2,27].

Dilated Cardiomyopathy

The guidelines do not mention congestive heart failure but it is implied. They specify that pacing as a class IIb indication is appropriate in patients with "symptomatic drug-refractory dilated cardiomyopathy with prolonged

PR interval when acute hemodynamic studies have demonstrated hemodynamic benefit of pacing". This is a highly controversial recommendation because it is not supported by data. Indeed conventional dual-chamber pacing benefits very few patients with marked depression of left ventricular systolic function even those with a long PR interval and QRS prolongation[27]. The selection criteria are discussed in the chapter "Cardiac pacing in patients with marked first-degree AV block" (IE. Ovsyshcher and SS. Barold).   In the text of the guidelines is a statement that "preliminary data...suggest that simultaneous biventricular pacing may improve cardiac hemodynamics and thus lead to subjective and objective symptom improvement". Biventricular or left ventricular pacing is more promising but still investigational.

Prevention of Paroxysmal Atrial Fibrillation
The guidelines give drug-refractory paroxysmal atrial fibrillation (AF) a class IIb indication for prevention by pacing. Importantly the guidelines do not specify whether this recommendation refers to patients with or without bradycardia. Although acute studies suggest that 2 site atrial pacing may prevent AF inducibility[27], there is no real evidence so far that long-term single-site or multisite pacing prevents AF in the absence of underlying *bradycardia.*

REFERENCES

1. Gregoratos G; Cheitlin MD; Conill A, et al. ACC/AHA guidelines for implantation of cardiac pacemakers and antiarrhythmia devices: a report of the American College of Cardiology/American Heart Association Task Force on Practice Guidelines (Committee on Pacemaker Implantation). J Am Coll Cardiol 1998; 31:1175-1209.
2. Hayes DL, Barold SS, Camm AJ et al. Evolving indications for permanent pacing. An appraisal of the 1998 American College of Cardiology/ American Heart Association guilines. Am J Cardiol 1998; 82:1082-1086.
3. Zipes DP, Gettes LS, Akhtar M et al. Guidelines for clinical intracardiac electrophysiologic studies. A report of the American College of Cardiology/American Heart Association Task Force on assessment of diagnostic and therapeutic cardiovascular procedures (Subcommittee to Assess Clinical Intracardiac Electrophysiological Studies). J Am Coll Cardiol 1989;14:1827-1842.
4. Zipes DP, DiMarco JP, Gillette PC, et al. Guidelines for clinical intracardiac electrophysiological and catheter ablation procedures. A report of the American College of Cardiology/American Heart

Association Task Force on Practice Guidelines (Committee on Clinical Intracardiac Electrophysiologic and Catheter Ablation Procedures), developed in collaboration with the North American Society of Pacing and Electrophysiology. J Am Coll Cardiol 1995; 26:555-573.

5. WHO/ISC Task Force.Definition of terms related to cardiac rhythm. Am Heart 1978; 95:796-806.

6. Surawitz B, Uhley H, Borun R et al. Optimal Electrocardiography. Tenth Bethesda Conference co-sponsored by the American College of Cardiology and Health Resourses Administration of the Department of Health, Education, and Welfare. Task Force 1. Standardization of terminology and interpretation. Am J Cardiol 1978;41:130-144.

7. Ursell S, Habbab MA, El-Sherif N. Atrioventricular and intraventricular conduction disorders. Clinical aspects. In El-Sherif N, Samet P, (Eds), Cardiac Pacing and Electrophysiology, 3rd Edition, Philadelphia PA, W.B. Saunders 1991;140-169.

8. Barold SS, Barold HS. Pitfalls in the characterization of second-degree AV block. *Heartweb* (Internet) 1997; Article #97040001.

9. Barold SS. ACC/AHA guidelines for implantation of cardiac pacemakers: how accurate are the definitions of atrioventricular and intraventricular conduction blocks? PACE 1993;16:1221-1226.

10. Rardon DP, Miles WM, Mitrani RD, et al. Atrioventricular block and dissociation in Zipes DP, Jalife J. Cardiac Electrophysiology: From Cells to Bedside, 2nd Edition, Philadelphia, Saunders, 1995:935-942.

11. Wolbrette DL, Naccarelli GV. Bradycardias. Sinus nodal dysfunction and AV conduction disturbances, In Topol EJ (Ed), Comprehensive Cardiovascular Medicine, Philadelphia, Lippincott 1998:1803-26.

12. O'Keefe JH Jr, Hammil SC, Zolnick MR et al. Electrocardiography study guide. Scoring criteria and definitions. In Murphy JG (Ed), Mayo Clinic Cardiology Review, Armonk NY, Futura 1997:427-445.

13. Narula OS. Clinical concepts of spontaneous and induced atrioventricular block. In Mandel WJ (Ed), Cardiac Arrhythmias 3rd Edition, Their Mechanisms, Diagnosis and Management. Philadelphia PA, J.B. Lippincott, 1995:441-459.

14. Puech P, Grolleau R, Guimond C. Incidence of different types of A-V block and their localization by His bundle recordings. In Wellens HJJ, Lie KI, Janse MJ (Eds), The Conduction System of the Heart. Structure, Function, and Clinical Implications, Leiden The Netherlands H.E. Stenfert Kroese B.V. 1976:467-484.

15. Barold SS. Indications for permanent pacing in first-degree block. Class I, II, or III ? PACE 1996;19:747-751.

16. Rosenbaum MB, Elizari MV, Lazzari JO. Clinical evidence of hemiblock: syndrome of RBBB and intermittent LAH and LPH.

Trifascicular block. In: Rosenbaum MB, Elizari MV, Lazzari JO, (Eds.). The Hemiblocks. Oldsmar, FL, Tampa Tracings:1970:55-69.

17. Josephson ME. Clinical Cardiac Electrophysiology: Techniques and Interpretation, 2nd Edition, Philadelphia: Lea& Febiger, 1993:117-149.

18. Wellens HJJ, Conover MB. The ECG in Emergency Decision Making. Philadelphia, WB Saunders, 1992:115-128.

19. Barold SS. Indications for pacing in acquired atrioventricular block. The 1991 ACC/AHA guidelines should be revised. In Barold SS, Mugica J.(Eds), Recent Advances in Cardiac Pacing. Goals for the 21st Century, Armonk NY, Futura 1998:115-134.

20. Petrac D, Radic B, Birtic K, et al. Prospective evaluation of infrahisal second-degree AV block induced by atrial pacing in the presence of chronic bundle branch block and syncope. PACE 1996;19:784-792.

21. Englund A, Bergfeldt L, Rosenqvist M. Pharmacological stress testing of the His-Purkinje system in patients with bifascicular block. PACE 1998;21:1979-1987.

22. Sumiyoshi M, Nakata Y, Yasuda M, et al. Clinical and electrophysiologic features of exercise-induced atrioventricular block. Am Heart J, 1996;132:1277 -1281.

23. Stegman SS, Burroughs JM, Henthorn RW. Asymptomatic bradyaarhythmias as a marker for sleep apnea. Appropriate recognition and treatment may reduce the need for pacemaker therapy. PACE 1996;19:899-904.

24. Ryan TJ, Antman EM, Brooks NH, et al. 1999 update: ACC/AHA Guidelines for the Management of Patients With Acute Myocardial Infarction: Executive Summary and Recommendations: A report of the American College of Cardiology/American Heart Association Task Force on Practice Guidelines (Committee on Management of Acute Myocardial Infarction). Circulation 1999;100:1016-1030.

25. Barold SS. American College of Cardiology/American Heart Association guidelines for pacemaker implantation after acute myocardial infarction. What is persistent advanced AV block at the atrioventricular node? Am J Cardiol 1997;80:770-774.

26. Barold SS, Barold HS. Infranodal AV block in acute inferior myocardial infarction. Heartweb 1997 (on internet) Article No. 97040002.

27. Barold SS. New indications for pacing. In Singer I, Barold SS, Camm AJ, (Eds), Nonpharmacological Therapy of Arrhythmias for the 21st Century. The State of the Art, Armonk NY, Futura 1998:775-817.

28. Saksena S, Delfaut P,Prakash A et al. Multisite electrode pacing for prevention of atrial fibrillation. J Cardiovasc Electrophysiol 1998:9 (8 Suppl):S155-162.

39.
THERAPY CONCEPT AND CLINICAL RELEVANCE OF CLOSED LOOP STIMULATION

M. Schaldach[1], M. Schier[1], T. Christ[2], M. Hubmann[3], K. Malinowski[4]

[1]Department of Biomedical Engineering, Friedrich-Alexander-University Erlangen-Nuremberg, Germany
[2]Institute for Pharmacology, Technical University Dresden, Germany
[3]Department of Internal Medicine, Waldkrankenhaus Erlangen, Germany
[4]Department of Cardiology, Helios-Clinics Aue, Germany

Introduction

The treatment of pathologic limitations of the cardiovascular system has changed from simply eliminating particular symptoms to a more general support of the cardiac, vascular, and neurohumoral control mechanisms. This important evolution was initiated with the introduction of Closed Loop Stimulation (CLS) as a therapeutic concept for electrostimulation of the heart. In the meanwhile, this management method has been established as a standard therapy for the treatment of various diseases of the cardiovascular system, which are not limited to forms of sick sinus syndrome. The basis for the development of this therapeutic strategy and the realization of the clinical applicability was a detailed understanding of the physiology of the cardiovascular system. This understanding has taken into account the physical, technical, as well as medical aspects, thereby building the prerequisite for an interdisciplinary process of research and evaluation.

Physiology of the Cardiovascular System

The basis for a discussion of the complex structure of the cardiovascular system is the definition of its main task and the corresponding parameters. In order to ensure a continuous supply of all body cells with nutriments, oxygen, other substances, and the disposition of metabolic products, a stable and appropriate perfusion pressure has to be provided by the cardiovascular system.[1] Within that regulation process, mean arterial blood pressure (MABP) and total peripheral resistance (TPR) play a major role, since local metabolic changes directly respond to the vasomotors, while the baroreceptors assess the appropriate perfusion by continuously measuring blood pressure. MABP as a central parameter of cardiovascular regulation, is influenced by numerous factors. These include physiologic variations due to changing organic requirements, as well as the consequences of pathologic structural or cellular changes (Figure 1).

From Ovsyshcher IE. *Cardiac Arrythmias and Device Therapy: Results and Perspectives for the New Century.* Armonk, NY: Futura Publishing Company, Inc., © 2000

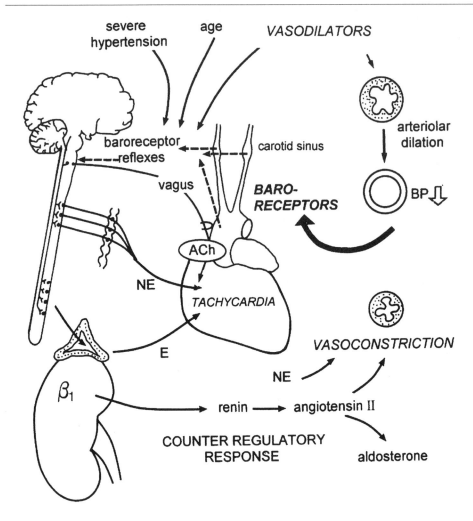

Figure 1. Interaction of mechanisms in cardiovascular control.

Various activities of daily life are coupled with numerous individual requirements to the organism, which cause local and global constriction or dilation of the vessels. Increasing workload of certain parts of the organism initially causes vasodilation, in order to ensure an elevated blood flow through the corresponding tissue. With the help of neural and humoral control mechanisms, the heart starts to counteract the decreasing blood pressure by increasing the cardiac output.[2] As these regulation processes act continuously and mostly delay-free the blood pressure remains stable or shows a slight increase during phases of increased workload despite the significantly decreasing TPR. The baroreceptors, which are continuously monitoring the blood pressure, are the most important natural sensor for providing hemodynamic stability on a beat-to-beat basis.[3] Sudden changes in the TPR are immediately responded by antagonistic variations in the heart rate. This behavior is reflected in the cardiac response to provoked blood pressure changes during Valsalva maneuvers,[4-5] as well as in the characteristic heart rate variability,[6-7] which indicates continuous pressure stabilizing short-term regulations.. A detailed analysis of the neurohumoral mediation of necessary compensatory variations in cardiac output essentially leads to a discussion of the important role of myocardial and circulating catecholamines and their effect on cardiovascular parameters. Changing load stages cause variations in the dynamics of catecholamine release via the medullary circulation center. Hence, a decreased TPR, triggered by higher metabolic needs, initiates a pronounced release of catecholamines and adapts the cardiac output with the help of the known cardiac mechanisms: chronotropy, inotropy , and dromotropy. Pathologic limitations of the cardiovascular system significantly impact the main parameters, such as blood pressure. The main difference between pathophysiologic and physiologic effects is the lack of balance in pathologic situations and, thus, the inability of the system to appropriately counteract deviations in the perfusion pressure. This limitation can be caused by malfunctions of cardiovascular sensors, neurohumoral balance, or vascular and cardiac mechanisms.

Thermodynamic description
Although the functioning and interaction of the various cardiovascular mechanisms, as well as the wide range of pathologic changes give the impression of incalculable complexity, the system can be described in a very compact way using the terminology of thermodynamics. Based on mechanical explanation of the heart cycle, the efficiency of the heart can be defined as the "relationship between cardiac work output (which mainly depends on stroke volume and mean arterial blood pressure), and myocardial energy consumption, which can be quantified by analyzing the cardiac oxygen uptake." Proceeding to the thermodynamic refinement of the physical description, discussed by Cesarman et al., the entropy of the heart becomes the parameter of global interest, which is indirectly proportional to cardiac efficiency.[8-10] The entropy describes the spontaneous movement of energy towards the random distribution of matter and heat. Hence, the main aim of myocardial as well as all other biological cells is to continuously reduce entropy, thereby maximizing the ability to perform work in a highly effective way. The various mechanisms and subsystems of the cardiovascular system permanently balance all entropy- determining factors, including the availability of glucose, lipides, ATP, oxygen, catechol-

amines and workload. This occurs in order to counteract the natural tendency of physical systems to approach a random distribution of matter and energy (Figure 2). In this description, the inclusion of periodic cardiac contractions leads to the thermodynamic separation of systole and diastole. The minimization of entropy and, thus, the restoration of excitability and contractility, is subject to mechanical diastole; whereas systole is consuming these energy resources and simultaneously increasing entropy. The knowledge of these thermodynamic aspects enables new possibilities in understanding pathologic limitations within the cardiovascular system. The majority of known pathologic anomalies of the heart, the vascular system and the neurohumoral regulation, can be defined as an inability of the system to appropriately balance the entropy- determining factors, leading to reduced entropy disposition and decreased cardiac efficiency. The resulting pathological biochemical and structural changes draw the system towards a suboptimal working point with the absence of a stable minimum energy production. The analysis of different clinical manifestations emphasize the applicability of thermodynamic theories for the functionality of the cardiovascular system, as discussed in the two examples above. In patients with congestive heart failure the attenuation of the cellular ability to minimize entropy causes structural changes, which again amplify the initial process of pathologic cellular modifications. In cases of neurocardiogenic syncope, the system's ability to reduce entropy is intact, but the sudden neurohumoral imbalance disables the necessary transfer of minimum entropy into effective cardiac work. With respect to this knowledge, a more global approach for developing and providing therapeutic measures is necessary. Supporting the cardiovascular system is the main task of minimizing entropy production rather than simply treating particular symptoms. This might significantly improve the effectiveness of therapy by initiating remodeling of the structural changes and offering preventative measures.

Concept and technology of Closed Loop Stimulation

The practical way of supporting the cardiovascular system in this global manner is CLS, which is based on the principle of disturbance variable feedforward. Typical pathologic changes limit the dynamic range of one of several control mechanisms, thereby causing significant delays and deviations in the cardiovascular regulation. The continuous stabilization of an appropriate perfusion is disabled and the metabolic requirements can be fulfilled only within certain limits. As in some physiologic control loops (especially if the control is acting with long reaction times), the disturbance variable feedforward is a method to eliminate these restrictions.

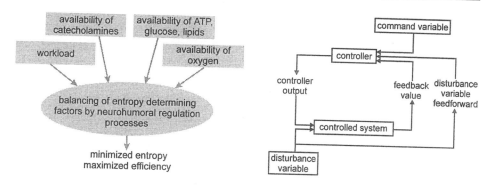

Figure 2. Left: Thermodynamic aspect of cardiovascular regulation. Right: Principle of disturbance variable feedforward for the acceleration of slowly reacting control loops.

The direct transmission of information (about disturbance variables in the control center) significantly accelerates the control and avoids deviations of the controlled variable due to sudden changing requirements (Figure 2). The CLS pacemaker has direct access to the disturbance variable, i.e. the hemodynamic requirement, by monitoring the inotropic mechanism of contraction dynamics. The pacemaker bypasses the diseased sinus node reaction by providing appropriate heart rates. In this way, the continuous and immediate balancing of the different mechanisms is reestablished and the system is able to periodically reduce entropy and perform effective work. This ensures the permanent adequate supply of the organism.

During several years of interaction between technical development and clinical research, a technology for the realization of this principle was designed and validated. Clinical consequences, benefits, and applicability have been analyzed within numerous investigations. Technically, changes in the inotropic state are assessed via unipolar intracardiac impedance measurements. Biphasic subthreshold pulses are injected between the tip of the ventricular lead and the pacemaker housing. The resulting potential difference is measured between the same points. Changes in myocardial contractility result in varying morphology of the measured unipolar intracardiac impedance curve.[11-12]

Validation of the System

Based on the known correlation between unipolar impedance changes and inotropic drive,[13] the realization of a CLS pacemaker based on the monitoring of contraction dynamics is possible. As a consequence of the pacemaker integration into the circulatory regulation system, it is expected that the heart rate for patients with CLS systems is influenced by changes in the level of circulating catecholamines. During a pharmacological stress test using the catecholamine dobutamine, heart rates of patients with CLS pacemakers were examined. The increase in myocardial contractility was measured using an echocardiographic method for dP/dt determination. The patients showed a significantly increased stimulated heart rate during dobutamine infusion. A few minutes after the end of the infusion, all patients reached their original resting heart rate. The inotropic parameter dP/dt_{max} increased in parallel during infusion. These results confirm the hypothesis of a chronotropic reaction to increased catecholamine levels with the CLS pacemaker, by re-synchronizing inotropic and chronotropic control mechanisms.[14]

Clinical Implications

A closed loop system, which forwards the disturbance variable input to the cardiac control mechanisms, should continuously provide adequate organic perfusion. As a consequence, it shows the same reactions on external influences and comparable behavior of the cardiovascular parameters as in the healthy organism, as previously discussed. Performing the Valsalva maneuver in patients with the CLS pacemaker yields the characteristic curves of blood pressure and heart rate during the forced expiration, against the pressure of 30 mmHg (Figure 3).[15] This typical behavior can only be observed, if the pacing rate is controlled by the baroreceptor reflex. Thus, the CLS pacemaker controls the heart rate based on neurohumoral regulation, and establishes a continuous feedback loop between pacemaker and cardiovascular system.

The analysis of heart rate variability confirms the active rate- controlling role of the baroreceptors for patients with CLS pacemaker therapy. Parasympathetic and sympathetic activities cause characteristic fluctuations in heart rate that are related to special frequency ranges. In 16 patients with CLS pacemakers and in a control group of 16 chronotropically competent subjects, a high quality ECG was performed at rest and during exercise. The data regarding heart rate variability was automatically deducted from ECG recordings by using special software for analysis. Power spectral density 1 week after automatic CLS initialization consisted of a well-pronounced LF-part and HF-part indicating parasympathetic and sympathetic influence. No difference in the normalized power values was found in the comparison between CLS and control group, indicating a strong correlation of heart rate variability between CLS and sinus node functionality (Figure 3).[16]

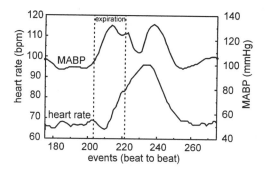 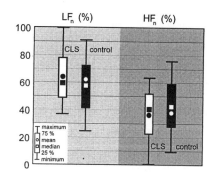

Figure 3. Left: Response of mean arterial blood pressure (MABP) and heart rate of a CLS patient to Valsalva maneuver. Right: Statistics of normalized power spectral density HF$_n$-part and LF$_n$-part of heart rate variability at rest for CLS patients and control group.

Conclusion

The presented investigations of CLS therapy demonstrate the successful integration of the pacemaker into the natural cardiovascular control loop. The above described effects of different physiologic processes on cardiovascular mechanisms, and the resulting behavior of the mean arterial blood pressure are similarly observed in patients with CLS therapy. This indicates the optimal support of the system in maintaining efficient supply to the organism. Returning to the thermodynamic description of the cardiovascular system, CLS can be characterized as an auxiliary mechanism for balancing entropy- determining factors in cases of pathologic limitations of one or more natural regulation modules.

References

1. Schmidt RF, Thews G (Hrsg). Physiologie des Menschen. Springer, Berlin, 1995.
2. Opie LH. The Heart: Physiology, from Cell to Circulation. Lipincott-Raven, Philadelphia, 1998.
3. Roddie IC, Shepherd JT. Receptors in the high-pressure and low-pressure vascular systems. Their role in the reflex control of the human circulation. Lancet 1958: 493-496.
4. Porth CJ, Bamrah VS, Tristani FE, et al. The Valsalva maneuver: mechanisms and clinical implications. Heart Lung. 1984; 13 (5): 507-518.
5. Smith SA, Stallard TJ, Salih MM, et al. Can sinoaortic baroreceptor heart rate reflex sensitivity be determined from phase IV of the Valsalva manoeuvre? Cardiovasc Res. 1987; 12 (6): 422-427.

6. Malliani A, Pagani M, Lombardi F, et al. Cardiovascular neural regulation explored in the frequency domain. Circulation. 1991; 84: 482-492.

7. Lombardi F, Malliani A, Pagani M, et al. Heart rate variability and its sympatho-vagal modulation. Cardiovasc Res. 1996; 32: 208-216.

8. Cesarman E, Brachfeld N. Thermodynamics of the Myocardial Cell. A Redefinition of its Active and Resting States. Chest, 1977, 72, 296.

9. Cesarman E, Brachfeld N. Bioenergetics and Thermodynamics of the Cardiac Cycle. In: New Horizons, Cardiovascular Disease. Part 1. Kones, RJ (ed). Futura, New York Mount Kisko, 1980.

10. Cesarman E. The Four Diastoles. A Cardiac Cycle Model. Acta Cardiol, 1990, XLV, 15.

11. Schaldach M, Hutten H. Intracardiac Impedance to determine sympathetic activity in rate responsive pacing. PACE. 1992; 15: 1778-1786.

12. Schaldach M. Automatic adjustment of pacing parameters based on intracardiac impedance measurements. PACE. 1990; 13: 1702-1710.

13. Osswald S, Hilti P, Cron T, et al. Correlation of Intracardiac Impedance and Right Ventricular Contractility During Dobutamine Stresstest. Prog Biomed Res. 1999; 4 (3): 166-170.

14. Christ T, Brattström A, Kühn H, et al. Effects of Circulating Catecholamines on the Pacing Rate of the Closed Loop Stimulation Pacemaker. Prog Biomed Res 1998; 3 (3): 143-146.

15. Hubmann M, Thaufelder H, Vestner J, et al. Particularities of Pacemaker Therapy in Elderly Patients. Prog Biomed Res. 1999 4 (2): 130-135.

16. Malinowski K. Heart Rate Variability in Patients with Closed Loop Stimulation. Prog Biomed Res. 199; 4 (4): 445-448.

40.

OUTCOME OF PATIENTS WITH SICK SINUS SYNDROME TREATED BY DIFFERENT PACING MODALITIES.

Lene Kristensen, MD, Jens Cosedis Nielsen, MD, Henning Rud Andersen, MD, D.MSc.

Department of Cardiology, Skejby Sygehus, Aarhus University Hospital, Aarhus, Denmark.

Introduction

Sick sinus syndrome (SSS) is the indication for pacemaker implantation in 40-50% of all patients undergoing primary pacemaker implantation.[1] It is well recognized, that cardiac pacing is effective in abolishing bradycardia-related symptoms in patients with SSS, the most optimal pacing mode is, however, still debated.

Patients with SSS and normal atrioventricular (AV) conduction and no bundle branch block can be treated with either single lead atrial pacing (AAI), single lead ventricular pacing (VVI), or dual chamber pacing (DDD). AAI pacing preserves both AV synchrony and the normal ventricular activation pattern, but if AV block occurs, a re-operation is needed. DDD pacing also preserves AV synchrony, but disturbs the ventricular activation pattern, whereas VVI pacing disturbs both AV synchrony and the ventricular activation pattern. Both DDD and VVI pacing confer protection against bradycardia in case of AV block. Despite growing evidence, that AAI and DDD pacing are both clinically superior and cost effective as compared with VVI pacing, VVI pacing is still used in most countries in approximately 50% of the patients with SSS.

The present review will focus upon the impact of different pacing modes on the clinical outcome in patients with SSS.

Atrial Fibrillation

Atrial fibrillation (AF) is a part of the natural history of SSS.[2] The impact of different pacing modalities on the development of chronic AF has been reported in several studies. In an observational study, Rosenqvist et al.[3] reported, that after 4-years of follow up, the incidence of chronic AF was 47% in the VVI group and 6.7% in the AAI group. Santini et al. reported AF in 47% of patients treated with VVI pacing, 13% in patients treated with DDD pacing, and 4% in those treated with AAI pacing after 5 years of follow-up.[4] In another large observational study of 507 patients treated with AAI/DDD pacemaker (n=395) or VVI pacemaker (n=112), Sgarbossa et al. observed chronic AF in 17% of the patients after a mean follow-up

From Ovsyshcher IE. *Cardiac Arrythmias and Device Therapy: Results and Perspectives for the New Century.* Armonk, NY: Futura Publishing Company, Inc., © 2000

of 59 months.[5] Independent predictors of chronic AF were: prior history of paroxysmal AF (p<0.001); use of preimplant antiarrhythmic drug (p<0.001); VVI pacing mode (p=0.003); age (p=0.005); and valvular heart disease (p<0.001). In patients without a history of paroxysmal AF, the incidence of chronic AF was 0% during the first 5 years of follow up for both pacing modalities.

In 1994 Andersen et al.[6] reported the first randomized trial comparing AAI and VVI pacing in 225 patients with SSS. After a mean follow-up of 40 months, 23% of the VVI paced patients had AF at one or more ambulatory visits compared with 14% in the AAI group. Chronic AF developed in 13% of the patients in the VVI group and in 7% of the patients in the AAI group. In 1997, after an extended follow-up to a mean of 5.5 years, the differences between the AAI and VVI groups had enhanced substantially in favor of AAI pacing.[7] Both AF and chronic AF were significantly reduced in the AAI group (relative risk 0.54, p=0.012 and relative risk 0.35, p=0.004, respectively).[7]

Recently, the PASE (Pacemaker Selection in the Elderly) trial, which is the first randomized trial of VVI-R versus DDD-R pacing, was published.[8] A total of 407 patients aged at least 65 years were included, 175 had SSS. Concerning AF, a strong trend favoring DDD-R pacing was seen after 30 months of follow-up in the subgroup of patients with SSS (19% *vs.* 28%, p=0.06).

In the Pac-A-Tach (Pacemaker Atrial Tachycardia) trial, 198 patients with brady-tachy syndrome were randomized to DDD-R (n=100) or VVI-R pacing,[9] the primary endpoint was recurrence of AF. At 2 years follow-up, 48% of the patients in the DDD-R group and 43% of the patients in the VVI-R group had recurrence of AF (p=0.09).

In the first large-scale, randomized trial, CTOPP (Canadian Trial Of Physiological Pacing),[10] comparing VVI (n=1474) and physiological pacing (n=1095), AF was the only endpoint in which a significant difference occurred between the treatment groups after 3 years of follow-up. The Kaplan-Meier curves of AF separated after 2 years of pacing and a 19% risk reduction was observed in the physiological paced group (p=0.036).[11] The CTOPP trial included both patients with AV block and SSS, thirty-four percent of the patients had SSS.

Thus, based on these results, it seems evident, that VVI pacing is associated with an increased risk of AF in patients with SSS as compared with AAI pacing. DDD pacing also seems to cause less AF than VVI pacing although the documentation for this superiority of DDD pacing is less clear than for AAI pacing.

Thromboembolism

There is a definite risk of thromboembolism in patients with SSS, both before and after implantation of a pacemaker.[5, 12] In observational studies, the incidence of thromboembolic events is higher after implantation of a VVI pacemaker than after implantation of an AAI pacemaker[3] or a DDD pacemaker.[4]

In a review by Sutton and Kenny,[2] the incidence of thromboembolism in SSS patients with VVI pacemakers was 13% (n=532) and only 1.6% in those with AAI pacemakers (n=321) (p<0.001). Sgarbossa et al. did a follow-up on 507 patients paced for SSS (22% VVI, 4% AAI, 74% DDD). Thirty-two patients developed stroke (mean follow up 65 months). By multivariate analysis, history of cerebrovascular disease and ventricular pacing mode were the strongest predictors for stroke.[5]

In the randomized trial by Andersen et al.,[6] arterial thromboembolism occurred in 17.4% of patients in the VVI group versus in 5.5% of patients in the AAI group during a mean follow-up of 40 months (p=0.0083). After an extended follow-up to a mean of 5.5 years,[7] thromboembolic events were significantly reduced in the AAI group (relative risk 0.47, p=0.023).[6] Multivariate analysis identified randomization to VVI-pacing and brady-tachy syndrome at the time of randomization as the only variables significantly associated with risk of thromboembolism during follow-up (p=0.04). This finding may partly reflect the higher frequency of AF observed with ventricular pacing.

In the Pac-A-Tach trial[9] comparing VVI-R and DDD-R pacing, thromboembolism occurred in 11 patients in the VVI-R group and in 4 patients in the DDD-R group. In the CTOPP trial, comparing VVI-R and DDD-R pacing,[10] there was no difference in the incidence of arterial thromboembolism after 3 years of follow-up.[10] Thus, based on these trials, it seems evident that VVI pacing is associated with an increased risk of thromboembolism compared with AAI and DDD pacing.

Heart Failure

Many experimental studies have demonstrated, that cardiac output is higher during AAI pacing than during DDD pacing and further decreases during VVI pacing, where AV synchrony is lost.[13, 14] Right ventricular apical pacing during VVI and DDD pacing causes an asynchronous and prolonged ventricular electrical activation and an abnormal mechanical contraction of the ventricles, which is associated with a reduced global left ventricular ejection fraction as compared with normal sinus rhythm or AAI pacing.[14] Furthermore, experimental data have indicated that chronic ventricular pacing may be harmful to the left ventricular function.[13, 15]

In several observational studies of patients with SSS, single chamber ventricular pacing (VVI) has been associated with a higher incidence of congestive heart failure (CHF) than single chamber atrial pacing (AAI).[3, 16-18] In the study by Rosenqvist et al., CHF occurred in 23% after 2 years and in 37% after 4 years in the VVI paced patients, whereas in the AAI paced patients, CHF occurred in only 7% and 15% of patients after 2 and 4 years, respectively.[3, 16] In contrast Sgarbossa et al.[19] found no difference in congestive heart failure between patients with VVI pacemakers (n=112) and patients with physiological pacemakers (AAI: n=19 and DDD: n=376) during long term follow up. In that study impairment of the ventricular function owing to right ventricular pacing may have occurred in both groups, because 95% of the patients in the "physiological" group were treated with DDD pacing and therefore actually stimulated in the ventricle. In the prospective study by Andersen et al.[7] comparing VVI and AAI pacing in 225 patients with SSS, there was no significant difference in congestive heart failure after a mean follow up of 40 months. During extended follow-up to a mean of 5.5 years, NYHA functional class increased in 10 patients in the AAI group versus in 35 patients in the VVI group (p<0.0005), use of diuretics increased in the VVI group, but not in the AAI group, and dyspnea and crural oedema were more common in the VVI group. These findings were associated with a decreased left ventricular fractional shortening due to an increase in left ventricular end-diastolic volume and an excess dilatation of the left atrium in the VVI group as compared with the AAI group.[20] Death due to CHF occurred in 7 patients in the VVI group (1.1% per year) versus in 3 patients in the AAI group (0.5% per year) p=0.18. Thus, the prospective findings support findings from observational studies, that VVI pacing is associated with excess CHF and CHF mortality as compared with AAI pacing in patients with SSS.

In the PASE trial[8] and in the Pac-A-Tac[9] trial, CHF was not an end point. In the CTOPP trial, there was no significant differences between the physiological paced group and the VVI paced group in "hospitalization for CHF" or "functional capacity" estimated by 6 min. walk test, which were secondary endpoints.[21]

Therefore, in patients with SSS, VVI pacing increases the incidence of CHF as compared with AAI pacing. Apparently, the harmful effects of VVI pacing takes years to become clinically important. At present there is no convincing evidence, that DDD pacing causes less CHF than VVI pacing.

Mortality

A few observational studies comparing VVI pacing with no pacemaker treatment indicate that the survival rate among paced patients with SSS is similar to the survival rate of the non-paced population. In the study comparing VVI and AAI pacing by Rosenqvist et al.,[3] mortality was significantly higher during VVI pacing (23%) than during AAI pacing (8%) after 4-years of follow-up. In contrast, in the largest, long-term observational study comparing DDD pacing and VVI pacing in SSS, Sgarbossa et al. found no significant influence of pacing mode on mortality after 59 months of follow up.[22]

In the randomized trial by Andersen et al.,[7] the total mortality, after follow-up to a mean of 5.5 years, was significantly less in the AAI group (relative risk 0.66, p=0.045), and the excess mortality in the VVI group was due to cardiovascular deaths.[7]

The three trials comparing VVI-R and DDD-R pacing modes have reached different results on mortality. In the PASE trial,[8] there was a strong trend favoring DDD-R pacing in the secondary endpoint "all-cause death" (12% *vs.* 20%, p=0.09) in the subgroup of patients with SSS after 30 months of follow-up. In the large CTOPP trial,[10] there was no difference in the primary combined endpoint "cardiovascular death or stroke" after 3 years of follow-up. In the Pac-A-Tach trial,[9] mortality, which was a secondary endpoint, was 21% in the VVI-R group versus 5% in the DDD-R group (p=0.001) at 2 years follow-up. Cardiovascular death occurred in 14 patients in the VVI-R group and in 1 patient in the DDD-R group.

In conclusion AAI pacing seems to improve survival as compared with VVI pacing. It is still unclear whether DDD pacing and VVI pacing differs with respect to mortality in SSS.

Atrioventricular conduction defects

The most important problem in the use of AAI pacing in SSS is the risk of later development of AV block. In a review by Sutton and Kenny, progression of AV conduction disturbances was found in 8% of the patients with an annual incidence of 3%.[2] However, these authors considered a PR interval over 0.24 seconds, complete bundle branch block, a Wenckebach block point of $\leq$120 bpm., His-ventricular prolongation or second- and third-degree AV block as progressive AV conduction disturbance, and most of the electrocardiographic changes were non-symptomatic. In 1989, Rosenqvist and Obel reviewed data on a total of 1878 patients.[23] Only patients with progression in AV conduction disease requiring replacement of the AAI pacemaker were considered as AV block. The total prevalence of progression was 2.5% during a median follow up of 36 months. The median annual incidence was 0.65%. They thus found a low risk for developing a clinically important AV conduction disturbance, and concluded that AAI pacing was a safe treatment.[23]

In the randomized trial by Andersen et al.[7] patients were excluded from randomization if a standard ECG showed first-degree AV block (PQ interval > 0.22 seconds in patients ≤ 70 years and a PQ interval > 0.26 seconds in patients > 70 years), second- or third-degree AV block, left bundle branch block or bifascicular block, or during atrial fibrillation RR interval > 3 seconds or a QRS rate < 40 bpm for 1 minute. During implantation an atrial pacing test was performed and a Wenckebach block point ≥100 bpm was required for an AAI implant. After follow up to a mean of 5.5 years, AV block occurred in only 4/110 patients in the AAI group (0.6% annual incidence).[24] Two of these four patients had right-bundle-branch block at randomization. Therefore, it seems conclusive, that the risk of AV block requiring re-operation with upgrading of the pacing system is low.

It is obvious that ventricular bradycardia due to AV block could be avoided by implantation of a VVI or DDD pacemaker, but the potential disadvantages of the ventricular pacing should be considered and weighed against a risk less than 1 % per year for developing AV block.

Pacemaker syndrome

Overt CHF[25] or clinical symptoms, which may be interpreted as CHF can be precipitated by the so-called pacemaker syndrome, which is defined as "symptoms and signs present in the pacemaker patient which are caused by inadequate timing of atrial and ventricular contraction".[26] The pacemaker syndrome is most common in VVI pacing, but can occur also during DDD or AAI pacing. The pathophysiology of the VVI pacemaker syndrome is complex and not fully understood, but atrial contraction against closed atrioventricular valves producing increased atrial pressure, so-called cannon A waves, appears essential for the syndrome to develop. The increased atrial pressure may lead to systemic and pulmonary venous congestion and a concomitant drop in arterial blood pressure. Associated symptoms may include syncope or near syncope, dyspnea, limitation of exercise capacity, induction of CHF and pulmonary venous congestion. The true incidence of pacemaker syndrome in VVI pacing is not known. In the trial by Andersen et al., only 2% of the patients in the VVI group needed upgrading of the pacing system due to pacemaker syndrome. In contrast, in the PASE and Pac-A-Tach trials, 26% and 28% of the patients in the VVI-R groups crossed over to DDD-R pacing mode because of pacemaker syndrome. In these trials cross-over was easily done by reprogramming. One study indicates, that 75% of patients with VVI pacemakers benefits from upgrading to DDD pacing, suggesting the existence of "subclinical" pacemaker syndrome in these patients.[27]

Pacemaker syndrome during DDD pacing is less common and most often can be solved by pacemaker reprogramming. During AAI-R pacing, a paradoxical prolongation of the spike-R interval during exercise occurs in a minority of patients, and may be associated with symptoms as chest pain, dyspnea, and light-headedness, the so-called "AAI-R pacemaker syndrome". This phenomenon is probably the result of an inadequate balance between the pacemaker sensor activity and the level of sympathetic tone during initial exercise, most often occurs in patients on drugs depressing AV conduction, and tend to correct itself as sympathetic tone progressively increases during exercise.[28] The risk of AAI-R pacemaker syndrome is low, especially if the maximum sensor rate is programmed to approximately 100-110 bpm, which is appropriate in most elderly patients during normal daily activities.

Ongoing trials and remaining questions

Currently, 3 trials of mode selection in SSS are ongoing. The MOST (Mode selection Trial in Sinus Node Dysfunction), in which DDD-R and VVI-R pacing modes are compared in 2000 patients,[29] STOP-AF (Systematic Trial Of Pacing for Atrial Fibrillation), testing VVI versus DDD or AAI in 350 patients,[30] and DANPACE, comparing AAI-R and DDD-R pacing in 1900 patients.[31] These trials probably will add further important knowledge regarding the impact of pacing modes on clinical outcome.

Lately there has been some focus on multisite atrial pacing in prevention of AF.[32, 33] However, the long-term benefit of these new approaches in patients with SSS and brady-tachy syndrome remains to be documented.

Moreover, it still has to be evaluated whether there are any differences between DDD and VVI pacing during follow-up beyond 3 years. The ongoing extended follow-up in the CTOPP trial might help answer this question. Last, any differences between rate adaptive pacing and fixed rate demand pacing remain to be elucidated. In an observational study, rate adaptive pacing was associated with better survival than fixed rate demand pacing.[34]

Conclusion

AAI pacing, preserving both AV synchrony and the normal ventricular activation pattern, causes less AF, thromboembolism, death, and CHF than VVI pacing in SSS. When the patients are carefully selected, the risk of

AV block during follow-up is less than 1% per year. Also DDD pacing seems superior to VVI pacing. DDD pacing causes less AF and thromboembolism than VVI pacing but has not yet been found advantageous with respect to CHF or mortality. Therefore, AAI pacing should be considered first choice treatment for isolated SSS with DDD pacing being an acceptable alternative.

References

1. Bernstein AD, Parsonnet V. Survey of cardiac pacing and defibrillation in the United States in 1993. *Am J Cardiol* 1996; 78:187-196.
2. Sutton R, Kenny RA. The natural history of sick sinus syndrome. *Pacing Clin Electrophysiol* 1986; 9:1110-1114.
3. Rosenqvist M, Brandt J, Schuller H. Long-term pacing in sinus node disease: effects of stimulation mode on cardiovascular morbidity and mortality. *Am Heart J* 1988; 116:16-22.
4. Santini M, Alexidou G, Ansalone G, et al. Relation of prognosis in sick sinus syndrome to age, conduction defects and modes of permanent cardiac pacing. *Am J Cardiol* 1990; 65:729-735.
5. Sgarbossa EB, Pinski SL, Maloney JD, et al. Chronic atrial fibrillation and stroke in paced patients with sick sinus syndrome. Relevance of clinical characteristics and pacing modalities. *Circulation* 1993; 88:1045-1053.
6. Andersen HR, Thuesen L, Bagger JP, et al. Prospective randomised trial of atrial versus ventricular pacing in sick-sinus syndrome. *Lancet* 1994; 344:1523-1528.
7. Andersen HR, Nielsen JC, Thomsen PE, et al. Long-term follow-up of patients from a randomised trial of atrial versus ventricular pacing for sick sinus syndrome. *Lancet* 1997; 350:1210-1216.
8. Lamas GA, Orav J, Stambler BS, et al. For the Pacemaker Selection in the Elderly Investigators. Quality of life and clinical outcomes in elderly patients treated with ventricular pacing as compared with dual-chamber pacing. *N Engl J Med* 1998; 338:1097-1104.
9. Wharton JM, Sorrentino RA, Campbell P, et al., the PAC-A-TACH Investigators: Effect on pacing modality on atrial tachyarrhythmia recurrence in the tachycardia-bradycardia syndrome: preliminary results of the pacemaker atrial tachycardia trial. *Circulation* 1998; 98:I-494. Abstract.

10. Connolly SJ, Kerr C, Gent M, et al. Dual-chamber versus ventricular pacing. Critical appraisal of current data. *Circulation* 1996; 94:578-583.

11. Skanes AC, Krahn AD, Yee R, et al., for the CTOPP Investigators: Physiologic pacing reduces progression to chronic atrial fibrillation. *Pacing Clin Electrophysiol* 1999; 22:728. Abstract.

12. Santini M, Ansalone G, Auriti A. Sick sinus syndrome: Natural history before and after pacing. *Eur J C P E* 1993; 3:220-231.

13. Lee MA, Dae MW, Langberg JJ, et al. Effects of long-term right ventricular apical pacing on left ventricular perfusion, innervation, function and histology. *J Am Coll Cardiol* 1994; 24:225-232.

14. Leclercq C, Gras D, Le Helloco A, et al. Hemodynamic importance of preserving the normal sequence of ventricular activation in permanent cardiac pacing. *Am Heart J* 1995;129:1133-1141.

15. Tse H-F, Lau CP. Long-term effect of right ventricular pacing on myocardial perfusion and function. *J Am Coll Cardiol* 1997; 29:744-749.

16. Rosenqvist M, Brandt J, Schuller H. Atrial versus ventricular pacing in sinus node disease: a treatment comparison study. *Am Heart J* 1986; 111:292-297.

17. Zanini R, Facchinetti AI, Gallo G, et al. Morbidity and mortality of patients with sinus node disease: comparative effects of atrial and ventricular pacing. *Pacing Clin Electrophysiol* 1990; 13:2076-2079.

18. Sasaki Y, Shimotori M, Akahane K, et al. Long-term follow-up of patients with sick sinus syndrome: a comparison of clinical aspects among unpaced, ventricular inhibited paced, and physiologically paced groups. *Pacing Clin Electrophysiol* 1988; 11:1575-1583.

19. Sgarbossa EB, Pinski SL, Trohman RG, et al. Single-chamber ventricular pacing is not associated with worsening heart failure in sick sinus syndrome. *Am J Cardiol* 1994; 73:693-697.

20. Nielsen JC, Andersen HR, Thomsen PE, et al. Heart failure and echocardiographic changes during long-term follow-up of patients with sick sinus syndrome randomized to single chamber atrial or ventricular pacing. *Circulation* 1998; 97:987-995.

21. Ishikawa T: Evolution of left atrial diameter in patients implanted with physiological pacemakers. *Eur.J.C.P.E.* 1999; 3:140-144. Abstract.

22. Sgarbossa EB, Pinski SL, Maloney JD. The role of pacing modality in determining long-term survival in the sick sinus syndrome. *Ann Intern Med* 1993; 119:359-365.

23. Rosenqvist M, Obel IW. Atrial pacing and the risk for AV block: is there a time for change in attitude? *Pacing Clin Electrophysiol* 1989; 12:97-101.

24. Andersen HR, Nielsen JC, Thomsen PE, et al. Atrioventricular conduction during long-term follow-up of patients with sick sinus syndrome. *Circulation* 1998; 98:1315-1321.

25. Curzi G, Purcano A, Molini E, et al. Deleterious clinical and haemodynamic effects of V-A retroconduction in symptomatic sinus brady-arrhythmias (S.S.B.) treated with VVI pacing: their regression with AAI pacing., in Steinbach K (ed): *Cardiac pacing. Proceedings of the VII. world symposium on cardiac pacing.* Steinkopff Verlag, Darmstadt, 1983, pp 127-134.

26. Schuller H, Brandt J. The pacemaker syndrome: old and new causes. *Clin Cardiol* 1991; 14:336-340.

27. Sulke N, Dritsas A, Bostock J, et al. "Subclinical" pacemaker syndrome: a randomised study of symptom free patients with ventricular demand (VVI) pacemakers upgraded to dual chamber devices. *Br Heart J* 1992; 67:57-64.

28. Linde C, Nordlander R, Rosenqvist M. Atrial rate adaptive pacing: what happens to AV conduction? *Pacing Clin Electrophysiol* 1994; 17:1581-1589.

29. Lamas GA. Pacemaker mode selection and survival: a plea to apply the principles of evidence based medicine to cardiac pacing practice. *Heart* 1997; 78:218-220.

30. Charles RG, McComb JM. Systematic trial of pacing to prevent atrial fibrillation (STOP-AF). *Heart* 1997; 78:224-225.

31. Andersen HR, Nielsen JC. Pacing in sick sinus syndrome - Need for a prospective, randomized trial comparing atrial with dual chamber pacing. *Pacing Clin Electrophysiol* 1998; 21:1175-1179.

32. Daubert C, Mabo P, Berder V, et al. Permanent dual atrium pacing in major interatrial conduction blocks: A four years experience. *Pacing Clin Electrophysiol* 1993; 16:885. Abstract.

33. Saksena S, Prakash A, Hill M, et al. Prevention of recurrent atrial fibrillation with chronic dual- site right atrial pacing. Prevention of recurrent atrial fibrillation with chronic dual- site right atrial pacing. *J Am Coll Cardiol* 1996; 28:687-694.

34. Fletcher R, Karasik P, McManus C, et al. Patient survival improved with rate-responsive and dual-chamber pacing. *Pacing Clin Electrophysiol* 1999; 22:728. Abstract.

41.
CLINICAL TRIALS OF PACING MODE SELECTION

Stuart J. Connolly, M.D.

Faculty of Health Sciences, McMaster University, Hamilton, ON Canada

Advances in pacemaker technology have resulted in availability of different types of pacemakers with quite different modes of pacing available and different costs. One of the more important distinctions between pacemakers is that some pace (and sense) both atrium and ventricle and others only pace (and sense) the ventricle. Dual chamber pacing requires a second lead and more complex programs but has the theoretical advantage over single chamber pacing in that it maintains the normal synchrony of atrial and ventricular contraction, as well as dominance of the sinus node. Atrial pacing has been advocated by some investigators as a safe and cost effective mode of pacing in patients with sinus node dysfunction[1-3]. Atrial pacing also maintains a normal synchrony of AV node conduction. Physiologic pacing has been suggested as a general term for those modes of pacing (either atrial or dual chamber) which preserve atrio-ventricular synchrony and maintain sinus node dominance. While observational studies have suggested an advantage of physiologic pacing, such investigations have been flawed by lack of randomization. It is obvious that considerable physician selection occurs when choosing the type of pacemaker to implant. Therefore, even though most non-randomized trials have reported a benefit of physiologic pacing over single chamber pacing, it is clear that these studies cannot be relied upon to provide a true measure of the benefits of physiologic pacing[4].

There are a number of potential mechanisms by which dual chamber pacing might improve patient outcomes. Retrograde atrioventricular nodal conduction may cause asynchronous atrial contraction, which in turn may lead to atrial stretch and hypertrophy. These may be predisposing factors for the development of atrial fibrillation. Asynchronous atrial activation and persistent sinus bradycardia may also predispose to atrial fibrillation. Loss of the atrial contribution to ventricular filling could result in a greater likelihood of development of congestive heart failure in susceptible patients.

Randomized Controlled Trials Already Reported
Two randomized controlled clinical trials of pacemaker mode selection have been reported. One of these, the Danish Study[5,6], has been reported at two different points in follow-up. In this study 225 patients with sinus node

From Ovsyshcher IE. *Cardiac Arrythmias and Device Therapy: Results and Perspectives for the New Century.* Armonk, NY: Futura Publishing Company, Inc., © 2000

dysfunction were randomized to receive either an atrial or ventricular pacemaker. Study outcomes were stroke, atrial fibrillation and death. The two patient groups were similar at baseline. During follow-up there was no significant difference in the risk of atrial fibrillation or death. Stroke events were significantly higher in the ventricular group. The Danish Study published a second report when the mean follow-up in these patients was 5.5 years, with some patients followed as long as eight years. At this point in time there was a significantly lower risk of atrial fibrillation in the atrial paced group with a relative risk reduction of 0.54 (95% confidence interval 0.33, 0.89, p=0.012). Thromboembolic events were also reduced by atrial pacing, relative risk 0.47 (95% confidence interval 0.24, 0.92 p=0.023). Cardiovascular death was also significantly reduced with a relative risk of 0.47 (95% confidence interval 0.27, 0.82 p=0.0065). These data would appear to provide strong evidence for a benefit from atrial pacing, however, they need to be interpreted cautiously as the study is rather small and more prone to chance variation. All of the statistical power of the trial was attributed to the first analysis in the study making the second analysis at five years exploratory and hypothesis generating rather than definitive.

The other randomized trial of pacemaker mode selection to have been reported is the Pacemaker Selection in the Elderly Study (PASE), reported in 1998[7]. This was the first randomized controlled trial evaluating the effect of pacing mode on health related quality of life. This multi-center study was performed in 29 American centers and randomized patients to receive ventricular pacing or dual chamber pacing. All patients received a dual chamber pacemaker and the randomization effected only the type of programming. Four hundred and seven patients were enrolled and evenly randomized to the two pacing modes. The primary study outcome was quality of life as measured by the Short Form 36 and the Specific Activity Scale, two well-validated measures of health related quality of life. Between baseline and three months, there was a marked improvement in quality of life in all patients enrolled in the study irrespective of pacing mode. There were however, no differences between the two pacing modes groups in either of the quality of life measures. There was no significant difference between treatment groups in the risk of atrial fibrillation, stroke or death.

A sub-group analysis did show the patients with sinus node dysfunction, but not those with AV block, had a trend towards a lower risk of atrial fibrillation and death that did not meet nominal levels of statistical significance. The results of PASE indicate that implantation of any kind of permanent pacemaker improves health-related quality of life, but the quality of life measures are not effected by pacing mode. There is no trend in the overall patient population towards improvement in atrial fibrillation or survival.

In 1998 Mattioli et al.[8] reported a randomized trial of 210 patients who received either physiologic or single chamber ventricular pacing from management of symptomatic bradycardia. Patients in the two groups were similar in terms of baseline characteristics. During follow-up the incidence of chronic atrial fibrillation was higher in patients with ventricular pacing then in those with physiologic pacing (p<0.05). There was also a significantly lower incidence of cerebral ischemia in those randomized to physiologic pacing. During two years of follow-up the risk of cerebral ischemia in the single chamber pacing patients was 19 events in 105 patients compared to 10 events in 105 patients with physiologic pacing. The relatively high risk of cerebral ischemia in these patients may be partly explained by their advanced age (79±9 years). The risk of cerebral ischemia is, however, much higher than would be expected. This unusually higher risk of cerebral ischemia makes interpretation of this small study somewhat problematic.

Completed but Unpublished Studies

The Pacemaker Atrial Tachycardia (PAC-A-TACH) trial is a recently completed small scale multi-center randomized study in which 198 patients with sick sinus syndrome were randomized to rate responsive dual chamber or rate responsive single chamber pacing[9]. The primary outcome was the development of atrial tachy-arrhythmias. Secondary end-points were death, congestive heart failure, stroke, embolic events and quality of life. There was no significant difference in the recurrence of atrial tachy- arrhythmia between dual chamber and single chamber pacing. There was a significant reduction in mortality with dual chamber pacing (3.2%) compared to ventricular pacing (6.8%), p=0.007.

The Canadian Trial of Physiologic Pacing (CTOPP) is the first large scale multi-center randomized trial which compares physiologic to ventricular pacing. A total of 2,568 patients with symptomatic bradycardia were randomized to receive either a physiologic pacemaker or a single chamber ventricular pacemaker. Rate adaptive pacing used in patients with chronotropic incompetence in both groups. The primary study outcome was the first occurrence of either cardiovascular death or stroke. Secondary end-points were all-cause mortality, atrial fibrillation or hospitalization for congestive heart failure. The study was powered to be able to detect a 30% reduction in the relative risk of the primary end-point.

The trial was completed in 1998. Complete results have not yet been published, however, they have been reported at the Scientific Sessions of the North American Society of Pacing Electrophysiology in Toronto, Canada in May 1999. There was no significant difference in cardiovascular death or stroke between physiologic pacing and ventricular pacing. It was reported that there was a significant reduction in the risk of atrial fibrillation.

Ongoing Trials
The Systematic Trial of Pacing to Prevent Atrial Fibrillation (STOP-AF) is an ongoing small multi-center randomized trial designed to assess whether atrial-based pacing reduces the incidence of chronic and paroxysmal atrial fibrillation[10]. A total of 350 patients with sick sinus syndrome or other atrial arrhythmias who require pacemaker implantation will be enrolled. Patients will all receive dual chamber pacemakers and will then be randomized to have these programmed into ventricular or dual chamber modes.

The United Kingdom Pacing and Cardiovascular Events (UKPACE) Trial is a large scale randomized trial designed to evaluate dual chamber pacing compared with single chamber ventricular pacing in patients aged >70 years who also have high degree atrio-ventricular block[11]. For this study a total of 2000 patients requiring their first pacemaker implantation will be enrolled. The primary outcome measure is all-cause mortality and a variety of secondary outcome measures will also be assessed, including atrial fibrillation, quality of life and exercise capacity.

The Mode Selection Trial (MOST) is a large randomized multi-centered trial designed to assess whether rate modulated dual chamber pacing improves survival compared to rate modulated ventricular pacing in patients with sick sinus syndrome. Two thousand patients will be enrolled from approximately 100 American centers. All patients will receive a dual chamber pacemaker and then will be randomized to have the pacemaker programmed to DDDR or VVIR modes. The primary end-point will be the first occurrence of death or stroke. Secondary end-points include quality of life, total mortality, stroke and congestive heart failure requiring hospitalization (personal communication, Dr. G. A. Lamas).

Conclusion
It is likely that within the next few years, the results from completed and ongoing randomized controlled trials will provide a fairly clear picture of the benefits and cost effectiveness of dual chamber pacing. At present it appears that these benefits are of a much smaller magnitude then was

originally anticipated. At present it appears that for many patients requiring a pacemaker there is little to be gained from dual chamber pacing. There may be sub-groups of patients, such as those entirely pacemaker dependent or at high risk of atrial fibrillation, who will benefit. Undoubtedly the results of meta-analysis of the randomized trials will help us to delineate sub-groups who can derive the significant benefit from physiologic pacing.

REFERENCES:
1. Berstein SB, Van Natta BE, Ellestad MH: Experiences with atrial pacing. Am J Cardiol. 1988; 61:113-116.
2. Brandt J, Anderson H, Fahraeus T, et al: Natural history of sinus node disease treated with atrial pacing in 213 patients: implications for selection of stimulation mode. J Am Coll Cardiol. 1992; 20:633-639.
3. Clarke KW, Connelly DT, Charles RG: Single chamber atrial pacing: an underused and cost-effective pacing modality in sinus node disease. Heart. 1998; 80:387-389.
4. Connolly SJ, Kerr C, Gent M, et al: Dual chamber versus ventricular pacing. Critical appraisal of current data. Circulation. 1996;94:578-583.
5. Anderson HR, Thuesen L, Bagger JP, et al: Prospective randomized trial of atrial versus ventricular pacing in sick-sinus-syndrome. Lancet 1994; 344:1523-1528.
6. Andersen HR, Nielsen JC, Thomsen PE, et al: Long-term follow-up of patients from a randomized trial atrial versus ventricular pacing for sick-sinus-syndrome. Lancet. 1997; 350:1210-1216.
7. Lamas GA, Orav EJ, Stambler BS, et al: Quality of life and clinical outcomes in elderly patients treated with ventricular pacing as compared with dual chamber pacing. Pacemaker Selection in the Elderly Investigators. N Engl J Med. 1998; 338:1097-1104.
8. Mattioli AV, Castellani ET, Vivoli D, et al: Prevalence of atrial fibrillation and stroke in paced patients without prior atrial fibrillation: a prospective study. Clin Cardiol. 1998; 21:117-122.
9. Wharton JM, Sorentino RA, Campbell P, et al: Effect of pacing modality on atrial tachyarrhythmia recurrence in the tachycardia-bradycardia syndrome: preliminary results of the Pacemaker Atrial Tachycardia Trial (Abstract). Circulation 1998; 98:1-494.
10. Charles RG, McComb JM: Systematic trial of pacing to prevent atrial fibrillation (STOP-AF) (Editorial). Heart. 1997; 78:224-225.
11. Toff WD, Skehan JD, de Bono DP, et al: The United Kingdom pacing and cardiovascular events (UKPACE) trial. Heart. 1997; 78:221-223.

42.

CLINICAL EXPERIENCE WITH DUAL CHAMBER VENTRICULAR AUTOCAPTURE

Paul A. Levine, M.D.

St. Jude Medical CRMD, Sylmar, CA, USA
Loma Linda University Medical Center, Loma Linda, CA, USA

There are two conflicting variables in cardiac pacing - one is patient safety while the other is maximizing device longevity. This has led to the concept of a "safety margin" which is an output setting which is likely to exceed the highest possible capture threshold thus protecting the patient while still keeping the output level as low as possible thus minimizing the battery current drain effectively extending device longevity. An additional factor driving the need to reduce outputs has been continuing requests by the medical professions for smaller and smaller devices which, in most cases, means a smaller battery with a reduction in its overall energy capacity. To some degree, increased efficiencies in the device circuitry has reduced the housekeeping current of these device but the major factor in battery current drain is the delivered output energy with each and every paced beat. Improvements in electrode design decreasing the actual energy needed for capture (unique geometry and materials) in conjunction with techniques to minimize the threshold rise associated with lead maturation (steroid elution) allow for lower chronic outputs but still do not absolutely preclude late threshold rises(1). Another is the ability of the pacemaker to monitor the presence or absence of capture, run the output as low as possible, provide a higher output back-up pulse in the setting of noncapture and automatically adjust the output based on the beat-by-beat capture threshold. This has been a goal of both the profession and industry since 1973 when first proposed by both Drs. Preston (2) and Mugica (3) in separate papers. Although there have been a number of attempts, each has fallen short of the mark until the introduction of the single chamber rate modulated Microny® (4) pacemaker in 1995 with an effective AutoCapture® Pacing System algorithm (Pacesetter, St. Jude Medical CRMD, Sylmar, CA). In 1998, this technology was transferred to the ventricular channel of a dual chamber pacing system, Affinity DR® (Pacesetter, St. Jude Medical CRMD, Sylmar, CA). This paper will describe the features of the AutoCapture™ Pacing System algorithm and early clinical experience with Affinity DR.

From Ovsyshcher IE. *Cardiac Arrythmias and Device Therapy: Results and Perspectives for the New Century.* Armonk, NY: Futura Publishing Company, Inc., © 2000

Evoked Response/Polarization Detection:

The AutoCapture algorithm is based upon the successful detection of the evoked response (ER) following the output pulse. In a standard pacing system, this signal coincides with the absolute portion of the standard refractory period precluding its being sensed. As such, a special detection circuit needed to be developed for these devices. A 15 ms blanking period is triggered by delivery of the ventricular output pulse followed by an alert period extending to 64 ms following the output pulse. If a signal is not detected within this 46 ms Evoked Response Detection Window, the output pulse is labeled as ineffective and a 4.5 Volt back-up pulse is delivered at 100 ms after the primary output pulse. This is termed Capture Verification.

The other known signal that will occur within this same window is the polarization artifact. Polarization is the residual charge at the electrode-tissue interface that follows the output pulse, a signal that would normally be covered by the standard refractory period precluding its being detected. However, with the unique ER Detection Window, if the polarization signal is too large, it may be detected resulting in the labeling of an ineffective output pulse as being effective. In earlier attempts to effect a totally automatic threshold tracking system, a variety of mechanisms have been employed to minimize the polarization signal including recharge pulses (charge balancing), changes to the internal circuit of the pacemaker and, as in these devices, intentional utilization of a low polarization electrode. To determine whether or not AutoCapture can be safely enabled, the system must be able to measure the amplitude of both the evoked response signal and the polarization artifact (Figure 1), a form of device-based testing. Since the largest polarization signal is associated with the higher output pulses, testing is performed at a 4.5 Volt output setting. If there is a sufficient difference between the two, an Evoked Response sensitivity setting can be programmed that will promote the detection of the ER signal while precluding recognition of the polarization signal. Experience with factors that may impact the amplitude of the ER signal is limited as the ability to measure this signal is new, the degree of fluctuation that has been demonstrated to date is usually minimal (5,6) with the recommended ER Sensitivity settings providing a sufficient safety margin to assure appropriate system function. In Microny, the lowest polarization signal that could be measured was 1 mV while the smallest ER signal that would be allowed for AutoCapture was 4.0 mV. Affinity is able to measure even smaller polarization signals and uses a ratio of ER signal to Polarization signal such that AutoCapture is allowed over a wider range. In addition, the clinician is given the option of enabling AutoCapture even if the system recommends otherwise.

Working Margin vs Safety Margin:

Once the capture threshold is assessed, the system sets the output to 0.25 Volts above the measured capture threshold. This is the working margin, not a safety margin and it is set automatically. It reflects the absolutely lowest output possible for any given system effectively minimizing battery current drain and maximizing device longevity. However, it is also know that there are multiple factors which cause the capture threshold to wax and wane during the course of the day (1,7,8) which is the rationale behind the concept of a safety margin. The only way this narrow a working margin would be safe is for the system to monitor capture

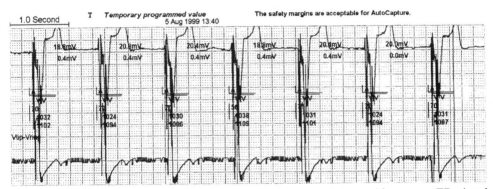

Figure 1: Evoked Response/Polarization Sensitivity Test printout with a mean ER signal amplitude of 19.97 mV and a mean polarization signal amplitude of 0.39 mV.

on a beat-by-beat basis associated with every ventricular output pulse. If the system labels a complex as noncapture, a 4.5 Volt/0.5 ms pulse is delivered 100 ms after the primary "ineffective" output.

Thus the working margin is very close to the capture threshold while the safety margin is the 4.5 Volt output. The pulse duration of the back-up pulse is either 0.5 ms or the programmed pulse duration if set wider than 0.5 ms. For most patients, the Safety Margin is far greater than the accepted 2:1 or 100% industry standard and often greater than the 150% to 200% which has been recently recommended by Danilovic and Ohm(1).

Loss of Capture Recovery

While capture thresholds are known to fluctuate, even in a stable system, there is a design feature to minimize the repeated delivery of higher output back-up pulses. The system's definition of a threshold rise is "noncapture" on two consecutive primary ventricular outputs. In addition to the back-up pulse that follows each ineffective primary pulse, the output of the third primary pulse in this sequence is increased by 0.25 Volts. Assuming that this output continues to be ineffective, the system continues to increment the amplitude of the primary output, a process called Capture Recovery. If the progressive increased outputs continue to be read as noncapture until reaching 3.825 Volts, the system defaults to 4.5 Volts for 128 cycles after which it resumes another search. Except in the setting of lead dislodgment in which case the required output is likely to exceed the highest output in the pacemaker, capture will be established at a significantly lower level. When two consecutive primary pulses are identified as demonstrating capture, this is the new Capture Threshold.

Automatic Capture Threshold Assessment

Following either a loss of capture recovery sequence, a period of intentional disabling of the AutoCapture algorithm as with noise mode function or associated with magnet application as might occur during a routine follow-up evaluation as well as every 8 hours during the course of the day, the system will automatically reassess the capture threshold. If the capture threshold is identified as having decreased which is most likely to be identified at the time of the routine periodic capture threshold assessments, the delivered output can be reduced. This Automatic Capture Threshold test can also be initiated using

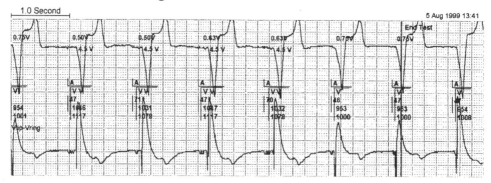

Figure 2 - Capture Threshold Test with loss of capture occurring at 0.50 Volts and the capture threshold being 0.75 Volts at a 0.6 ms pulse duration.

the programmer at a routine follow-up evaluation (Figure 2). In the performance of this test, the system performs the test at the functional paced rate but shortens the paced and sensed AV delay to 50 and 25 ms respectively. This precludes possible fusion beats in the setting of intact AV nodal conduction. It then begins reducing the output in 0.25 Volt steps on consecutive pairs of beats. When loss of capture occurs on two consecutive primary output pulses, each of which is then followed by the higher output back-up pulse, the system begins to increase the output in 0.125 Volt steps. Thus, the defined capture threshold is an "up-threshold" which is often higher than that defined by the output setting just prior to loss of capture when the output is progressively decreased from the point of capture to noncapture (Wedensky Effect). The capture threshold requires that two consecutive primary outputs be associated with capture at which point the system terminates the test, adds the 0.25 Volt working margin to the threshold value termed Output Regulation and restores the pacing system to its other pretest values.

Fusion Beats and the Fusion Avoidance Algorithm

Fusion beats in combination with the AutoCapture Pacing System algorithm can create the situation where the implanted device will have difficulty detecting the ER signal and be unable to verify capture. In this setting, patient safety is considered paramount and although a back-up pulse is not required as there actually is a heart beat, the pacemaker doesn't know this and a back-up pulse is delivered. Occurring approximately 100 ms after the primary pulse, the back-up pulse has the potential for engendering a confusing rhythm on the surface ECG but will not trigger any adverse rhythms in patients as it will be delivered at a time of physiologic refractoriness. While fusion beats can be minimized by changes in the paced rate in single chamber pacing systems, dual chamber systems may predispose to repeated fusion in the setting of intact AV nodal conduction.

In any sequence involving a ventricular output pulse in the dual chamber mode, noncapture associated with the ventricular output may be either true noncapture, a fusion or a pseudofusion beat. In each case, a back-up pulse will be delivered. However, the system will attempt to determine if the loss of capture was due to fusion or true noncapture. As such, it extends the paced or sensed AV delay by 100 ms on the next cycle. If it was "true" noncapture associated with a capture threshold rise and the next cycle also demonstrates noncapture, the system returns to the programmed AV delay and proceeds with Capture Recovery and then a reassessment of the capture threshold. If conduction is intact and the extended AV delay allows a native R wave to be recognized, the basic output level is not incremented while the functionally increased AV delay is allowed to remain in place, a form of AV/PV hysteresis. The rationale behind this decision is based on the studies of Rosenqvist (9) and LeClercq (10) demonstrating that AAI pacing with intact AV nodal conduction and a normal ventricular activation sequence is associated with improved hemodynamics over AV sequential pacing. Ventricular output inhibition will also further reduce battery current drain increasing the potential device longevity.

However, there are situations where the intentional goal is ventricular pacing even though AV nodal conduction is intact. A prime example would be first degree AV block or when pacing is used in the management of hypertrophic obstructive cardiomyopathy or dilated cardiomyopathy. Unless the Fusion Avoidance Algorithm were able to be disabled, the AutoCapture algorithm would be counterproductive in these subgroups of patients. The fusion avoidance feature can be disabled by intentionally programming Negative AV/PV Hysteresis. This is an algorithm first introduced in the Trilogy family of dual chamber pacemakers where the paced and sensed AV delays will shorten by a programmable interval in response to an R wave which is detected before completion of the programmed AV delay. Enabling even 10 ms of Negative AV/PV hysteresis will effectively cancel the Fusion Avoidance Algorithm enabling the effective use of AutoCapture in the presence of intact AV nodal conduction where one intentionally wants to usurp control from the normal AV node.

Long Term Threshold Record

An essential component of any new feature or algorithm is the ability of the system to provide information as to how the algorithm functioned between scheduled visits. Integral to Affinity is a Long Term Threshold Record (LTTR) which will record the threshold measurements for 128 consecutive measurements. At a sampling rate of every 6 hours, detailed information as to threshold fluctuations are provided over a period of approximately 1 month (Figure 3). Once all the bins are filled with data, the system automatically deletes the oldest data while adding the newest results. Selecting a less frequent sampling rate will provide an overview of threshold performance over a longer period of time. After the early lead stabilization period, I reduce the sampling frequency to once daily which will then provide an overview of the threshold performance over the previous 4 months when the patient is seen in follow-up.

Clinical Experience

Although the CE mark for Affinity was received in August 1998, general release of the device was deferred until after a careful prospective multicenter clinical monitoring study(11) was performed between centers in Europe and Canada. A total of 94 devices were implanted in 93 patients (one was replaced due to infection). A variety of leads were used including the Membrane series of leads which are available in Europe and the Tendril DX and Passive Plus DX series of leads available in both North America and Europe. AutoCapture was able to be enabled in 96% of the patient at the moment of implant and in 98% of patients by one month post-implant using device-based testing as the guide.

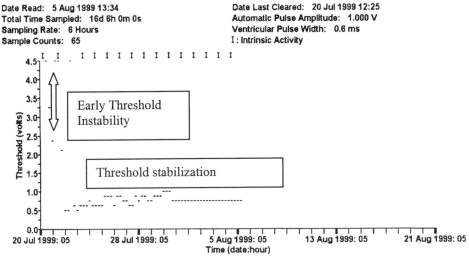

Date Read: 5 Aug 1999 13:34
Total Time Sampled: 16d 6h 0m 0s
Sampling Rate: 6 Hours
Sample Counts: 65

Date Last Cleared: 20 Jul 1999 12:25
Automatic Pulse Amplitude: 1.000 V
Ventricular Pulse Width: 0.6 ms
I : Intrinsic Activity

Figure 3 - Long Term Threshold Record showing early threshold instability

The capture thresholds, evoked response and polarization signal amplitudes were stable and are detailed in this Table.

	Pre-Discharge	**1 Month**	**3 Months**
Polarization (Mean ± SD)	0.5 ± 0.5 mV	0.7 ± 0.6 mV	0.7 ± 0.7 mV
Evoked Response (Mean ± SD)	14.1 ± 6.0 mV	15.5 ± 6.0 mV	14.4 ± 6.5 mV
Capture Threshold (Mean ± SD)	0.5 ± 0.2 V	0.8 ± 0.3 V	0.9 ± 0.3 V
Automatic Amplitude (Mean± SD)	0.7 ± 0.2 V	1.1 ± 0.3 V	1.1 ± 0.3 V

As of March 2000, Affinity has been implanted over 1 year in only a relatively small number of patients. Estimates of projected longevity must be based on calculations made from recorded battery current drains in functioning devices With AutoCapture enabled and the ventricular output under 1.5 Volts, the projected longevity of Affinity will exceed 10 years assuming 100% pacing.

Post Study Experience:

A number of observations have been made as increasing numbers of patients receive Affinity in association with a primary implantation or as a replacement device connected to chronic leads.

(1) Although low polarization leads have been recommended, many of these devices have been connected to chronic leads or leads from other manufacturers. In many cases, there was a sufficient difference between the amplitude of the polarization and evoked response signals that would allow AutoCapture to be enabled.

(2) Virtually all the standard algorithms that are otherwise available in Affinity continue to be active in the presence of AutoCapture (Figure 4).

(3) The present iteration of AutoCapture requires a bipolar lead with a unipolar output pulse. On occasion, the higher output back-up pulse is detected by the patient and in some cases, this has been sufficiently bothersome to cause the physician to disable the algorithm. Normally, most patients will not feel even a 5 Volt unipolar output pulse as this was standard with the earlier generation of pacemakers.

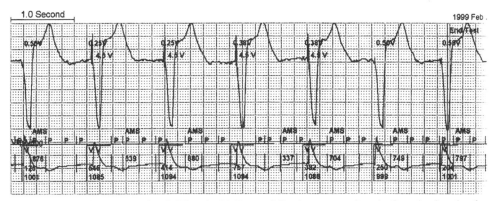

Figure 4 - Performance of AC Threshold Test while the pacemaker is functioning in the nontracking mode associated with Automatic Mode Switch

In a study by Dorian et al (12), unipolar stimulation was rarely associated with bothersome sensations in comparison to outputs of 7.5 Volts in which case local muscle stimulation was relatively common. In my own patient experience, I have had one patient who complained of an awareness of local stimulation although there was no visible or palpable local muscle contractions. I suspect that this may be due to abrupt change between the low output and the higher output back-up pulses which trigger this awareness.

Development is presently in process with respect to a bipolar back-up pulse and a totally bipolar system for both the primary as well as back-up pulses.

(4)   AutoCapture is not presently recommended for use on the atrial channel and is not accessible when the AAI mode is enabled in either the dual or single chamber system. However, there have been anecdotal reports of physicians who have implanted a single chamber Affinity pacing system connected to an atrial lead and have been able to successfully activate AutoCapture. Active work is in progress on detecting the atrial evoked response (13).

Summary:
The concept of AutoCapture was first suggested over 25 years ago. First enabled in Microny introduced into Europe in 1995, it has now been incorporated on the ventricular channel of a dual pacing system. The present algorithm requires the use of a bipolar lead with a further recommendation that the lead be low polarization however active research is underway to enable the algorithm to be used with any lead, bipolar or unipolar, be used in a dedicated unipolar or bipolar configuration and on the atrial channel. Based on the experience to date, the algorithm as implemented in the Microny, Regency and Affinity family of pacemakers provides the combined values of both safety and longevity in a relatively small device.

Bibliography:
1. Danilovic D, Ohm OJ, Pacing threshold trends and variability in modern tined leads assessed using high resolution automatic measurements: Conversion of pulse width into voltage thresholds, PACE 1999; 22: 567-587
2. Preston TA, Bowers DL, The automatic threshold tracking pacemaker, Med Instr 1974; 8: 352-355
3. Mugica J, Lazarus B, Buffet J, Catte M, Pacemaker with automatic adaptation to the pacing threshold, Cardiac Pacing, Van Gorcum Assen, 1973: 150-155
4. Clarke M, Liu B, Schüller H, et al, Adjustment of pacemaker stimulation output correlated with continuously monitored capture thresholds, a multicenter study, PACE 1998; 21: 1567-1575
5. Schüller H, Kruse I, Svensson O, Mortenson P, Long-term benefit of AutoCapture, Four years of follow-up, PACE 1999; 22: 807
6. Schuchert A, Meinertz T, AutoCapture: Is reprogramming of the evoked response sensitivity necessary after hospital discharge, PACE 1999; 22: 872
7. Preston TA, Fletcher RD, Lucchesi BR, Judge RD, Changes in myocardial threshold. Physiologic and pharmacologic factors in patients with implanted pacemakers, Amer Heart J 1967; 74: 235-242
8. Syed J, Lau C, Nishimura SC, Circadian and unexpected changes in stimulation threshold, PACE 1999; 22: 757
9. Rosenqvist M, Isaaz K, Botvinick EH, et al, Relative importance of activation sequence compared to atrioventricular synchrony in left ventricular function, Amer J Cardiol 1991; 67: 148-156
10. LeClercq C, Gras D, Le Helloco A, et al, Hemodynamic importance of preserving the normal sequence of ventricular activation in permanent cardiac pacing, Amer Heart J 19995; 129: 1133-1141

11. St. Jude Medical CRMD, Final Report Affinity DR Model 5330 and SR model 5130 Clinical Monitoring Study, 1999 (on file with St. Jude Medical CRMD, Sylmar, CA)
12. Davies T, Dorian P, Yao J, et al, Do permanent pacemakers need an insulative coating? Results of a prospective randomized double-blind study, PACE 1997; 20: 2394-2397
13. Bradley K, Sloman L, Bornzin GA, Florio J, An atrial autothreshold algorithm using the atrial evoked response, PACE, 1999; 22: A5

43.
DIAGNOSTIC VALUE OF THE 12 LEAD ECG DURING CARDIAC PACING

S.Serge Barold, Helen S. Barold, Robert S. Fishel

Boca Raton and Palm Beach, Florida, USA.

Introduction

The importance of the 12 lead ECG in pacemaker follow-up has been eclipsed by sophisticated ECG/marker systems linked to programmers. However the 12 lead ECG is undergoing a renaissance spurred by new indications for pacing. ECG interpretation can be challenging because of unipolar stimuli, fusion beats, metabolic problems, latency (and its mimicry), interatrial conduction delays and the cardiac memory phenomenon.

Normal QRS Patterns Mimicking Myocardial Infarction

A number of patterns can mimic myocardial infarction (MI) during ventricular pacing. Pacing from the right ventricular (RV) outflow tract produces a dominant R wave in the inferior leads and may generate qR, QR, or Qr complexes in leads I and aVL. Occasionally with slight displacement of the pacing lead from RV apex to outflow tract, leads I and aVL may register a qR complex in conjunction with the typical negative complexes of RV apical stimulation in the inferior leads[1]. This qR pattern must not be interpreted as a sign of MI. RV pacing from any site does not produce qR complexes in V_5 and V_6. A qR (Qr) complex in the precordial or inferior leads is always abnormal in the absence of ventricular fusion.

Dominant R wave in Lead V_1

A dominant R wave in V_1 during ventricular pacing has been called a right bundle branch block (RBBB) pattern of depolarization but this terminology is misleading because this pattern is often not related to RV activation delay (Table I).

Table I   Causes of a Dominant R wave in Lead V_1

- Ventricular fusion.
- Pacing in the myocardial relative refractory period.
- Pacing from the coronary venous system.
- Lead perforation of RV or ventricular septum with left ventricular (LV) stimulation.
- LV endocardial or epicardial pacing.
- Uncomplicated RV pacing.

From Ovsyshcher IE. *Cardiac Arrythmias and Device Therapy: Results and Perspectives for the New Century.* Armonk, NY: Futura Publishing Company, Inc., © 2000

A dominant R wave in the right precordial leads occurs in approximately 8-10% of patients with uncomplicated RV stimulation[2-4]. The position of V_1 and V_2 should be checked because a dominant R wave can be sometimes recorded at the level of the third intercostal space during uncomplicated RV pacing. The pacing lead is almost certainly in the RV (apex or distal septal site) if V_1 and V_2 are negative when recorded one space lower (5th intercostal space). A dominant R wave is not eliminated at the level of the 5th interspace if pacing originates from the midseptal region[5]. Furthermore the "RBBB" pattern from pacing at the RV apical and distal septal sites results in a precordial vector change[5] from positive to negative by V_3. The ECG pattern with a truly posterior RV lead has not been systematically investigated as a potential cause of a high voltage R wave in V_1 during pacing.

Left Ventricular Pacing

Passage of a pacing lead in the LV occurs via the subclavian artery or an atrial septal defect. The access sites to the LV can be easily identified by the RBBB pattern during pacing, standard chest radiographs and echocardiography[4,6]. During LV pacing the frontal plane axis can indicate the site of pacing. As a rule with a RBBB configuration the frontal plane axis cannot differentiate precisely a LV site from one in the coronary venous system. A LV lead is a potential source of cerebral emboli. Most patients with neurologic manifestations do not exhibit echocardiographic evidence of thrombus on the pacing lead. In symptomatic patients, removal of the lead after a period of anticoagulation should be considered[7,8]. A chronic LV lead in asymptomatic patients is best treated with long-term anticoagulant therapy.

Old Myocardial Infarction

Table II outlines the difficulties in the diagnosis of old myocardial infarction (MI) and Table III lists a number of signs of no value in the diagnosis of MI.

Anterior Myocardial Infarction

1) St-qR Pattern. Because the QRS complex during RV pacing resembles (except for the initial forces) that of spontaneous left bundle branch block (LBBB), many of the criteria for the diagnosis of MI in LBBB also apply to MI during RV pacing[1,9-11]. RV pacing almost invariably masks a relatively small anteroseptal MI. During RV pacing, as in LBBB, an extensive anteroseptal MI close to the stimulating electrode will alter the initial QRS vector, with forces pointing to the right because of unopposed activation of the RV. This causes (initial) q waves in leads I, aVL, V_5, and

V_6. Castellanos et al.[10] have called this sign "St-qR pattern" (St-stimulation spike). The abnormal q wave is usually 0.03 sec or more but a narrower one is also diagnostic. Occasionally the St-qR complex is best seen in leads V_2-V_4 and it may even be restricted to these leads. Finding the (initial) q wave may sometimes require placing the leads one intercostal space higher or perhaps lower.

The sensitivity of the St-qR pattern varies from 10-50% according to the way data are analyzed[12,13]. Patients who require temporary pacing in acute MI represent a preselected group with a large MI, so that the overall sensitivity is substantially lower than 50% in the patient population with implanted pacemakers. The specificity is virtually 100%. Only one group[14] has claimed that q waves in leads I, aVL and V6 are not diagnostically useful but their conclusions are questionable because of problematic methodology: 1. Only q waves lasting > 0.03 sec were examined. MI can produce q waves > 0.03 sec during ventricular pacing. 2. The number of "abnormal" patients with q waves in the two frontal plane leads and not in

Table II   Difficulties in the Diagnosis of MI During Ventricular Pacing

1. Large unipolar stimuli may obscure initial forces, cause a pseudo Q wave and false ST segment current of injury.
2. Fusion beats may cause a pseudoinfarction pattern (qR/Qr complex or notching of the upstroke of the S wave).
3. Retrograde P waves.
4. MI vs ischemia.
5. Acute MI vs old or indeterminate age MI.
6. Signs in QRS complex are not useful for the diagnosis of acute MI.
7. Recording QRS signs of MI may require different sites of the left V leads.
8. ST segment changes usually but not always indicate an acute process.
9. Cardiac memory. Repolarization ST-T wave abnormalities (mostly T wave inversion) in the spontaneous rhythm may be secondary to RV pacing per se and not related to ischemia or non Q wave MI.
10. Many but not all criteria are similar to those of MI in LBBB.
11. QRS abnormalities have low sensitivity (but high specificity).

Table III   QRS Criteria of no Value in Diagnosis of MI

- QS complexes V_1 to V_6
- RS or terminal S wave in V_5 and V_6
- QS complexes in the inferior leads
- Notching of R waves

V_6 was not specified. 3. The protocol called for an LBBB pattern with left axis deviation (more negative than −30 degrees). Normal subjects might have been included in the "abnormal" group because a pacing lead somewhat away from the RV apex can cause left-axis deviation with q waves in I and aVL.

2) Late Notching of the Ascending S wave (Cabrera's Sign)

As in LBBB, during RV pacing an extensive anterior MI may produce notching of the ascending limb of the S wave in the precordial leads usually V_3 and V_4 - Cabrera's sign ∞ 0.03 sec and present in 2 leads[1]. The sign may occur together with the St-qR pattern in anterior MI. The sensitivity varies from 25 to 50 % according to the size of MI but the specificity is close to 100% if notching is properly defined[1,12]. Interestingly the workers[14] that placed little value on q waves (as already discussed) found a 57% sensitivity for Cabrera's sign (0.04 sec notching) in the diagnosis of extensive anterior MI. Table IV outlines the causes of "false" Cabrera's signs and the highly specific variants of Cabrera's sign.

Table IV   Cabrera' s Sign
  1. *Specific Cabrera Variants*
   - Small, narrow r wave deforming the terminal QRS[1].
   - Series of tiny notches giving a serrated appearance along the ascending S wave[1].
   - Similar notches on QRS during epicardial pacing.

   Notches are probably due to a gross derangement of intraventricular conduction.
  2. *False Cabrera's Signs*
   - Slight notching of the ascending S wave in V leads is normal during RV apical pacing. It is usually confined to 1 lead and usually <0.03sec. No shelflike appearance of true Cabrera's sign.
   - Fusion beats.
   - Early retrograde P waves.

Inferior Myocardial Infarction

The QRS complex is often unreaveling. During RV pacing in inferior MI diagnostic Qr, QR or qR complexes provide a sensitivity of 15% and specificity of 100%[12]. The St-qR pattern must not be confused with an overshoot of the QRS complex due to massive ST elevation creating a diminutive terminal r wave. Cabrera's sign in leads III and aVF is very specific but even less sensitive than its counterpart in anterior MI[15].

MI at Other Sites

A posterior MI should shift the QRS forces anteriorly and produce a dominant R wave in the right V leads but the diagnosis cannot be made during RV pacing because of the many causes of a dominant R wave in V_1. An RV MI could conceivably be reflected in V_{3R} with prominent ST elevation[4].

Acute Myocardial Infarction

Sgarbossa et al.[16,17] recently reported the value of ST segment abnormalities in the diagnosis of acute MI during ventricular pacing and their high specificity. ST elevation ≥ 5 mm in predominantly negative QRS complexes is the best marker with a sensitivity of 53% and specificity of 88% and was the only criterion of statistical significance in their study. Other less important ST changes with high specificity include ST depression ≥ 1 mm in V_1, V_2, and V_3 (sensitivity 29%, specificity 82%), and ST elevation ≥ 1 mm in leads with a concordant QRS polarity. So-called primary T wave abnormalities are not diagnostically useful during RV pacing[16].

Cardiac Ischemia

Marked discordant ST elevation (>5mm) described above for the diagnosis of myocardial infarction[16], could also be used for the diagnosis of severe reversible transmural myocardial ischemia. Only two cases of ischemia with discordant ST elevation during ventricular pacing have been published[18,19]. Both affected the *inferior* wall.

Impact of Recent Advances

1. In hypertrophic obstructive cardiomyopathy, selection of the longest AV delay that achieves complete ventricular capture by QRS criteria may not be optimal. Lack of improvement may require repositioning of the RV lead with echocardiography to ensure a distal apical position because fluoroscopy and QRS morphology during pacing are imprecise markers of lead position.
2. The configuration, duration and delay (and degree of atrial latency) of the paced P waves should be carefully evaluated for evidence of interatrial conduction delay that may require reprogramming of the AV delay or the addition of a second atrial lead for biatrial pacing to provide optimal mechanical AV synchrony on the left side of the heart.
3. The advent of multisite pacing has added a new dimension to ECG

follow-up. The patterns of pacing from the coronary venous system need reevaluation. In heart failure patients, QRS morphology and duration must be correlated with hemodynamic response. Multisite atrial pacing must be shown to capture both atria simultaneously by fusion without reliance on capture data during sequential single site atrial testing.

REFERENCES

1. Barold SS, Falkoff MD, Ong LS et al. Electrocardiographic diagnosis of myocardial infarction during ventricular pacing. Cardiol Clin 1987; 5:403-417

2. Barold SS, Falkoff MD, Ong LS, et al. Electrocardiographic analysis of normal and abnormal pacemaker function. In Dreifus LS (Ed), Pacemaker Therapy, Cardiovascular Clinics, Philadelphia, F.A.Davis, 1983:97-134.

3. Klein HO, Becker B, Sareli P et al. Unusual QRS morphology associated with transvenous pacemakers. The pseudo RBBB pattern. Chest 1985;87:517-52111.

4. Klein HO, Becker B, DiSegni E et al. The pacing electrogram. How important is the QRS complex configuration? Clin Prog Electrophysiol 1986;4:112.-136.

5. Coman JA, Trohman RG. Incidence and electrocardiographic localization of safe right bundle branch block configurations during permanent ventricular pacing. Am J Cardiol 1995;76:781-784.

6. Sharafi M, Sorkin R, Sharifi V et al. Inadvertent malposition of a transvenous-inserted pacing lead in the left ventricular chamber . Am J Cardiol 1995;76:92-95.

7. Trigano JA, Paganelli F, Fekhar s et al. Pocket infection complicating inadvertent transarterial permanent pacing. Successful percutaneous explantation. Clin Cardiol 1999;22:492-493.

8. Orlov MV, Messenger JC, Tobias S et al. Transesophageal echocardiographic visualization of left ventricular malpositioned pacemaker electrodes:Implications for lead extraction procedures. PACE 1999;22:1407-1409.

9. Hands ME et al. Electrocardiographic diagnosis of myocardial infarction in the presence of complete left bundle branch block. Am Heart J 1988;116:23-31.

10. Castellanos A Jr, Zoble R, Procacci PM et al. St-qR pattern. New sign of diagnosis of anterior myocardial infarction during right ventricular pacing. Br Heart J 1973;35:1161-1165.

11. Brandt RR, Hammil SC, Higano ST. Electrocardiographic diagnosis of acute myocardial infarction during ventricular pacing. Circulation

1998;97:2274-2275

12.Kafka W. ECG and VCG diagnosis of infarction in pacemaker dependent patients (Abstract). PACE 1985;8:A-16.

13.Kaul U, Anand IS, Bidwai PS et al. Diagnosis of myocardial infarction in patients   during right ventricular pacing. Indian J Chest Dis Allied Sci 1981;23:68-72.

14.Kindwall KE, Brown JP, Josephson ME. Predictive accuracy of criteria for chronic myocardial infarction in pacing-induced left bundle branch block. Am J Cardiol 1985;57:1255-1260

15. Barold SS. Unpublished obvservations.

16.Sgarbossa EB, Pinski SL, Gates KB, Wagner GS, for the Gusto-1 Investigators.Early electrocardiographic diagnosis of acute myocardial infarction in the presence of a ventricular paced rhythm. Am J Cardiol 1996;77:423-424.

17. Sgarbossa EB. Recent advances in the electrocardiographic diagnosis of myocardial infarction: left bundle branch block and pacing. PACE 1996;19:1370-1379.

18. Manyari DE, Klein GJ, Kostuk WJ. Electrocardiographic recognition of variant angina during permanent pacing. PACE 1983;6:99-103.

19. Mery D, Dagran O, Bailly E, Grolleau R, Puech P. First and second degree blocks (Wenckebach type) during right ventricular stimulation in the course of Prinzmetal's angina. Arch Mal Coeur Vaiss 1979;72:385-390.

44.

PACING LEADS FOR THE NEW MILLENIUM.

Harry G Mond MD, FRACP, FACC.

Physician to the Pacemaker Clinic, Royal Melbourne Hospital, Australia.

Introduction

The cardiac pacemaker lead, the Achilles heel of pacing hardware, is a relatively fragile cable of insulated conductor wire implanted into the hostile environment of the human body. Its function is to interface the power source and sophisticated electronics of the pulse generator with the heart. In comparison with the marked advances in pulse generator and sensor technology, concomitant advances in pacing leads have occurred relatively slowly. This chapter will review some of the deficiencies in pacemaker lead design, currently being addressed with bold and exciting engineering developments. The pacing lead of the twenty-first century will be safe, thin and long life with reliable sensing and low stimulation threshold pacing.

Lead Polarity

A controversy has continued unabated for more than 30 years with respect to which lead system, unipolar or bipolar is superior.[1] Unlike early designs, modern bipolar leads approximate unipolar designs in size, ease of insertion and reliability.[2] Although unipolar pacing leads remain popular in selected areas of Europe, the use of bipolar, silicone rubber insulated leads is gradually increasing in both the atrium and ventricle.

The Pacing Electrode
Electrode Size

The earliest transvenous pacing leads had a large stimulating cathode, low pacing impedance and an excessive current drain.[3] In addition, a large electrode surface area dispersed the electron flow over a large area, resulting in a low current density and hence a high stimulation threshold. By reducing the cathodal surface area, high current densities and lower stimulation threshold levels were achieved, together with improved longevity of the power source.[4,5] Today, leads with $<2mm^2$ cathode electrodes and $>1000\ \Omega$ impedance have extremely low stimulation thresholds and are safe for long term pacing and sensing.[6]

Polarization and Electrode Porosity

Polarization results from an intense chemical reaction at the electrode-tissue interface when current flows from the electrode to the tissues. The flowing away of the negatively charged ions leaves behind an alignment of oppositely charged particles attracted by the emerging electrons. Like the

From Ovsyshcher IE. *Cardiac Arrythmias and Device Therapy: Results and Perspectives for the New Century.* Armonk, NY: Futura Publishing Company, Inc., © 2000

resistance effect of the electrode, the electrochemical polarization effect increases as the geometric electrode surface area is reduced and this in turn can reduce pacing efficiency. The trade-off between low stimulation thresholds resulting from small surface area electrodes and the effects of polarization has been addressed by designing electrodes with a complex porous structure. The original macroporous electrode consisted of sintered platinum-iridium fibers, giving the appearance of a fine wire mesh. More recently microporous electrodes have been developed. This may involve surface treatment of a solid electrode such as sintering or electroplating a metal powder or micro-spheres onto a metal substrate. A recent development has been fractal coating.[7] The titanium electrode is totally covered with iridium hemispheres. On top of these hemispheres, smaller hemispheres are applied again and again, enlarging the active surface area many thousand folds.

Electrode Composition

The composition of the electrode is critical to its long-term function. Some metals, such as stainless steel and zinc exhibit excessive corrosion, thus causing an excessive foreign body reaction and a thick peri-electrode fibrous capsule. Platinum is relatively non-reactive and alloying it with 10% iridium increases its mechanical strength without altering its electrical performance. Other materials used as cathode materials include Elgiloy (an alloy of cobalt, iron, chromium, molybdenum, nickel and manganese) and vitreous carbon, which demonstrates, low stimulation thresholds and relatively low polarization properties.[8] In recent years, titanium, titanium oxide, titanium alloys, iridium-oxide coated titanium and especially titanium nitride, have become very popular for use as cathode materials.[9,10]

Electrode-Tissue Interface

The rise in stimulation threshold that normally follows lead implantation results from inflammation at the electrode-tissue interface.[11] Physical methods, such as reducing the stiffness of the distal part of the lead [12] or keeping the electrode clean with an ion exchange membrane [13] may partially overcome this problem. The most effective way to prevent the rise in stimulation threshold is to use steroid at the electrode-tissue interface.[14] The original and most common design uses an internal chamber containing a plug of silicone rubber compounded with ≤ 1mgm dexamethasone sodium phosphate, lying immediately behind a porous electrode.[11]

Tined passive fixation leads with steroid-eluting electrodes have demonstrated very low acute and chronic stimulation thresholds in both the atrium and ventricle with virtual elimination of the early post-operative peak.[15,16,17] The author has demonstrated low stimulation thresholds even at 16-years post implantation. Patients implanted with small, high impedance, porous, steroid-eluting cathode electrodes can be safely paced from the day of implantation at or less than 2.5 volts.[18] The ability to safely use these low voltages has important ramifications for pulse generator longevity and size.

Another steroid-eluting electrode, particularly for active-fixation screw-in leads designs uses a steroid impregnated silicone rubber or ceramic collar positioned immediately behind the cathode.[19,20,21] Steroid-eluting epicardial electrodes using a platinized porous-platinum button behind, which lies a steroid-eluting silicone rubber plug are also available.[22]

Lead Conductor

With the re-emergence of bipolar pacing as the preferred form of pacing, attention has centered on the development of thin bipolar leads comparable in diameter to unipolar designs. The helically coiled conductor wound around an empty core has stood the test of time, particularly as it allows the passage of a stainless steel stylet to aid implantation. Such leads are prone to fracture at stress points and to some extent this can be overcome with a multi-filar coil arrangement, which allows redundancy.

Bipolar transvenous leads require two conductors. Rather than the original parallel arrangement of conductors in bi-lumen insulation tubing, the coaxial design created a much smaller circumference lead body with a single inner lumen for stylet control. Such leads are thicker than unipolar designs and because of complexity, the long-term reliability may be less than for unipolar leads. A new novel design, marginally thicker than a standard unipolar lead has a multi-filar helical cathodal coil which accepts the stylet, whereas the anode is a very small diameter cabled nickel alloy wire, which has very little impact on the overall lead diameter.[23]

The development of *coated wire technology* has allowed bipolar leads to have the same diameter as unipolar leads. The technique involves the coating of single strands of conductor wire with a very thin layer of polymer insulation. Two or more conductors can be grouped together into a multi-filar, single coil, which is then placed within an insulative tube. The flexibility and handling characteristics are identical to a unipolar lead.[9]

Lead Insulation

Silicone rubber was replaced by thin polyurethane insulation in the late 1970's, because of its low tear strength and consequently the need to create thick insulation tubing. The polyurethanes exhibit very high tensile and tear strengths, flexibility and a low coefficient of friction when wetted with blood making them easier to insert and pass along venous channels. The material introduced was Pellethane 2363® (Upjohn Co., CPR Division, Torrance CA.).

By the early 1990's, a number of disturbing reports appeared, describing in-vivo degradation of implanted polyurethane with surface cracking and subsequent insulation failure.[24,25] Some of these failures could be attributed to manufacturing processes. The cracking and crazing caused during manufacture and exacerbated at stress points such as ligature sites and between the clavicle and first rib can continue in the biologically corrosive environment of the human body in a process referred to as *environmental stress cracking (ESC)*. This may eventually lead to insulation failure. Another problem encountered by polyurethane insulation is *Metal induced oxidation* (MIO). This probably results from hydrogen peroxide released by inflammatory cells and the catalyst is thought to be a conductor corrosion product, which accumulates following ingress of body fluids from the insulation breakdown.[26] In order to minimize MIO, conductors can be barrier coated with a submicroscopic layer of inert platinum.[2] These problems are more common with bipolar leads.

Pellethane® 55D, which is stiffer and harder than Pellethane® 80A, has improved biostability, but the stiffness may result in perforation of the right ventricle. New varieties of polyurethane are continually being investigated and combinations of silicone rubber and polyurethane may be clinically acceptable. For instance a polyurethane lead may have a silicone rubber distal end. Another alternative is to place a barrier of silicone rubber, between the polyurethane and the conductor. A novel design uses a thin polymer layer of insulation and then coated with a tough material such as expanded Polytetrafluoroethylene (ePTFE or Gore-Tex®) (WL Gore and Associates Inc. Flagstaff, AZ., USA).

During the late 1970's, a stronger and tougher extra tear resistance silicone rubber (ETR) was introduced, but this material demonstrated stretching at implantation. A further development was high performance silicone rubber (HP) which had improved tear strength, but demonstrated, creep. This results from the movement of molecules over areas of stress such as ligature sites resulting in insulation thinning. Recently, thin leads using a hybrid silicone rubber, Med 47190, which encompasses the best features of all the previous silicone rubbers, has become popular.[27]

Atrial Pacing Leads

The development of a transvenous atrial lead presents specific challenges. Because the right atrial appendage is heavily trabeculated, passive fixation atrial endocardial leads are J shaped to allow cathode positioning within or close to the atrial appendage. Because of the concern with lead dislodgement, endocardial screw-in leads became popular, although it was soon recognised that high-energy outputs were necessary to overcome high stimulation thresholds.[20] As experience was obtained with both active and passive fixation leads, lead dislodgement was found to be very low and high volume implanters report an incidence of 1 to 4% with no clear preference for either design.[20,23] The recent introduction of steroid-eluting screw-in leads demonstrates stimulation thresholds comparable to tined leads, thus allowing a choice of lead designs in the atrium.[28] Active fixation leads may be J shaped or straight and can be positioned anywhere in the atrium. However, an area close to or within the right atrial appendage is desirable to prevent far field sensing. Recently steerable stylets for active fixation leads have been introduced and have been found to be extremely useful in patients with enlarged atria, difficult anatomy, congenital abnormalities or the need for positioning in unusual locations in either the atrium or ventricle.[29]

Single Pass Leads

With the popularity of dual chamber pacing, it was not surprising that a single lead pacing system would be developed to overcome the need for two separate leads. The main limiting factor of a single pass lead is the necessity for the atrial electrode to make contact with the atrial wall to allow atrial pacing. Consequently such systems can only provide VDD pacing which limits patient selection, to atrio-ventricular block with normal sino-atrial function. A normal right atrial size is desirable.

The search for a single pass lead with atrial pacing capabilities (DDD) continues. A single pass tined lead with an atrial J component activated by stylet withdrawal, after the ventricular component is positioned is under evaluation.[30] The question remains, whether an intra-atrial floating bipolar electrode can be used for DDD(R) pacing? A new stimulation technique involves a novel form of overlapping biphasic pulses on a bipolar two-ring atrial electrode.[31] The first unipolar square wave pulse is applied to the distal electrode and is positive. The second pulse, which is negative, is applied to the proximal electrode and the delay between the two pulses is programmable. Early results indicate chronic stimulation thresholds in excess of that desirable for chronic long-term atrial pacing.[32]

Coronary Sinus Leads

Atrial pacing from the coronary sinus using specialized pacing leads was reported as early as the 1960's, but interest in such leads waned with the development of more reliable right atrial leads. With the recent interest in bi-atrial pacing, there has been a resurrection of coronary sinus pacing. One recent design uses a distal cathode with a double 45° angulation, one behind the anode and the other immediately behind the tip of the cathode.[33] The purpose of these angles is to enable close contact of the cathode with the coronary sinus wall. The coronary sinus has also been used for left ventricular pacing.[34] Using a standard ventricular lead, a modified atrial J lead or a coronary sinus lead, distal cathodal pacing with the lead pushed as far as possible into the coronary sinus will result in left ventricular pacing via the great cardiac or more distal cardiac veins. This can be used in conjunction with a lead at the apex or outflow tract of the right ventricle for bi-ventricular pacing. Such pacing has been recommended in patients with a wide QRS and severe cardiac failure to resynchronize the wave of depolarization and improve cardiac output.[35] New lead designs to improve the cardiac vein position and to lower the stimulation thresholds are currently being evaluated. One concept uses a work-station and introducer to position a thin floppy guide wire into a distal coronary venous tributary on the lateral left ventricular wall. The thin lead has a central orifice in the electrode, which communicates with the lumen of the lead. This lead can then be threaded like a coronary angioplasty catheter over the guide wire for positioning. Also being considered is the angioplasty monorail design with an external guide wire.

Because current dual chamber pulse generators cannot cater for more than two pacing leads, the use of complicated dual chamber pacing systems with three or four transvenous leads introduces a number of yet unresolved problems with pacing hardware. Specialized Y connectors to join the cathodes and anodes of the two leads in the same chamber have recently been used. The real answer awaits the design of new complicated pulse generator connector blocks able to accept three or four pacing leads.

Concluding Remarks

In recent years, there have been remarkable advances in cardiac pacing leads. The most important changes have been the establishment of safe bipolar leads with small, porous, steroid-eluting electrodes that provide extremely low chronic stimulation threshold and low polarization characteristics. It is important not to forget the less heralded advances in conductor and insulation technology. Currently, there is considerable research on left ventricular pacing via the cardiac veins in patients with heart failure which may provide a major new non-bradycardia indication for cardiac pacing.

References ⎯⎯⎯⎯⎯⎯⎯⎯⎯⎯⎯⎯

1. Mond H G: Unipolar versus bipolar pacing - Poles apart. PACE 1991;14:1411-1424.
2. Medtronic, Inc. Product performance report. Medtronic, MN. February 1998.

3. Mond H: The Cardiac Pacemaker. Function and Malfunction. New York, Grune and Stratton 1973, pp 60-66.

4. Schuchert A and Kuck KH: Influence of internal current and pacing current on pacemaker longevity. PACE 1994;17:13-16.

5. Bradycardia pacemaker longevity. Tech Memo, Sulzer Medica, Sept. 1997.

6. Ellenbogen KA, Wood MA, Gilligan DM, et al. Steroid eluting high impedance pacing leads decrease short and long term current drain: Results from a multicenter clinical trial. PACE 1999;22:39-48.

7. Schaldach M, Hubman M, Weikl A, et al: Sputter-deposited TiN electrode coatings for superior sensing and pacing performance. PACE 1990;13:1891-1895.

8. Elmqvist H, Schueller H, Richter G: The carbon tip electrode. PACE 1983;6:436-439.

9. Tang C, Yeung-Lai-Wah JA, Qi A, et al.: Initial experience with a co-radial bipolar pacing lead. PACE 1997;20:1800-1807.

10. DelBufalo AGA, Schlaepfer J, Fromer M et al: Acute and long-term ventricular stimulation thresholds with a new, Iridium oxide-coated electrode. PACE 1993;16:1240-1244.

11. Mond H and Stokes KB: The electrode-tissue interface: The revolutionary role of steroid elution. PACE 1992;15:95-107.

12. Cameron J, Ciddor G, Mond H, et al: Stiffness of the distal tip of bipolar pacemaker leads. PACE 1990;13:1915-1920.

13. Guerola M and Lindegren U: Clinical evaluation of membrane-coated 3,5 mm^2 porous titanium nitride electrodes. In Aubert AE, Ector H and Stroobandt R (Eds) Euro-pace '93. Monduzzi Editore 1993 pp 447-450.

14. Stokes K, Bornzin G: The electrode - biointerface: Stimulation. In Barold SS (ed): Modern Cardiac Pacing. New York: Futura Publishing, 1985, pp 33-77.

15. Mond H, Stokes KB: The steroid-eluting electrode: A 10-year experience. PACE 1997;19:1016-1020.

16. Mond HG: Development of low stimulation-threshold, low-polarization electrodes. In: New Perspectives in Cardiac Pacing. 2. Edited by Barold SS and Mugica J. 1991, Futura Publishing Company, Inc., Mount Kisco, New York P133-162.

17. Hua W, Mond HG, and Strathmore N: Chronic steroid eluting lead performance: A comparison of atrial and ventricular pacing.PACE 1997;20:17-24.

18. Hiller K, Rothschild JM, Fudge W et al: A randomized comparison of a bipolar steroid-eluting lead and a bipolar porous platinum coated titanium lead (Abstract). PACE 1991;14:695.

19. Mathivanar R, Anderson N, Harman D et al. In vivo elution of drug eluting ceramic leads with a reduced dose of dexamethasone sodium phosphate. PACE 1990;13:1883-1886.

20. Mond HG, Hua W and Wang CC: Atrial Pacing Leads:The clinical

contribution of steroid elution. PACE 1995;18:1601-1608.

21. Greco OT, Ardito RV, Martinelli M et al: Sweet Tip Rx – A new type of atrial active fixation lead (Abstract). PACE 1997: 20;1462.

22. Karpawich PP, Hakimi M, Arciniegas E: Improved chronic epicardial pacing in children: Steroid contribution to porous platinised electrodes. PACE 1992;15:1151-1157.

23. Grammage MD, Swoyer J, Moes R et al: Initial experience with a new design parallel conductor, high impedance, steroid-eluting bipolar pacing lead (Abstract). PACE 1997;20:1229.

24. Scheuer-Leeser M, Irnich W, Kreuzer J: Polyurethane Leads: Facts and Controversy. PACE 1983;6:454-458.

25. Timmis GC, Westveer DC, Martin R et al: The significance of surface changes on explanted polyurethane pacemaker leads. PACE 1983;6:845-857.

26. Stokes K, Urbanski P, Upton J: The in vivo auto-oxidation of polyether polyurethanes by metal ions. J.Biomatr.Sc., Polymer 1990;1:207.

27. Medtronic family of Novus® Leads. Medtronic, Minneapolis, MN.

28. Crossley GH, Brinkler JA, Reynolds D et al: Steroid elution improves the stimulation threshold in an active-fixation atrial permanent pacing lead. Circ. 1995; 92:2935.

29. Locator Steerable Stylet. A product of Pacesetter, AB Jarfalla Sweden.

30. Morgan K, Bornzin GA, Florio J et al: A new single pass DDD lead (Abstract). PACE 1997;20:1211.

31. Hartung WM, Strobel JP, Taskiran M, et al: "Overlapping bipolar impulse" – Stimulation using a single lead implantable pacemaker system first results (Abstract). PACE 1996;19:601.

32. Lucchese F, Halperin C, Strobel J et al. Single lead DDD pacing with overlapping biphasic atrial stimulation – First clinical results (Abstract). PACE 1996;19:601.

33. Daubert C, Leclercq C, Le Breton H et al: Permanent left atrial pacing with a specifically designed coronary sinus lead. PACE 1997;20:2755-2764.

34. Bai Y, Strathmore N, Mond H, Grigg L, Hunt D: Permanent ventricular pacing via the great cardiac vein. PACE 1994;17:678-683.

35. Leclercq C, Cazeau S, Le Breton H et al: Acute hemodynamic effects of bi-ventricular DDD pacing in patients with end-stage heart failure. JACC 1998;32:1825-1831.

45.

ELECTROMAGNETIC INTERFERENCE AND IMPLANTABLE DEVICES

David L. Hayes, MD

Mayo Clinic, Rochester, MN, USA

Pacemakers are subject to interference from many sources. Most sources of electromagnetic interference (EMI) are nonbiologic, but in addition, biologic sources of interference such as myopotentials and extremes of temperature or irradiation may cause pacemaker malfunction. In general, modern pacemakers are effectively shielded against electromagnetic interference (EMI), and the increasing use of bipolar leads has reduced the problem even further. There has always been some concern about EMI that patients may encounter in the non-hospital environment, with improvements in pacemaker protection, i.e. shielding and design changes, EMI is now of less concern. The principal sources of interference that affect pacemakers are in the hospital environment.

The portions of the electromagnetic spectrum that may affect pacemakers are *radio-frequency waves* with frequencies between 0 and 10^9 Hz, including alternating current electricity supplies (50 or 60 Hz) and electrocautery, and *microwaves* with frequencies between 10^9 and 10^{11} Hz.[1] Higher frequency portions of the spectrum, including infrared, visible light, ultraviolet, x-rays, and gamma rays, do not interfere with pacemakers because their wavelength is much shorter than the pacemaker or lead dimensions. However, therapeutic radiation can damage pacemaker circuitry directly.

The contemporary pacemaker is immune from most sources of interference because the circuitry is shielded inside a stainless steel or titanium case. In addition, the body tissues provide some protection by reflection or absorption of external radiation. Therefore, in vitro studies of pacemaker interference may at times demonstrate a disturbance of pacemaker function, whereas in vivo exposure may not result in any abnormalities.

Bipolar leads sense less conducted and radiated interference because the electrode distance, and thus the antenna, is smaller than for unipolar leads. Bipolar sensing has effectively eliminated myopotential inhibition and crosstalk as pacemaker problems. In addition, studies have shown that with bipolar sensing there is considerably less sensing of external electric fields[2-3] and less effect from electrocautery during surgery.

Sensed interference is filtered by narrow bandpass filters to exclude noncardiac signals. However, this still leaves signals in the 5- to 100-Hz

From Ovsyshcher IE. *Cardiac Arrythmias and Device Therapy: Results and Perspectives for the New Century.* Armonk, NY: Futura Publishing Company, Inc., © 2000

range, which overlap the cardiac signal range and are not filtered. These signals can give rise to abnormal pacemaker behavior if they are interpreted as cardiac signals and inhibit or trigger pacemaker output inappropriately.

The possible responses to external interference include:

- inappropriate inhibition of pacemaker output
- inappropriate triggering of pacemaker output
- asynchronous pacing
- reprogramming, usual to a back-up mode
- damage to the pacemaker circuitry

In the hospital environment, MRI remains the most controversial issue. When a pacemaker is near a MRI scanner with the electromagnet "on," the reed switch closes, and asynchronous pacing occurs, which may compete with the underlying cardiac rhythm. Measuring the effect of the MRI scanner on pacemakers is made difficult because the radio-frequency pulses cause electrocardiographic artifacts. However, several studies have demonstrated the potential effects using pacemakers connected to resistances and oscilloscopes, and in dogs. In some pacemakers there was no effect except asynchronous pacing.[4] In other pacemakers, however, a signal of approximately 20V was induced in the lead,[5] which can cause cardiac pacing at the same frequency or a multiple of the frequency of the radio-frequency current. Thus, cardiac pacing may occur at the frequency of the pulsed energy, 60 to 300bpm. In the case of a dual-chamber pacemaker, this may affect the atrial channel or the ventricular channel, or both. The radiofrequency signal is detected by the leads acting as an antenna and is then amplified by the pacemaker circuitry to produce sufficient energy to pace the heart. The lead must be attached to a pacemaker for pacing to occur, so it is not simply related to the radio-frequency energy in the lead.[4] However, the lead does not necessarily have to be in use, as has been demonstrated in a canine study that a dual-chamber pacemaker with both atrial and ventricular leads attached but programmed to the AAI mode produced rapid ventricular pacing in the presence of an MRI scanner.[4]

Pacemaker response to MRI may also vary by manufacturer and also by model from an individual manufacturer. Some companies comment on MRI in the individual technical manuals. Some advocate that MRI be a firm contraindication in the patient and others suggest that MRI may be used with caution. In general, patients with pacemakers should not routinely undergo MRI scanning until further studies are available.

Reported problems of pacemakers in MRI scanners include: magnet-activated asynchronous pacing, inhibition by the radio-frequency signal, rapid pacing induced by the radiofrequency signal, discomfort at the pacemaker pocket, and death in an unmonitored patient.[5-7] In the canine model, transient reed switch malfunction has also been seen.[4] There are no published reports of pacemaker reprogramming or of permanent component damage by MRI.

In phantom studies, Achenbach and colleagues[6] demonstrated significant heating of the electrode tip during MRI exposure. The documented temperatures at the electrode tip as high as 88.8°C, or an increase of 63.1°C from the starting temperature of 25.7°C. They warn that although clinical complications from electrode heating have not been reported, it is a potential adverse effect of which clinicians should be aware.

Although there are multiple reports of MRI being performed in patients with pacemakers and ICDs, MRI remains a relative contraindication. Reported problems of pacemakers patients undergoing MRI include: inhibition by the radio-frequency signal, rapid heart rate, discomfort at the pacemaker pocket, and death in an unmonitored patient[1]. If MRI is attempted, the patient must be given a thorough explanation regarding the relative contraindication of performing an MRI, potential adverse outcomes and the inability to predict adverse outcomes.

For any other potential source of EMI in the hospital, the most important clinical step is to review the programmed settings of the device prior to and after exposure to any procedure where EMI is a potential concern.

In the industrial environment, conventional wisdom has been to advise patients to avoid "arc-welding" and close contact with combustion engines. This advice needs to be reexamined as pacemakers become more resistant to external interference. However, pacemakers of unipolar sensing configuration remain more susceptible to EMI than pacemakers in a bipolar sensing configuration.[8] For patients whose livelihood involves equipment with potential for EMI, a pacemaker with committed bipolar sensing configuration should be implanted.

Industrial environments with significant potential for clinically significant EMI include industrial-strength welding, i.e. welding equipment of ≥500 amperes, degaussing equipment and induction ovens.[8]

In the non-hospital environment there are many potential sources of single beat inhibition but very few sources that are of clinical significance. There are no reports of normally functioning domestic appliances having any significant effect on modern pacemakers. Despite the safety of microwave ovens, warning signs still exist inappropriately in many public places. Potentially, an electric shaver moved over a unipolar pacemaker may cause temporary asynchronous pacing. There are no reports of interference from portable non-cellular telephones or portable computers, but if this technology changes, the potential for EMI should be reassessed.

Metal detectors are frequently mentioned as a potential problem and warning signs are often seen at airport security stations. However, the only realistic adverse effect would be transient asynchronous pacing, transient oversensing or single-beat inhibition, and these should not result in ill effect to the patient. The major reason to warn patients about metal detectors is that the detector may be activated by the implanted device.

The potential for interference from cellular phones and electronic article surveillance equipment have been of intense interest because of the potential public health issues. Prior studies have demonstrated the potential for clinically significant EMI during cellular phone use.[9] However, in a large multi-center study testing a variety of commercially available phones used in the United States, there was no clinically significant interference that occurred when phones were tested in a normal use position, i.e. phone at the ear.[10] EMI is more likely to occur if an activated phone is held over an implanted pacemaker. Therefore, patients with pacemakers and ICDs should avoid carrying a cellular phone in the "on" mode, such that it would be over the device. Ideally the phone should be used on the ear contralateral to the implanted device. Among varieties of cellular phones, phones of the analog variety displayed the least interference, even in "worst-case" applications, and of digital varieties tested, the least interference was noted with the (Personal Communication System variety.) There is less information available regarding cellular phone interference with ICDs.[11] Nonetheless, no significant interactions have been reported. ICD patients should follow the same basic rules of cellular phone use described for pacemaker patients.

Interference from electronic article surveillance (EAS) systems has been the source of recent controversy. Antitheft devices (electronic article surveillance equipment), in many department stores consist of a tag or marker that is sensed by an electromagnetic field as the individual walks through or by a "gate." Most systems consist of a "deactivator" that a cashier may use to remove or deactivate the tag following the purchase of an item. This allows the individual to purchase an item and leave the store without activating an alarm. These electronic antitheft devices consist of multiple technologies that generate electromagnetic fields in various ranges and include devices using the radio-frequency range of 2 to 10 mHz, magnetic material in the 50 to 10 kHz-range, pulsed systems at various frequencies, and electromagnetic fields in the microwave range. In vitro testing of pulse generators as well as "in vivo" studies of patients with permanent pacemakers and/or ICDs have been performed.[12-13] In an earlier study[12] the authors studied 32 volunteers with 26 different pacemaker models and demonstrated that 1 of 22 patients with a single-chamber pacemaker experienced inhibition, whereas 7 of 10 patients with dual-chamber generators experienced inhibition of output, with long pauses being seen in the majority of pacemaker-dependent patients. Inhibition occurred when patients were in regions of low- and high-intensity magnetic fields at 10 kHz and at 300 Hz, or both. Radio-frequency and pulsed electromagnetic fields did not affect pacemaker function. Alterations in pacing thresholds or programmed parameters were not noted. The authors concluded that electronic antitheft devices can be dangerous to pacemaker patients, particularly if a unipolar DDD generator is implanted.[12]

In a "Study of pacemakers and implantable cardioverter defibrillator triggering by electronic article surveillance devices" or "SPICED TEAS", 33 patients implanted with a total of 35 devices, 18 pacemakers and 17 ICDs, were exposed to 6 different electronic article surveillance (EAS) detectors.[13] Of the 6 EAS equipment, 3 were radiofrequency devices, 1 was magneto-acoustic and 2 were magnetic devices. No reprogramming or damage of pulse generators was noted. Sixteen of the pacemakers demonstrated noise reversion and/or inhibition when they were exposed to a magneto-acoustic system at a close range, i.e. <18 inches. Reprogramming the sensitivity of the pacemaker could not abolish this effect. In addition, one epicardial, unipolar pacemaker exhibited inhibition or noise reversion in each magnetic device. No EMI effects on any of the ICDs were demonstrated. No EMI was detected in any patients during exposure to the radiofrequency system.

Another abstract details 53 patients with pacemakers exposed to two security systems, one anti-theft device and an electromagnetic access device.[14] The difference between these devices is not detailed in the abstract. They note pacemaker malfunction in 13% of the monitored patients exposed to the first security system. They go on to describe one patient with a VVIR pacemaker that was reprogrammed to a back-up VOO mode. (It is not clear if the single patient accounts for the 13% malfunction rate.) With the second security system a malfunction was detected in 4% of the patients tested. In patients with pacemakers with bipolar sensing configurations no malfunctions were seen with exposure to any of the equipment described. No patients, regardless of pacemaker sensing polarity demonstrated abnormalities with exposure to the anti-theft device or the electromagnetic access device. They recommended that patients with the potential for being near security systems should preferentially receive pacing systems with bipolar sensing configuration. McIvor[13] reported a study of 25 ICD patients and 50 pacemaker patients and demonstrated pacemaker interference, primarily from acousto-magnetic EAS equipment. Pacemaker interactions included asynchronous pacing, tachycardia due to atrial oversensing with ventricular tracking, inhibition via ventricular oversensing and extrasystoles hypothesized to be due to direct induction of a current in the pacemaker lead by the magnetic field. Asynchronous pacing was seen when 2 pacemakers were tested with a magnetic audio frequency EAS system.

No ICD interference was noted in their study but there is a subsequent case report of a patient with an ICD receiving inappropriate shocks due to oversensing of the pulsed electromagnetic signal.[15] An accompanying "letter to the editor" suggests that patients with devices should pass "quickly through the gates" of the EAS equipment and also promotes labeling of areas where a strong magnetic field may exist.[16] A more definitive study has been published that tested 170 patients with ICDS with exposure to EAS systems.[17] They concluded that it is safe for a patient with an ICD to walk through electronic article surveillance systems. Lingering in a surveillance system may result in an inappropriate ICD shock. The controversy has resulted in a mailing from the FDA warning clinicians of potential interactions between EAS systems and implanted devices.[18] Although larger studies are needed to provide clinicians and patients with definitive guidelines, it is reasonable to advise patients to pass rapidly through any obvious EAS equipment and avoid leaning on or standing "near" the EAS equipment.

Given the continued rapid advances in wireless technology, ongoing surveillance for potential sources of EMI and ongoing attempts to make implantable devices less vulnerable to EMI must continue. Medical professionals need to have a thorough understanding of potential sources of EMI and information regarding EMI should be part of patient education provided at the time of device implant.

References

1. Barold SS, Falkoff MD, Ong LS, et al: Interference in cardiac pacemakers: Exogenous sources. *In* El-Sherif N, Samet P (eds): Cardiac Pacing and Electrophysiology, 3rd ed. Philadelphia, WB Saunders, 1991, pp 608–632.
2. Toivonen L, Valjus J, Hongisto M, et al: The influence of elevated 50 Hz electric and magnetic fields on implanted cardiac pacemakers: The role of the lead configuration and programming of the sensitivity. PACE 14:2114-2122, 1991.
3. Astridge PS; Kaye GC; Whitworth S; Kelly P; Camm AJ; Perrins EJ. The response of implanted dual chamber pacemakers to 50 Hz extraneous electrical interference. PACE 1993; 16: 1966-1974.
4. Hayes DL, Holmes DR, Gray JE: Effect of 1.5 tesla nuclear magnetic resonance imaging scanner on implanted permanent pacemakers. J Am Coll Cardiol 10:782, 1987.

5. Fetter J, Aram G, Holmes DR, et al: The effects of nuclear magnetic resonance imagers on external and implantable pulse generators. PACE 7:720, 1984.

6. Achenbach S, Moshage W, Diem B, Bieberle T, Schibgilla V, Bachmann K. Effects of magnetic resonance imaging on cardiac pacemakers and electrodes. AHJ 1997;134:467 - 473.

7. Gimbel JR, Lorig JR, Wilkoff BL. Safe magnetic resonance imaging of pacemaker patients [abstract]. JACC 1995;25:11A.

8. Marco D, Eisenger G, Hayes DL. Testing of work environments for electromagnetic interference. PACE 15:2016-2022, 1992.

9. Hayes DL, Carrillo RG, Findlay GK, Embrey M.   State of the science: pacemaker and defibrillator interference from wireless communication devices PACE 1996;19:1419-1430.

10. Hayes DL, Wang PJ, Reynolds DW, Estes M 3rd, Griffith JL, Steffens RA, Carlo GL, Findlay GK, Johnson CM. Interference with cardiac pacemakers by cellular telephones. NEJM 1997; 336: 1473-1479.

11. Fetter J, Ivans V, Benditt DG, Collins J. Digital cellular telephone interaction with implantable cardioverter-defibrillators. JACC 1998;623-628.

12. Dodinot B, Godenir JP, Costa AB: Electronic article surveillance: A possible danger for pacemaker patients. PACE 16:46-53, 1993.

13. McIvor ME, Reddinger J, Floden E, Sheppard RC.   Study of pacemaker and implantable cardioverter defibrillator triggering by electronic article surveillance devices (SPICED TEAS). PACE 1998;1847-1861.

14. Wilke A, Kruse T, Funck R, Maisch B. Security systems: Interferences with pacemakers. Eur Heart J 1997; 18:482 (abstract).

15. Santucci PA, Haw J, Trohman RG, Pinski SL. Interference with an implantable defibrillator by an electronic antitheft-surveillance device. NEJM 1998;339:1371-1374.

16. McIvor ME, Sridhar S. Interactions between cardiac pacemakers and antishoplifting security systems (letter to the editor). NEJM 1998;1394-1395.

17. Groh WJ, Boschee SA, Engelstein ED, et al.   Interactions between electronic article surveillance systems and implantable cardioverter-defibrillators. Circulation 1999 100: 387-392.

18. Burlington DB: Important information on anti-theft and metal detector systems and pacemakers, ICDs, and spinal cord stimulators. Department of Health & Human Services, Rockville, MD. [Online]. Available: http://www.fda.gov/cdrh/safety.html [1998, September 28]

46.
INFLUENCE OF NEW PACING ALGORITHMS ON GENERATOR LONGEVITY

Dan Gelvan, PhD, [1]Eugene Crystal, MD, [2]Barbaros Dokumaci, MD, [1]I. Eli Ovsyshcher, MD, PhD

Arrhythmia Service, Cardiology Department, Soroka University Medical Center & Faculty of Health Sciences, Ben Gurion University, BeerSheva, Israel[1], Cardiology, SSK Hospital, Eskisehir, Turkey[2], Medtronic, Israel

Introduction

Device longevity has been on the agenda ever since the first pacemakers were implanted, and it has remained a central issue in pacemaker design and in the clinician's choice of devices. The drive for maximization of pacemaker longevity is fuelled by the desire to reduce the need for replacement procedures and the long term cost of pacing therapy. This quest, however, is constantly at odds with the need for downsizing the devices, the incorporation of sophisticated functionalities that increase the current drain, and with the need to meet the safety requirements of the pacing therapy.

Contributions to the solution of this conflict have been made from both hardware and software development. Thus, batteries with higher current density have been developed, and high impedance, high efficiency leads, reduce pacing-current drain, and have been shown to extend pacemaker longevity[1-3]. Steroid eluting electrodes[4] and the high impedance, high efficiency electrodes[1-3] have contributed to the reduction of the pacing threshold, which could translate into lower battery drain and extended longevity if the devices are programmed accordingly[5-6]. Software-based reduction in pacing energy may be obtained from reductions in the amount of pacing, the output and the pulse width (PW). Thus, algorithms that decrease the amount of pacing by giving preference to intrinsic cardiac activity serve not only a potential therapeutic purpose, but may also extend the battery life of the device. The reduction of output and pulse width may be obtained when the threshold is reduced, or when safety features allow the reduction of safety margins.

To reduce safety margins, safety features must provide a closer follow up of the patient, such as a frequent periodic determination of the pacing threshold (*e.g.* Medtronic, Kappa 700 and Biotronic, Logos[7]) or beat-to-beat monitoring of the evoked response (Pacesetter, Microny)[8]. The optimization of the output parameters and therapeutic modes also require

From Ovsyshcher IE. *Cardiac Arrythmias and Device Therapy: Results and Perspectives for the New Century.* Armonk, NY: Futura Publishing Company, Inc., © 2000

appropriate programming of the devices. However, this is often not performed, and it has been estimated that more than half the pacemakers implanted in the US remain at the nominal settings from the time of implant[6]. In consequence, in this patient population, optimal therapy and extended device longevity can only be obtained if the pacemaker is able to make the appropriate adjustments automatically.

Medtronic, Kappa 700 pacemakers feature three distinct automatic algorithms, designed to provide improved pacing therapy, which may also affect pacemaker longevity. "Capture Management" (CM) periodically performs a strength-duration threshold test, and adjusts pacing output according to prespecified safety margins. "Sinus Preference" (SP) allows the sinus rate to prevail when it drops below the sensor rate within a prespecified range, and, when pacing, will actively search for an underlying sinus rate within the defined range. "Search A-V" allows an extension of the A-V interval beyond the programmed value, to give preference to intrinsic conduction within a prespecified range, and will periodically search for such conduction. Thus, CM serves to decrease the pacemaker output by improving safety due to close autonomic follow up and a reduction of the safety margin. SP and Search AV, while therapeutic in design, serve to reduce the amount of pacing therapy delivered[9].

The present study investigates the contribution of these three algorithms to pacemaker longevity, separately and combined. The study is retrospective and uses data obtained during the premarketing clinical evaluation of the pacemaker series.

Patients and Methods

We studied a population of 22 patients implanted in two centers. All patients received DDDR devices. Of these eight were programmed to DDDR and fourteen were operated in the VDD mode. One VDD patient crossed over from VDD to DDDR before the 6 months follow up and was considered as a DDDR patient for the purpose of this analysis. The patients were followed for one year.

In order to minimize the effects of random fluctuations, the 6 and 12 months data points were averaged for each patient before data analysis. One patient died before the 12 months follow up and only the 6 months data point was used. Another patient had his CM programmed "Monitor Only" at 6 months and "adaptive" at 12 months. Consequently, only the 12 months data point was used. One patient died before the 6 months follow up and was excluded from the analysis.

Data analysis and calculations: The data collected was analyzed for the contribution of the three algorithms to pacemaker longevity, using an equation provided by manufacturer, which is a slight simplification of the intrinsic calculation made by the pacemaker programmer. Calculations using this equation differed from the intrinsic calculation by less than 5%. The equation for Medtronic, Kappa 700 devices:

$$L = 1800/(N - 7.02)$$

Where L is longevity expressed in months and $N = 2.27 \times (K + I'_A + I'_V)$,

where $K = 9.87$

$$I'_A = (Rate\ fraction_A/60) \times (amplitude_A) \times M_A \times (1-e^{-[200*A\ PW/(A\ impedance+20)]})$$

$$I'_V = (Rate\ fraction_V/60) \times (amplitude_V) \times M_V \times (1-e^{-[200*V\ PW/(V\ impedance+20)]}),$$

where Rate fraction = Mean rate x paced fraction (e.g. mean rate 75, paced 60 % of time = 75 x 0.6) and M = 0.65 + amplitude.

The effect of CM on longevity was calculated as the difference in longevity at the actual settings (*actual longevity*) and the longevity at a commonly used standard setting of 2.5V and 0.4 msec or the actual settings if higher (*nominal longevity*). The rationale for these settings is presented in the Discussion. The effects of SP and Search AV was calculated at the actual output parameters, as the difference between the actual amount of pacing and the pacing that would have occurred without these features.

Statistics: The data are presented as mean ± SD. The data were statistically analyzed by Students t-test. Tests of hypotheses were conducted at the probability level 0.05.

Results:
The mean longevity reported by the pacemaker and the calculated values are presented in Table 1. The equation used was an excellent approximation for most devices, but was less accurate at very long longevity values. The discrepancy was less than 5%, and was sufficiently small to allow the use of the equation as a good approximation.

Table 1: A comparison of calculated and reported longevity[1]

Longevity (n)		Reported (m)	Calculated (m)	Discrepancy (m)	Discrepancy (%)
All	(21)	106.0±13.1	100.6±10.3	5.3±3	4.6±6.5

[1] Reported longevity is the value reported by the programmer 6 months post implant.

Capture management (CM): CM was activated in all nine DDDR patients and in 11 of the VDD patients. A moderate saving in battery life was observed in the group as a whole (Table 2A). However, the potential saving is directly dependent on the freedom given to the algorithm to adjust the pacemaker output and PW in accordance with the threshold measurements, while providing acceptable safety margins (SM). Eleven of the patients were kept on the basic CM settings, as provided by the manufacturer (Voltage SM x 1.5; Pulse Width SM x 1.5; minimum output 1.5V; minimum PW 0.34 msec), whereas nine were reprogrammed to higher minima, higher safety margins, or both. The longevity gain in the pacemakers where CM was left at the basic settings was 5.4 months, whereas pacemakers that were reprogrammed to limit the intended freedom of CM showed no significant gain (Table 2A).

Table 2A: The effect of Capture Management on pacemaker longevity.

Category (n)	Output (V)	PW (msec)	Actual Lty* (m)	Nominal Lty** (m)	Gained (m)	p-value[#]
All (20)	2.03±0.49	0.38±0.05	106.9±6.8	103.7±7.1	3.2	0.004
At Basic (11)	1.70±0.40	0.36±0.02	108.9±6.4	103.5±7.4	5.4	0.001
Reprogrammed (9)	2.43±0.21	0.40±0.07	104.4±7.4	104.0±7.4	0.4	0.68

*at the CM adapted settings;
**at 2.5V and 0.4 msec, or at the actual setting if higher,;
[#] p-values for comparison between actual and nominal longevity

SP and Search AV are algorithms that serve to reduce the amount of pacing in the atrium and ventricle, respectively, when the appropriate conditions prevail. Since CM reduces the energy of each delivered pulse, a decrease in the number of pulses delivered may partially mask the true potential of CM. This potential was extracted by eliminating the effects of SP and Search AV in the calculation. Table 2B presents the longevity of the pacemakers when these contributions were eliminated. It may be seen that the contribution of the CM algorithm is 40% higher when the sensing preference algorithms are eliminated.

Table 2B: The effect of Capture Management on pacemaker longevity, after elemination of contribution of SP and Search AV.

Category (n)	Actual Lty* (m)	Nominal Lty** (m)	Gained (m)	p-value[#]
All (20)	103.0±6.9	98.2±4.9	4.8	<0.001
At Basic (11)	105.7±6.0	98.2±5.7	7.5	<0.001
Reprogrammed (9)	99.7±6.7	98.2±4.4	1.5	0.03

*at the CM adapted settings; savings from SP and Search AV eliminated from
   the calculation
**at 2.5V and 0.4 msec, or at the actual output settings if higher. Savings from SP and
   Search AV eliminated from the calculation,
[#] p-values for comparison between actual and nominal longevity

Sinus Preference (SP): SP was activated in 4 of the DDDR patients at nominal settings (rate offset 10 bpm, search every 10 min). This feature is not available in the VDD mode. SP contributed to atrial sensing in all patients. Sensing was increased by 8 - 19.5 % of total time in the four patients in this group. The mean was 12.0±5.3. This decrease in pacing saved 1.5±0.45 months of battery life.

Search AV: Search AV was activated in 19 patients at the nominal setting (maximum offset = 110 msec), resulting in a moderate extension of longevity, Table 3. The purpose of the algorithm is to search for intrinsic AV conduction, within a prespecified range above the programmed AV delay (the maximum offset), and give priority to the intrinsic conduction over pacing. In our patient group, 11 had <2% sensing from Search AV, and were considered non-responders for the purpose of this analysis. Naturally, Search AV provided no longevity extension in this group. In the remaining 8 (42%) patients, Search AV activity resulted in increased ventricular sensing, amounting to 10.5 - 96.1 % of total time. The resultant increase in longevity was 8 months, Table 3 (Longevity gain). As discussed above, the concurrent activity of Search AV and CM will obscure the true potential of the former: Search AV eliminates part of the pacing pulses, while CM decreases the energy of the pacing pulses. Thus, the apparent saving, using the output settings as adjusted by CM, is smaller than the true potential of the Search AV algorithm in a manually programmed generator. Consequently, the true potential of Search AV was assessed by calculating the longevity gain in the absence of CM. The calculation used a nominal programming of 2.5V and 0.4 msec, or the actual value if it was higher. The results are presented in Table 3 (Nominal Lty gain). It is evident that Search AV is a powerful algorithm with CM on, and even more so when used for pacemakers without CM.

Table 3: The effect of Search AV on pacemaker longevity.

Category (n)	% V sense from Search AV	Longevity gain (m)	Nominal Lty gain* (m)
All (19)	31.2±40.3	3.3±-4.8	4.9±6.9
Responders** (8)	73.8±24.7	7.8±4.4	11.9±5.3
Non-responders (11)	0.3±0.5	0	0±0.1

*Nominal Lty gain is calculated for inactivated CM; output = 2.5V and PW = 0.4 msec, or actual values if higher.
** "Responders had > 2% V sensing from Search AV

Overall longevity: The overall actual longevity in this study was 106.3±8.4 months with all features as programmed, whereas the longevity without CM, SP and Search AV (Basic Lty) would have been 98.2±4.9 months. Thus, the combined features extended battery life by 8.1±5.8 months (range 0.3 - 18.3). The results are presented in Table 4.

Table 4: Total longevity gain by the combined battery saving algorithms.

Category (n)	Actual Lty[1] (m)	Basic Lty[2] (m)	Lty gain (m)	P values[3]
All (20)	106.3±8.4	98.2±4.9	8.1±5.8	<0.001
DDDR (9)	104.8±9.3	96.6±5.5	8.3±5.7	0.002
VDD (11)	107.5±7.8	99.5±4.2	7.9±6.2	0.002
Search AV responders (8)	113.0±3.4	98.5±3.3	13.6±3.7	<0.001
Search AV non-resp. (12)	101.8±7.7	97.4±5.7	4.4±3.6	0.001
CM at basic (11)	108.0±7.0	98.2±4.5	9.8±5.2	<0.001
CM reprogrammed (9)	104.1±9.8	98.2±5.7	6.0±6.1	0.02

[1]Longevity calculated at actual settings of the pacemaker.
[2]Longevity calculated without gains from CM, SP and Search AV.
[3]p values for the comparison of actual and basic longevity.

The highest saving of battery life was obtained in Search AV responders who experienced a saving of 13.6±3.7 months (12%). In this group there was only negligible difference between those with CM at nominal settings, and those who had been reprogrammed to more conservative values, likely due to the small residual fraction of pacing. Among Search AV non-responders, on the other hand, CM was an important factor, particularly when left at nominal values: Search AV non-responding patients with CM at nominal settings saved 6.7±3.6 months (6.4%), whereas those with reprogrammed CM saved only 2.1±1.8 months (2.1%).

Subdivision by CM status, shows more saving in the patients with CM at nominal values than in those with reprogrammed CM.

Discussion

The current study investigated the battery saving algorithms of Medtronic, Kappa 700. We have shown that a substantial saving of battery life can be obtained by the Capture Management and Search A-V algorithms, whereas Sinus Preference contributes only a minor saving.

A comparison of the reported and calculated longevity showed that the equation used for the calculation is accurate to within 5% of the reported longevity, which is calculated by the programmer. This makes the equation a valid tool for prediction of longevity, and was consequently used without reservation.

CM is designed to periodically measure the pacing threshold in the ventricle, and adjust the output and PW according to a set of prespecified safety margins. The primary function of this algorithm is the improvement of patient safety, by adjusting to changing threshold conditions. The daily measurement of the threshold and the consequent adjustment of the output parameters allowed a smaller safety margins for output and PW than those used in patients who receive only a routine annual or semiannual follow-up, since they have to accommodate only short term changes in the threshold. Thus, a safety factor of x1.5 was used by the manufacturer for both output and PW, and minima were set as low as 1.5V and 0.34 msec. In contrast, patients who receive only the periodic follow up are often given safety factors of x2-x4, depending on their dependence on pacing, and minima of 2.5V and 0.4 msec are commonly used. In calculating the savings provided by CM, the assumption was made that these values (or higher if required) would have been programmed in the absence of CM. Our results showed that in pacemakers kept at the manufacturers safety and minimum settings, CM extended battery life more than 5%, when seen in the context of other algorithms, and over 7.5% when isolated. CM provided no saving in pacemakers that had been reprogrammed to increase safety margins or set to higher minimum values, but would off course still meet its primary goal of improved safety. It should be borne in mind that many pacemakers are never reprogrammed to routine values (2.5V, 0.4 msec) and remain at shipping values of 3.5V and 0.4 msec. It has been suggested that this group may involve more than half the patient population[6]. Under such circumstances, CM could make a difference of an additional longevity extension of 10-12 months (data not shown).

Search AV is an algorithm primarily designed for improved therapy. The main goal is to maximize intrinsic AV conduction, with the resulting natural depolarization sequence. The primary value of this algorithm is in patients with intermittent AV block or with variable PR-intervals (responders), whereas patients with permanent complete AV block or consistent long PR (non-responders) will not benefit. In our study group 8 patients responded with 10.5-96.1% sensing ascribable to Search AV. These patients gained an average of 12 months of pacing when the effect of CM was eliminated. These results are consistent with a previously published report[9]. It might be argued that the AV interval in these patients should have been programmed permanently to longer values. However, this would have been inappropriate, since none of these patients reached 100% pacing, suggesting that all had a variable condition, best treated by a variable algorithm.

Sinus Preference is intended to give preference to the intrinsic sinus rhythm, when this rhythm is within a specified range of tolerance from the sensor rate. As with Search AV, the natural propagation sequence is preferred over the paced, whenever possible. The algorithm specifies a range of tolerance below the sensor rate (nominally 10 bpm), and an interval at which an active search will be performed (nominally 10 min). Patients in the VDD mode or patients with permanent bradycardia will not benefit from this algorithm. In our limited study group, the algorithm was activated only in four patients, who responded by saving 8-19.5% atrial pacing. The benefit in longevity was minor.

The overall longevity gain by the combination of all algorithms ranged between 0 - 18 months in individual patients, with a mean of 8 months. There was no difference between VDD and DDDR patients. Search AV responders had the highest gain, followed by patients with CM at basic values. The overall longevity extension reflects a trend of diminishing returns when algorithms are combined. Thus, CM and Search AV both reduce ventricular current drain. However, CM reduces current drain only on delivered pulses, and when Search AV decreases the number of delivered pulses, the incremental gain from CM decreases. When these algorithms are combined with other strategies for saving battery current, such as high impedance, high efficiency leads, the incremental gain is even smaller for each of the strategies employed, as the current drain approaches an asymptote at 0. Thus, Search AV reduces the number of pulses delivered, CM reduces the current of remaining pulses by decreasing output and PW, and the lead reduces the current of the delivered pulses further by increasing impedance. In the absence of atrial CM, the strategies for atrial current drain reduction are limited to SP, which had little impact in our study, and the combination with a high impedance, high efficiency electrode. Given the limited gain by SP, the choice of the atrial lead may have more impact on pacemaker longevity, as may the possible future development of an atrial CM algorithm.

The true value of the algorithms reviewed in this study goes beyond the straightforward gain in longevity. Major benefits to the patients are derived from the automaticity of the features, which allow the therapy to be constantly updated and adapted to the patient's needs. This is important in an optimally programmed patient, and even more so in patients who are programmed suboptimally or even never reprogrammed from factory settings.

Conclusions: In addition to their possible therapeutic value, CM, SP and Search AV can provide substantial savings in battery drain, extending the service life of the pacemakers significantly. However, as several battery saving strategies are employed concurrently, the contribution of each decreases. The automaticity contributes to the proper implementation of the battery saving functions.

References

1. Danilovic D, Ohm OJ, Breivik K. Clinical use of low output settings in 1.2-mm^2 steroid eluting electrodes: three years of experience. PACE 1998; 21:2606-15.
2. Ellenbogen KA, Wood MA, Gilligan DM, et al. Steroid eluting high impedance pacing leads decrease short and long-term current drain: results from a multicenter clinical trial. CapSure Z investigators. PACE 1999; 22: 39-48.
3. Moracchini PV, Cornacchia D, Bernasconi M, et al. High impedance low energy pacing leads: long-term results with a very small surface area steroid-eluting lead compared to three conventional electrodes. PACE 1999; 22: 326-34.
4. Klein HH, Steinberger J, Knake W Stimulation characteristics of a steroid-eluting electrode compared with three conventional electrodes. PACE 1990;3: 134-7.
5. Schwaab B, Frohlig G, Schwerdt H, et al. Telemetry guided pacemaker programming: impact of output amplitude and the use of low threshold leads on projected pacemaker longevity. PACE 1998; 21: 2055-63.
6. Crossley GH, Gayle DD, Simmons TW, et al. Reprogramming pacemakers enhances longevity and is cost-effective. Circulation 1996; 94 (Suppl.):II245-7.
7. Menezes AS, Queiros CFM, Cazorla FP, et al. Increased pacemaker lifetime due to ventricular capture control. HEARTWEB 1999; 4: NIL_76-NIL_80.
8. Antretter H, Bonatti J, Cottogni M, et al. A new cardiac pacemaker stimulation technology (autocapture) allows, with unchanged life expectancy, reduction of generator size by half. Acta Medica Austriaca 1996; 23:159-64.
9. Silverman R, Casavant D, Loucks S, et al.: Atrioventricular Interval Search: A Dual-Chamber Pacemaker Feature to Promote Intrinsic A-V Conduction. PACE 1999;22:873.

Part VIII.

New Indications for Cardiac Pacing: As We Approach the New Century

LONG-TERM EXPERIENCE WITH BIVENTRICULAR PACING IN REFRACTORY HEART FAILURE

J. Claude Daubert, MD, Christophe Leclercq, MD, Christine Alonso, MD, Serge S. Cazeau, MD.

Departement de Cardiologie et Maladies Vasculaires, Centre Cardio-Pneumologique, Hopital Pontchaillou – CHU, Rennes, France

Introduction

Despite pharmacological advances, the introduction of ACE inhibitors and of beta-blockers in particular, the prognosis of patients with severe heart failure (grades III and IV of the NYHA classification) remains pejorative and their quality of life is poor. A number of non-pharmacological treatments have been proposed for this type of patients: heart transplantation remains the reference treatment although its application is restricted by donor shortage, among other factors. Left ventricular support devices are still at the evaluation stage and the results of cardiomyoplasty are highly controversial. In the early 90s, standard dual-chamber pacing with short AV delay was proposed as a supplementary treatment of drug-resistant heart failure[1,2]. Initial results were encouraging but were never confirmed[3,4]. These studies however made it possible to select a population of potentially responsive patients, especially those with a prolonged PR interval reflecting major atrioventricular asynchrony in the left heart[5]. That relative failure of standard dual-chamber pacing could be linked to the fact that by capturing the ventricle from the right apex, it increases, or at least it cannot correct the marked asynchrony of activation, contraction and relaxation which characterizes a number of patients with chronic left ventricular dysfunction. Such is the case in particular in patients with important QRS enlargement linked to major intraventricular conduction delay. Biventricular pacing, which simultaneously activates both ventricles, may contribute to correcting the asynchrony and thus improve cardiac performance.

Rationale of biventricular pacing: electromechanical correlates in Chronic Heart Failure

The purpose of multi-site biventricular pacing is to correct the sometimes major electromechanical abnormalities that result from conduction disorders associated with chronic left ventricular systolic dysfunction.

Conduction disorders in chronic LV systolic dysfunction

Anatomoclinical studies, especially the Wilensky's study[6], have shown the high prevalence of conduction disorders in patients with chronic LV systolic dysfunction, and their progression over time with an independent prognostic value. AV conduction and intraventricular conduction are particularly concerned. The PR interval increases progressively and is significantly prolonged (≥ 200 ms) in 60 % of patients at the end-stage of the disease. It has been shown that 1-st or 2-nd degree AV block was an independent risk factor of cardiac death in patients with

From Ovsyshcher IE. *Cardiac Arrythmias and Device Therapy: Results and Perspectives for the New Century.* Armonk, NY: Futura Publishing Company, Inc., © 2000

dilated cardiomyopathy[7]. In the same way significant increase of QRS duration is observed in the course of follow-up and reflects the development of progressive intraventricular conduction delay (IVCD). In the Wilensky's study[6] 27% of patients had QRS width ≥150 ms with peaks up to 200 ms on the last ECG recording before death. IVCD has also been shown as independent mortality risk factor in patients with chronic LV systolic dysfunction[8-11].

Electromechanical consequences

These conduction disorders have a significant impact on cardiac performance. The lengthening of the PR interval, be it apparent or concealed, induces atrio-ventricular desynchronization, hence shorter ventricular filling time and reduced or even suppressed left atrial contribution to ventricular filling, as often reflected by the single-pulse aspect of the mitral Doppler flow resulting from the superimposition of wave A and wave E[5]. The haemodynamic consequences of abnormal LV activation in patients with DCM have been explored in depth by Xiao et al.[12-13]. That study conducted in 50 patients revealed a positive correlation between QRS duration and Q wave delay at LV pressure peak and the interval between the Q wave and the peak +dP/dt. In contrast, QRS duration ant the + dP/dt value were negatively correlated. These data showed that the longer the QRS duration, the longer the duration of LV isovolumetric contraction and relaxing time, hence the more altered the LV pump function was. Also, the increased isovolumetric contraction and relaxation times of the left ventricle induced a shortening of filling time in patients whose QRS duration was particularly long. Finally, abnormal activation sequence may play a role in increasing mitral regurgitation : Xiao et al.[13] and Nishimura et al.[5] found a positive correlation between mitral regurgitation time and QRS duration on the one hand, and PR interval duration on the other hand. In addition, left diastolic atrio-ventricular gradient is a common occurrence in AV conduction disorders and may result in diastolic mitral regurgitation.

Acute studies with temporary pacing

The first hemodynamic study of the acute effects of biventricular pacing was conducted post-operatively immediately following coronary bypass surgery in 18 patients with LVEF > 40 %. Biventricular pacing significantly increased cardiac output and reduced systemic arterial resistance, by comparison with no pacing or right or left ventricular single site pacing[14]. Our group[15,16] reported their experience in 18 patients in class III or IV with advanced DCM and intraventricular conduction delay (mean QRS duration=170±36 ms). All these patients were in sinus rhythm, with a mean PR interval of 224±36 ms. Biventricular pacing induced a significant decrease in QRS duration on baseline (154±18 ms vs 170± 37 ms; p<0.01). The cardiac index was significantly improved by biventricular DDD pacing, when compared with no pacing or right ventricular, single chamber DDD pacing (2.7±0.7 l/min/m², 2±0.5l/min/m² and 2.4±0.6 l/min/m², respectively; p<0.01). In parallel, a significant decrease in mean pulmonary capillary pressure was observed with biventricular pacing. Other authors studied the effects of left ventricular pacing. Blanc et al.[17] compared biventricular pacing, single site left ventricular pacing, apical and outflow tract right ventricular pacing in 23 patients. Compared to baseline, biventricular pacing and LV pacing induced the same hemodynamic benefit, as assessed from the following criteria: systolic blood pressure, mean pulmonary capillary pressure and V-capillary wave; cardiac output was not considered in that study. Recently Kass et al.[18] published the results of extensive hemodynamic studies aimed to assess the acute effects of VDD pacing at varying sites (RV-apex, RV-midseptal, LV-paced transvenously and biventricular) and AV delays in 18 heart failure patients. He showed that RV pacing at any site had negligible contractile/systolic effects. However LV free-wall pacing increased dP/dt max by 23.7$\pm$19% and pulse-pressure by 18$\pm$18.4% (p< 0.01). Biventricular pacing yielded less change than LV pacing alone. In the same way pressure-volume curves analysis consistently revealed minimal changes with RV pacing but increased stroke work and lowered end-systolic volumes with LV and biventricular pacing. Finally Kass et al[18] showed that AV delay had less influence on LV function than pacing site.

<u>Which heart failure patients could be candidate for pacing therapy ?</u>

At the present stage of knowledge , we can postulate that optimal anidates should be patients i) with chronic and severe heart failure (Class IV or preferably III) related to LV systolic dysfunction whatever the etiology ii) non-or insufficiently improved by optimal drug treatment including at least diurectics, ACE inhibitors and when possible beta-blocking agents iii) with the clear evidence of electromechanical abnormalities linked to significant conduction disorders, especially wide QRS complex. The value of this last point was clearly shown in the Kass[18] study where a positive linear relationship was observed between the QRS duration during intrinsic conduction and the percentage of increase in LV + dp/dt during biventricular- or LV-VDD pacing as compared to baseline without pacing. Interestingly this correlation was missed above a cut-off QRS width of 150 ms. In summary this study showed that, within this limit, the wider was the QRS complex, the greater the acute hemodynamic benefit, iiii) finally the presence of a significant mitral regurgitation (grade$\geq$2) seems to be an additional predictive factor of positive response to pacing.

Technical requirements of permanent biventricular or left-ventricular based pacing

* How to pace the left ventricle permanently ?

Among the technical difficulties of multisite biventricular pacing, one is to chronically and safely pace the left ventricle at the optimal site. The first pacing experiments[15,20] were conducted using the <u>epicardial route</u>, and thoracotomy or thoracoscopy. However this method has two principal disadvantages. First, it incurs a non-negligible operative risk in such a severely diseased patient population. Second, the epicardial technique is associated with a poor quality of acute pacing thresholds and a high rate of delayed exit blocks resulting in LV pacing loss. However this route has the theoritical advantage to may place the pacing electrode at the optimal site in each patient. In a preliminary experience of acute intra-operative hemodynamic testing in 25 patients, Auricchio et al.[27] showed that the observed benefit was primarily dependent on the LV pacing site. From the different tested sites, the mid-part of the LV free wall provided the greater hemodynamic benefit in most patients. To eliminate the need of general anesthesia and to minimize the operative risk, our group introduced from 1994 a transvenous approach using a lead inserted in a tributary vein over the LV free wall through the coronary sinus[21]. The target location was a lateral or posterolateral coronary vein.If lateral vein catheterization failed or in case of poor pacing thresholds, the LV lead was inserted into the great cardiac vein to pace the anterobasal wall, or in the mid cardiac vein to pace the inferoapical area. From the beginning of our experiment until 1996, non-specific models of unipolar ventricular leads were used. The implantation success rate was low, only 54%. Since 1996, specifically designed coronary sinus leads have been used. The implantation success rate increased at 85% in the whole experience, and up to 92% in the last fifty patients. The target location i.e. a lateral or posterolateral vein in a mid position, could be reached in 72% of patients. No serious complications were observed during the implantation procedure, or could be related to the coronary sinus lead during the follow-up. At the end of follow-up with a mean time of 10.2±8 months, 97% of the implanted leads were fully functional.

Recently[23] LV endocardial pacing using a transeptal approach was proposed as an alternative to coronary venous pacing. This new technique is now under investigation with special focus to the potential risk of thrombo-embolism.

* RV lead placement (biventricular pacing)

The optimal pacing configuration is that which best corrects electromechanical disorders. At the present stage of knowledge, our observations[16,19] encourage to try and find the best RV and LV pacing sites according to patient, i.e., sites that would ensure the shortest QRS duration as possible and optimal QRS axis normalization in each patient, during simultaneous pacing at the two ventricles. In practice, it can be suggested to position the LV lead first, if possible in a lateral or posterolateral vein, and to secondarily determine the best RV site, based on continuous surface ECG analysis during biventricular pacemapping. The best RV and LV pacing sites usually correspond to the earliest and latest activation sites during intrinsic conduction in the individual patient.

* Devices for multisite biventricular pacing

In patients with normal sinus rhythm, AV synchrony has to be preserved and the patients are usually paced in a biventricular–DDD or VDD mode. In the early clinical experience[14], standard DDDR pacemakers were used with the atrial lead conventionnally placed at the high right atrium and the two ventricular leads connected to the ventricular port of the device through a Y bifurcarted or a parallel adapter. Many technical problems were related to the use of this external adapter with the need to pace one of the two ventricles in an anodal configuration. That resulted in high pacing treshold with a subsequent risk of exit-block. With the introduction of new, more sophisticated pacemakers dedicated to biventricular pacing and featuring a built-in connector inside the device, the technical difficulties should be considerably reduced. In those patients with normal sinus rhythm the programmed AV delay has to be optimized individually by using echo-doppler techniques. Patients with chronic atrial fibrillation have to be paced in a biventricular-VVIR mode. The LV and RV leads are connected to the atrial and the ventricular ports of a standard DDDR pacemaker, respectively.The device is programmed in the DDDR mode with the shortest programmable value of AV delay (0–30 ms) in order to activate both ventricles nearly simultaneously. To ensure full and permanent biventricular capture, the AV junction is systematically ablated at the time of implantation. In our personal esperience[19], 22% of the patients implanted with a biventricular-DDDpacemaker evolved towards persistent AF after a mean follow-up time of 14 months. The pacemaker was then reprogrammed in a biventricular-VVIR mode.

Long-term results with permanent biventricular pacing

At that time, the results of two prospective but non-randomized studies have been reported.
* The <u>French pilot study</u> started on 1994 in two centers, Rennes and Saint-Cloud[19]. Until December 1997, 50 patients, 45 males and 5 females, mean age 68 ± 8 years, were included in the study. Inclusion criteria were chronic heart failure Class III or IV with symptoms refractory to medical therapy including at least diuretics and ACE inhibitors at the maximal tolerated doses in each patient, LV systolic dysfunction as assessed on LVEF<35% and LV endiastolic diameter>60 mm, and finally intraventricular conduction delay with a QRS duration>150 ms during intrinsic conduction. At the time of inclusion 34 pts were in NYHA Class IV, including 17 in terminal phase, requiring permanent IV inotropic support, and 26 were in Class III. The mean LVEF was 20 ± 6%. CHF was of ischemic origin in 24 pts and non-ischemic in 26. The mean QRS duration was 197 ± 32 ms.14 pts with chronic AF were implanted with a biventricular-VVIR pacemaker and had the AV junction ablated at the same time. The other 36 pts were in stable sinus rhythm and received a biventricular-DDDR pacemaker. The mean duration of follow-up was 15.4 ± 10.2 months, ranging from 1 to 48 months. 20 pts died during the follow-up period within a mean of 8 ± 7.2 months after pacemaker implantation. All deceased pts but two were NYHA Class IV at the time of biventricular pacemaker implantation. Death causes were progressive pump failure (n=11), sudden cardiac death (n=6) and non cardiac (n=3). At the end of follow-up period, 55% pts were alive without heart transplant or any circulatory support. The survival rate differed significantly between pts who were NYHA Class III or IV at the time of implantation. In the course of follow-up, patient's functional status was significantly improved by permanent biventricular pacing. One month after implantation, the mean NYHA classification value was 2.37 ± 0.66 vs 3.7 ± 0.5 at the time of inclusion; p<0.001. This functional improvement persisted henceforth to the end of follow-up, when the mean functional class was 2.2 ± 0.6. In the subgroup of 16 patients who were able to exercise before pacemaker implantation,

a significant improvement in exercice tolerance was observed at 3 months, with significant increase in exercise duration (9 ± 3.4 min vs 6.3 ± 1.6 min ; p=0.01), in sustained workload (73 ± 13W vs 56 ± 19W; p<0.01) and in maximal O_2 consumption (15.5 ± 3.4 ml/kg/min vs 11.1 ± 3 ml/kg/min; p<0.01) when compared with the pre-implantation period. Simultaneous biventricular pacing induced a significant decrease in QRS duration (162 ± 29 ms vs 197 ± 32 ms; p<0.001). The variation in QRS axis was also significant with a clear trend to normalization. Finally echocardiographic data revealed a significant improvement of LVEF under biventricular pacing (24 ± 10% vs 20 ± 6% ; p<0.01).

The multicenter In-Sync study[34] involved 14 different centers in Europe and Canada, and was aimed to assess the technical feasibility, the safety and the clinical efficacy of transvenous atrioventricular-biventricular pacing in heart failure patients with stable sinus rhythm. Inclusion criteria were identical to those of the French pilot study. Over a 10-month period, 81 patients were enrolled and 68 or 84% could be successfully implanted. The study population consisted of 52 males and 16 females, with a mean age of 66 ± 10 years. The etiology was ischemic in 28 pts and non ischemic in 40. At the time of inclusion, 43 pts were in NYHA class III and 25 were in class IV. The mean 6-minute walking distance was 299 ± 121 ms. The mean LVEF was 21 ± 9 % and the mean QRS duration was 177 ± 29 ms. After the implantation, serial evaluations including functional status (NYHA class), quality of life (Minnesota Living with Heart Failure questionnaire), exercice tolerance (6-min walking distance), 12-lead surface ECG recording and doppler-echocardiography were planned at 1, 3, 6 and 12 months. During the follow-up period (1–12 months), 7 pts died from cardiovascular cause between 11 and 127 days after pacemaker implantation including cardiac sudden death in 4. A first analysis at 3 months follow-up (Tab.I) showed that DDD biventricular pacing was associated with a significant improvement in symptoms, in quality of life and in exercice tolerance when compared with the pre-inclusion period.

Table I

	T_O	M_3	P
NYHA class (*)	3.4 ± 0.5	2.1 ± 0.7	< 0.001
QOL score	55.2 ± 20	34 ± 23	< 0.01
6 min.W. D.(m)	299 ± 114	418 ± 127	< 0.01
LVEF (%)	20.9 ± 7	23.9 ± 11	NS

The mean QRS duration decreased from 177 ± 29 ms to 143 ± 18 ms ; p < 0.001, and finally there was a non significant trend to increased LVEF.

Conclusion

By correcting left ventricular asynchrony as well as left atrio-ventricular asynchrony, multisite biventricular pacing appears to significantly and durably improve the functional status, the quality of life and exercice tolerance of patients with drug-refractory heart failure secondary to chronic LV systolic dysfunction, and major intraventricular conduction delay, thus corresponding to 20 – 30 % of class III–IV patients. The technique appears highly promising as an adjuvant treatment of drug-refractory heart failure, in particular in class III patients, as mortality remains high in class IV patients. Technical advances should improve accessibility of that treatment in the near future. However, controlled and randomized trials will be necessary to validate this novel concept and better define responding patients. The results of a small german study (PATH-CHF) with use of the epicardial route to pace the left ventricle, are expected soon.The MUSTIC trial is ongoing in Europe, under the auspices of the European Society of Cardiology, with the primary objective to assess the actual impact of biventricular pacing on exercise tolerance and quality of life. Inclusion was completed on April 1999 and final results are expected in the early 2000. Other propective multicenter trials were recently started both in Europe and in North America (MERIDIEN, MIRACLE, PATH-CHF II, VIGOR-CHF...). Further and larger studies will be needed after, to assess the effect on morbidity, mortality and cost-effectiveness. Technical advances should be evaluated in parallel, especially the potential interest to combine in the same implantable device multisite pacing and ICD function. The objective should be to significantly decrease the risk of sudden cardiac death which accounts for 30% to 50% of total mortality in class III–IV patients. So, do we have reasons to be enthusiastic about multisite pacing ? Probably yes, but there is still a long way to go before validating definitively this new concept.

REFERENCES

1. Hochleitner M, Hortnagl H, Choi-Keung Ng, et al. Usefulness of physiologic dual-chamber pacing in drug- resistant idiopathic dilated cardiomyopathy.Am J Cardiol 1990; 66:198-202.

2. Brecker SJ, Xiao HB, Sparrow J, et al. Effects of dual-chamber pacing with short atrioventricular delay in dilated cardiomyopathy. Lancet 1992; 340:1308-11

3. Linde C, Gadler F, Edner M, et al. Results of atrioventricular synchronous pacing with optimized delay in patients with severe congestive heart failure. Am J Cardiol 1995;75: 919-23

4. Gold MR, Feliciano Z, Gotdieb SS, et al. Dual-chamber pacing with a short atrioventricular delay in congestive heart failure : a randomized study. J Am Coll Cardiol 1995; 26:967-73

5. Nishimura RA, Hayes DL, Holmes DR Jr, et al. Mechanism of hemodynamic improvement by dual-chamber pacing for severe left ventricular dysfunction:an acute Doppler and catheterization study. J Am Coll Cardiol 1995; 25:281-8.

6. Wilensky RL, Yudelman P, Cohen AI, et al. Serial electrocardiographic changes in idiopathic dilated cardiomyopathy confirmed at necropsy. Am J Cardiol 1988; 62: 276-83.

7. Schoeller R, Andresen D, Buttner P, et al. First or second degree atrioventricular block as a risk factor in idiopathic dilated cardiomyopathy. Am J Cardiol 1993; 71:720-6.

8. Cowburn P, Cleland J, Coast A, et al. Risk stratification in chronic heart failure. Eur Heart J 1998; 19 :696-710.

9. Aaronson K, Schwartz S, Chen T, et al. Development and prospective validation of a clinical index to predict survival in ambulatory patients referred for cardiac transplant evaluation. Circulation 1997; 95:2660-7.

10. Silverman M, Pressel M, Brackett J,et al. Prognostic value of the signal-averaged electrocardiogram and a prolonged QRS in ischemic and non ischemic cardiomyopathy. Am J Cardiol 1995; 75:460-4.

11. Likoff M, Chandler S, Kay H. Clinical determinants of mortality in chronic congestive heart failure secondary to idiopathic dilated or to ischemic cardiomyopathy. Am J Cardiol 1987; 59:634.

12. Xiao HB, Roy C, Gibson DG. Nature of ventricular activation in patients with dilated cardiomyopathy: evidence for bilateral bundle branch block. Br Heart J 1994; 72:167-74

13. Xiao HB, Brecker SJD, Gibson DG. Effect of abnormal activation on the time course of the left ventricular pressure pulse in dilated cardiomyopathy. Br Heart J 1992; 68:403-7.

14. Foster AH, Gold MR, McLaughlin JS. Acute hemodynamic effects of atrio-biventricular pacing in humans. Ann Thorac Surg 1995; 59: 294-300.

15. Cazeau S, Ritter P, Lazarus A, et al. Multisite pacing for end-stage heart failure: early experience. PACE 1996; 19 (part II): 1748-57.

16. Leclercq C , Cazeau S, Le Breton H, et al. Acute hemodynamic effects of biventricular DDD pacing in patients with end-stage heart failure. J Am Coll Cardiol 1998; 32:1825-31.

17. Blanc JJ, Etienne Y, Gilard M, et al. Evaluation of different ventricular pacing sites in patients with severe heart failure. Circulation 1997; 96:3273-77.

18. Kass DA, Chen CH, Curry et al. Improved left ventricular mechanics from acute VDD pacing in patients with dilated cardiomyopathy and intraventricular conduction delay. Circulation 1999; 99:1567– 73.

19. Leclercq C., Cazeau S., Victor F., et al. Long-term results of permanent biventricular pacing in refractory heart failure : comparison between class III and class IV patients.Eur Heart J 1998; 19 :573 (abstract).

20. Auricchio A., Stellbrink C, Sack S., et al. The pacing therapies for congestive heart failure (PATH-CHF) study: rationale, design and endpoints of a prospective randomized multicenter study. Am J Cardiol 1999; 83:130D–135D.

21. Auricchio A., Klein H., Tockman B,et al. Transvenous biventricular pacing for heart failure: can the obstacles be overcome ? Am J Cardiol 1999; 83:136D–42D.

22. Daubert J.C., Ritter P., Le Breton H., et al. Permanent left ventricular pacing with transvenous leads inserted into the coronary veins. PACE 1998; 21:239–45.

23. Jais P., Douard H., Shah D.C., Barold S ; Barat JL, Cl□menty J. Endocardial biventricular pacing. PACE 1998; 21:2128–31.

24. Gras D., Mabo P., Tang T., et al. Multisite pacing as a supplemental treatment of congestive heart failure : preliminary results of the Medtronic Inc. In Sync study. PACE 1998; 21:2249–55.

48.
IMPLANTABLE DEVICE THERAPY FOR PATIENTS WITH HYPERTROPHIC CARDIOMYOPATHY

David L. Hayes, MD and Paul A. Friedman, MD

Mayo Clinic, Rochester, MN, USA

Pacing in Hypertrophic Cardiomyopathy

The most recent ACC/AHA guidelines for pacing have included hypertrophic obstructive cardiomyopathy (HOCM) as a Class IIb indication for pacing.[1] The guidelines indicate that the patient should have a "significant" resting or provoked LV outflow obstruction gradient but they are vague in terms of what resting or provoked gradient is considered "significant". No firm consensus exists, but gradients "significant" enough to warrant consideration for pacing have been suggested to be a resting gradient 30 mm Hg and/or a provoked gradient of 50 mm Hg. [2]

Dual-chamber pacing is useful as a therapeutic modality for some patients with severe, symptomatic hypertrophic obstructive cardiomyopathy.[3] Multiple investigators have reported a significant reduction in the left ventricular outflow tract gradient and symptomatic improvement in patients with hypertrophic obstructive cardiomyopathy in whom dual-chamber pacemakers have been implanted.

Fananapazir reported on 84 patients with HCM who had drug-resistant symptoms were treated with dual-chamber pacemakers programmed to the DDD mode with atrioventricular intervals short enough to fully activate the ventricle from the pacing site at the right ventricular apex (according to electrocardiographic criteria).[3] After a mean of 2.3 years, symptoms resolved (28 patients) or improved (47 patients) in 89 percent of cases. This was associated with a significant improvement in mean NYHA functional class from 3.2 to 1.6 and a reduction in the left ventricular outflow tract gradient from 96 to 27 mmHg in patients with significant outflow obstruction. These benefits persisted after cessation of pacing during normal sinus rhythm, as did some changes on the surface electrocardiogram (T-wave morphology) and the signal-averaged electrocardiogram.

The most widely accepted hypothesis to explain the improvement in hemodynamics that may occur in patients with HCM when paced is that the altered septal activation caused by right ventricular apical pacing may result in less narrowing of the left ventricular outflow tract and a subsequent decrease in the Venturi effect, responsible for systolic anterior motion of the mitral valve.[4] However, the persistence of improvement after cessation of pacing in some series as well as the observation that

From Ovsyshcher IE. *Cardiac Arrythmias and Device Therapy: Results and Perspectives for the New Century.* Armonk, NY: Futura Publishing Company, Inc., © 2000

subjective and objective improvement may also be seen in some patients with left bundle branch block all suggest that the effect of long-term pacing can not be attributed solely to alteration of the septal activation sequence by ventricular pacing. There are hypotheses that permanent pacing in patients with hypertrophic cardiomyopathy may result in long-term remodeling of the left ventricle[5] but this is not well established.

Pacing in HCM has been the subject of several randomized single-center and multicenter trials. (Table 1) A single-center randomized crossover trial demonstrated symptomatic improvement in 63% of patients when paced in the DDD mode.[6] However, 42% of patients improved when programmed to a low pacing rate in the AAI mode, i.e. effectively no pacing, suggesting a significant placebo effect.

In the PIC (Pacing in Cardiomyopathy) study, a multicenter randomized crossover study[7] dual-chamber pacing resulted in reduction of the left ventricular outflow tract gradient by 50%, a 21% increase in exercise duration and improvement in NYHA functional class compared to baseline status. When clinical parameters including chest pain, dyspnea and subjective health status were compared being DDD and back-up AAI pacing, there was no significant difference, again suggesting a significant placebo effect.

In another randomized, double-blind crossover study, the M-PATHY (Multicenter Study of Pacing Therapy for Hypertrophic Cardiomyopathy) trial, with randomization, no significant differences were evident between pacing and no pacing, either subjectively or objectively when exercise capacity, quality of life score, treadmill exercise time or peak oxygen consumption were compared.[8] The investigators concluded that pacing should not be regarded as a primary treatment for HCM, and that subjective benefit without objective evidence of improvement should be interpreted cautiously.

When pacing is applied in the HCM patient, AVI programming is crucial to achieve optimal hemodynamic improvement. Ventricular depolarization must occur as a result of pacing. Therefore, the AVI must be short enough to result in depolarization via the paced event. However, the shortest AVI is not necessarily the most optimal.[6] Some experts have advocated AV nodal ablation to assure paced ventricular depolarization if rapid intrinsic AV nodal conduction prevents total ventricular depolarization via the pacing stimulus.[4]

Multiple methods have been used for AVI optimization. Hemodynamic measurements at various AVIs via echo/Doppler are the most widely used method for AVI optimization. Plethysmographic techniques have also been used but are not well validated against echo/Doppler. For patients with HCM, a simplistic approach, and not necessarily optimal for every patient, is to program the longest AVI that still results in complete paced ventricular depolarization.

ICD Therapy in Hypertrophic Cardiomyopathy

Patients with HCM have an increased risk for sudden death ranging from 3-6% annually, and approximately 50% of deaths are sudden.[9] Hypertrophic cardiomyopathy is the most common cause of sudden death in otherwise healthy young individuals. Symptoms such as palpitations or syncope may be difficult to assess in patients with HCM due to the potential presence of multiple etiologic factors including autonomic dysregulation, an outflow gradient, atrial fibrillation, and ventricular tachyarrhythmias. Moreover, these and other factors, such as subendocardial ischemia, enhanced AV nodal conduction of atrial fibrillation, conduction defects, and septal myocyte disarray have been proposed as triggers for sudden death. In light of the complexity of the pathogenesis of sudden death, it is not surprising that risk stratification is difficult. There no clear consensus in the literature regarding the predictive power of ambulatory monitoring and electrophysiologic study, and many studies suffer from small patient numbers or limited follow.[10-11] Given the known progressive phenotypic expression of HCM over time, assessment of the pathologic substrate at one point in time may have limited long-term predictive power. Ultimately, the best prognostic study may genotyping to determine the specific genetic defect present.

Despite the challenges in assessing patients with hypertrophic cardiomyopathy, there are several areas of broad consensus. The available data suggest that ventricular tachyarrhythmias are the cause of sudden death in most patients, even if initially triggered by one or several mechanisms. Patients fortunate enough to survive an episode of out of hospital cardiac arrest, or who have sustained ventricular tachyarrhythmias are at highest risk for sudden death and should generally undergo ICD implantation. Patients without a dramatic clinical event, i.e. OHCA or frank syncope, but with recurrent episodes of near-syncope or other risk factors, particularly a family history of sudden death, or a markedly thickened ventricular wall (i.e., >3 cm) are at increased risk.

Previously published data on the use of ICDs in patients with HCM have reported mixed results and suffer from small sample size. Our own experience indicates that patients with HCM that receive an ICD for primary prevention have high rate of appropriate therapies.[12] More recently, a large multicenter series pooled the outcome of 128 HCM patients treated with ICDs and followed them for a mean of 3.1 years.[13] During the follow up period, 23% of patients received appropriate shocks or antitachycardia pacing for VT or VF. The event rate for the 43 patients who received ICDs for secondary prevention following an episode of cardiac arrest or sustained VT was 11% per year. For the 85 patients in whom the device was implanted for primary prevention (i.e., prophylactically), the event rate was 4.5% per year. Although the patient selection for primary prevention was not well controlled, it is doubtful that a randomized prospective clinical trial will ever be performed in this patient group. The high frequency of appropriate discharges in patients without an antecedent clinical event pose a compelling argument for prophylactic ICD use in high risk patients. Given the low implant morbidity and insured compliance of ICD therapy, combined with the uncertain effectiveness of antiarrhythmic drugs in this population[10], we often offer device therapy to these patients, though the approach is highly individualized. The ACC/AHA guidelines now include a Class IIB indication for patients with familial or inherited conditions with a high risk for life-threatening ventricular tachyarrhythmias such as hypertrophic cardiomyopathy.[1]

A secondary benefit of ICD therapy in this population is the potential for dual chamber pacing to alleviate symptomatic gradients in a subset of patients, and the growing availability of devices with therapies specific for atrial arrhythmias, including atrial defibrillation. Although a clinical benefit of dual chamber pacing to alleviate symptoms in obstructive HCM is obtained in only a subset of patients that are paced, these patients are at increased risk for atrial fibrillation and may also benefit from the atrial sensing and possibly from atrial pacing for atrial fibrillation prevention. Atrial defibrillation capability and atrial rate stabilization algorithms may also provide benefit in the HCM population. In a study of patients with atrial arrhythmias who also had a ventricular ICD indication, we found that the atrial fibrillation burden was significant decreased with device therapy, often with painless high frequency burst intervention.[14] Patients (n=53) were randomized to atrial prevention and termination therapies ON or OFF for 3 months after implantation, then crossed over to the opposite arm. During the time atrial therapies were turned on, there was a 44% reduction in AF frequency (p=0.13) and a 77% (5.5 hour) reduction in total AF burden (duration/week, p=0.05, Table 2). This reduction persisted even when considering episodes treated with atrial pacing therapies only. Given that many HCM patients are highly symptomatic with the occurrence of atrial arrhythmias in light of their hemodynamic derangements, this therapy may prove particularly useful in that population.

In summary, based on current data, device therapy appears to have a role in a subset of patients with HCM. It remains controversial as to when pacing should be offered to patients with HCM and how to determine which patients are most likely to respond to permanent pacing. ICD therapy clearly has a role in HCM patients for the prevention of sudden death in the patient with a history of syncope and/or family history of sudden death. Application of atrial therapies in HCM patients may also offer clinical benefit.

Table 1: Clinical Trials in Pacing for HCM

Study	Patient Inclusion Criteria	Endpoint(s)	Treatment Arms	Key Results
Mayo-Pacing in HCM[6]	• Symptomatic HCM despite maximal medical regimen	• LVOT gradient • Quality of life • Exercise duration • Oxygen consumption	• Blinded crossover of DDD pacing vs • No pacing (AAI)	• Subjective improvement in ≈ 60% pts • Significant placebo effect from pacing • ↓ LVOT gradient of ≈ 40%
PIC[7]	• Refractory sxs from HCM despite stable drug regimen • NYHA Class II or III • Angina and/or dyspnea • LVOT > 30 mm HG	• Exercise tolerance • Dyspnea/angina symptom score • NYHA Class • Quality of life	• Blinded crossover of DDD pacing vs • No pacing (AAI)	• 50% reduction in LVOT gradient • 21% ↑ in exercise duration • 0.7 ↓ in NYHA class
M-PATHY[8]	• Symptomatic HCM despite maximal medical regimen • LVOT ≥ 50 mm Hg	• Quality of life • Treadmill ex duration • Peak O2 consumption • Δ LVOT gradient • Δ LV wall thickness	• Blinded crossover of DDD pacing vs • No pacing (AAI at 30 bpm)	• No significant subj. or obj. improvement with randomization • Significant placebo effect • ↓ LVOT gradient of 40%

Table 2

Atrial Fibrillation Frequency and Burden With Atrial Therapies (Rx) ON and OFF in Patients with a Ventricular ICD Indication and Atrial Arrhythmias

	Mean Rx "ON"	Mean Rx "OFF"	% Reduction OFF vs. ON	P Value
Frequency (episodes/mo)	3.5±11	6.2±17	44%	0.13
Duration (min/week)	97±259	427±1259	77%	0.05

References:

1. Gregoratos G, Cheitlin MD, Conill A, Epstein AE, Fellows C, Ferguson TB, Freedman RA, Hlatky MA, Naccarelli GV, Saksena S, Schlant RC, Silka MJ. ACC/AHA Guidelines for Implantation of Cardiac Pacemakers and Antiarrhythmia Devices: a report of the American College of Cardiology/American Heart Association Task Force on Practice Guidelines (Committee on Pacemaker Implantation). JACC 1998;31:1175-1206.

2. Symanski JD, Nishimura RA. The use of pacemakers in the treatment of cardiomyopathies. Current Problems in Cardiology 1996;21: 385-444.

3. Fananapazir L, Cannon RO III, Tripodi D, Panza JA. Impact of dual-chamber permanent pacing in patients with obstructive hypertrophic cardiomyopathy with symptoms refractory to verapamil and ß-adrenergic blocker therapy. Circulation 1992; 85:2149-61.

4. Jeanrenaud X, Goy JJ, Kappenberger L: Effects of dual-chamber pacing in hypertrophic obstructive cardiomyopathy. Lancet 1992;339:1318-23.

5. Fananapazir L, Epstein ND, Curiel RV, et al. Long-term results of dual-chamber (DDD) pacing in obstructive hypertrophic cardiomyopathy: Evidence for progressive symptomatic and hemodynamic improvement and reduction of left ventricular hypertrophy. Circulation 1994;90:2731-42.

6. Nishimura RA, Hayes DL, Ilstrup DM, Holmes DR, Tajik AJ. Effect of dual-chamber pacing on systolic and diastolic function in patients with hypertrophic cardiomyopathy. Acute Doppler echocardiographic and catheterization hemodynamic study. JACC 1996;27(2):421-30.

7. Kappenberger L, Linde C, Daubert C, et al. Pacing in hypertrophic obstructive cardiomyopathy. A randomized crossover study. Eur Heart J. 1997;18:1249-1256.

8. Maron BJ, Nishimura RA, McKenna WJ, et al. Assessment of permanent dual-chamber pacing as a treatment for drug-refractory symptomatic patients with obstructive hypertrophic cardiomyopathy. A randomized, double-blind, crossover study (M-PATHY) Circulation 1999(22):2927-2933.

9. McKenna W. Sudden death in hypertrophic cardiomyopathy: identification of the "high risk" patient. In: Brugada P, Wellens H, eds. Cardiac Arrhythmias: Where to Go From Here? Mount Kisco, NY: Futura, 1987:353-65.

10. Borggrefe M, Breithardt G. Is the implantable defibrillator indicated in patients with hypertrophic cardiomyopathy and aborted sudden death? [editorial; comment]. Journal of the American College of Cardiology 1998;31(5):1086-8.

11. Kuck KH. Arrhythmias in hypertrophic cardiomyopathy. Pacing & Clinical Electrophysiology 1997;20(10 Pt 2):2706-13.

12. Lobo TJ, Friedman PA, Rea RF, et al. Clinical outcome following cardioverter defibrillator implantation in patients with hypertrophic cardiomyopathy. Journal of the American College of Cardiology 1998;31(Supp. A):435A.

13. Maron BJ, Shen WK, Link MS, et al. Efficacy of the implantable cardioverter-defibrillator for the prevention of sudden death in hypertrophic cardiomyopathy. AHA 72nd Scientific Sessions Program 1999; p 83 (abstract).

14. Friedman PA, Stein KM, Wharton JM, et al. Reduced atrial fibrillation burden with prompt treatment by an implantable arrhythmia management device - evidence of reverse remodeling? AHA 72nd Scientific Sessions Program 1999; p 83 (abstract).

49

EASY AND SAFE PERMANENT LEFT ATRIAL PACING – CHALLENGE FOR THE BEGINNING OF THE NEW CENTURY

Andrzej Kutarski MD, PhD, Max Schaldach Prof. Dr*

University Medical Academy. Lublin; POLAND;
*Department of Biomedical Engineering, Friedrich-Alexander University, Erlangen, GERMANY

Coronary sinus (CS) plays recently growing role as a place for permanent atrial pacing. Indications for permanent CS pacing can be divided as: I. technical RA pacing difficulties: 1) impossible stable right atrium appendage (RAA) lead fixation, 2) second or next RAA lead dislodgement, 3) RAA exit block and very high RAA pacing threshold (PTh) on next lead implantation, and sometimes 4) severe RAA undersensing 5) difficulties with RA pacing sensing of transplanted heart. II. Indication for biatrial (BiA) pacing: a) hemodynamic prevention of pacemaker syndrome on DDD pacing in pts. with severe interatrial block, b) avoidance of ventricular capture in pts. DDD paced due to hypertrophic cardiomyopathy c) BiA for recurrent atrial arrhythmias prevention (1,2,3). Acute and long-term observation of Moss, Greenberg, Daubert and Kutarski (1,2,3,5,6) pointed two main problems of permanent CS pacing: high percentage of lead dislodgement (3-14%) and exit block (0-16%) with frequent re-operation necessity (5-20%).

I) How to prevent CS lead dislocation?
Two different ways were used in the past towards better CS lead fixation: **1)** Utility of standard screw-in system in it's proximal part (10), **2)** shape fixation concept – double lead angulation (3) or lengthening of the distal inactive part of lead (5,6)
We started with CS pacing in 1995 using standard BP leads and we were primary surprised finding lowest PTh values during ring CS pacing (table 1) (7).

Table 1. Acute values of CS pacing / sensing conditions obtained with ERA 300 in 204 pts

Pacing / sensing configuration	Prox UP (ring)	Distal UP (tip)	BP (tip-ring)
A-wave (mV)	2.6	2.4	3.0
Threshold(V)	2,26	4,16	2,93
Impedance	287	582	625

From Ovsyshcher IE. *Cardiac Arrythmias and Device Therapy: Results and Perspectives for the New Century.* Armonk, NY: Futura Publishing Company, Inc., © 2000

Our later modification of split BP BiA pacing system enables evaluation of lone ring CS pacing conditions (8) and it allowed for comparison of ring – and tip CS pacing conditions during long-term follow-up (table 2). The study showed utility of ring electrode for cathodal CS pacing in split BP BiA (hybrid) pacing system (distal part of standard CS BP lead, tip and tines play only role of anchoring strand) and obtained results indicated us the direction for permanent CS lead construction (8,9).

Conditions of permanent CS pacing / sensing (1,2,5,6,7,8)

Proximal CS:	Distal CS
• Lower PTh values	• Higher PTh values
• *The worst lead stability*	• *The best lead stability*
• No risk of V pacing	• The risk of V pacing
• No risk of phrenic nerve pacing	• The risk of phrenic nerve pacing

Our hitherto experience showed (2,7,8,9):

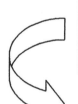

The lowest PTh in proximal CS
Utility of the ring of standard BP lead for CS pacing
Relatively low percentage of dislocation if the tines of standard lead were not removed

The concept of the new CS designed lead with ring electrodes and long anchoring strand in cardiac vein.

It brought to construction of special lead: the inactive part with (longer than the special ones) tines is lengthened up to 6 cm to reach the narrow cardiac vein and area of both rings were reduced

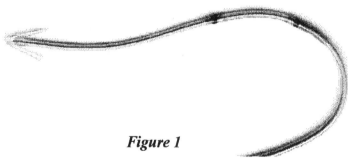

Figure 1

in following models (figure 1). We implanted the new special BIOTRONIK CS lead (figure 2) in **68** pts. All implantations were successful. X-ray scopy time ranged 1-**20** min and in half the number of pts did not exceed 5 min. Acute, subacute and chronic sensing conditions were satisfactory (LA wave over 2 mV).

Table 2. Tip and ring CS pacing

Leads and connection	Parameters	Acute	Months of observation						Dislo-cations
			1	2	3	4	5	6	
Tip pacing standard leads	No of pts	205	187	172	168	156	143	134	24/209 **11%**
	PTh	**4,2**	**4,2**	**4,1**	**4,1**	**3,9**	**3,8**	**3,8**	
	Impedance	582	548	584	612	611	616	628	
Ring pacing standard leads	No of pts	44	31	**31**	31	22	10	15	2/57 **3,5%**
	PTh	2,3	2,2	2,0	2,0	2,1	1,7	1,7	
	Impedance	282	289	275	322	328	349	337	
Ring pacing CS lead	No of pts	68	58	36	31	22	19	18	1/68 **1,4%**
	PTh	1,9	2,4	2,5	2,8	2,6	2,9	2,3	
	Impedance	283	386	360	371	391	429	408	

In none of the pts with CS lead ventricle, phrenic nerve pacing or exit block was observed. Our observations supported the concept of utility of ring electrode for permanent CS pacing and usefulness log anchoring strand for prevention of dislocation of CS lead (9); we hope that some modifications will further decrease PTh values.

II) How to improve effectiveness of LA pacing?

The second one unsolved finally problem of permanent LA pacing consist of its effectiveness. Relatively high LA PTh values and high energy consumption are frequent findings; the risk of loss of LA capture in BiA pacing system is real too, especially if standard pacemaker is used (1,3,5-9). Our long term experience (2) and a lot performed studies indicates five (parallel) ways towards improvement of LA pacing effectiveness:

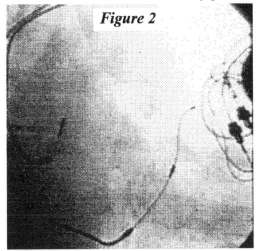

Figure 2

1) Pacing of proximal / middle part of CS (2,7-9); **2)** BP CS pacing (2,7-9); **3)** Utility of OLBI system for CS pacing (11-13); **4)** Application of optimal (for individual patient) pacing configuration in BiA pacing system (13-16); **5)** Optimal pacemaker output programming (17).

1. Ring mid/proximal CS pacing. The new BIOTRONIK CS lead permits for safe CS pacing in its optimal region (8,9).

2. BP CS pacing. In non-programmable pacemaker's era Moss' and Greenberg's groups used mainly standard BP leads or special CS Medtronic leads BP too (5,6). Comparison of conditions and effects of UP and BP CS pacing was impossible. 20 years later Daubert showed possibility of permanent CS pacing with standard "J" shaped BP leads connected classically with BP port of standard pacemaker but did not compare effectiveness of UP and BP CS pacing (1). Split BP pacing system (cathode and anode of the same channel of pacemaker paces both atria simultaneously) introduced by Daubert's group (1,3) makes impossible lone CS pacing and effects of BP CS pacing were not evaluated too. For permanent CS pacing we used standard leads (usually straight), classically connected to SSI pacemaker or to atrial or ventricular port of DDD pacemaker; it enabled CS pacing in UP and BP program (2,4,7-9,11,12,14).

Table 3. EPS effects of different energy CS pacing in 120 pts

| | | | Coronary Sinus pacing | |
| | Sinus rhythm | UP | BP pacing energy | |
			threshold (1-2,4 V)	max. (6,0-7,2 V)
P-Q (S-Q) (ms)	192,0	198,6	185,0	174,0
P (II) duration (ms)	**118,1**	**139,8**	**123,1**	**110,1**

We found that RAA and UP mid/distal CS pacing provides to PII wave prolongation (from 117 to 140 and from 148 to 155 in different groups of pts) and to prolongation of total atrial activation time (TAAT) (from 199 to 225 ms) in comparison to sinus rhythm. High energy BP CS pacing (18,19) shows reverse effects - PII wave shortening (to 109 ms) and reduction of TAAT (to 188 ms). It suggests possibility of real bifocal pacing (left atrium from tip of lead and basis of right atrium from ring of bipolar lead located in CS ostium or proximal part of coronary sinus). We found some antiarrhythmic effect of "high energy" BP CS pacing in recurrent atrial arrhythmias additionally (18,19).

3. OLBI CS pacing. OLBI system was invented for RA wall pacing from typical VDD floating lead. The new stimulation method - the overlapping biphasic impulse (OLBI) stimulation is based on simultaneous generation of two monophasic impulses with inverted polarity, each of them is delivered from one or two rings of atrial part of standard VDD lead. A number of studies reported effective atrial pacing in most of the pts due to deep impulse penetration; pacing thresholds of RA wall was 1,8-4,0 V. We found high utility of OLBI system for permanent CS pacing (11,12).

Table 4. Acute OLBI CS pacing

Acute parameters in 41 pts	Temporary pacing program			
	UP distal	UP prox.	BP	OLBI™
PTh (V)	3,8	2,2	2,8	1,3
Impedance (Ω)	542	339	609	604
Energy consumption (μA)	7,4	6,6	4,6	4,1

Table 5. Pacing/sensing conditions during permanent CS OLBI pacing; the comparison with UP program

Compared programs and parameters (telemetry)	after operation	month of FU		
		1	3	6
No. of pts.	24	20	15	6
Amplitude A on BP sensing	2,3	2,8	2,9	2,6
UP pacing threshold	4,3	4,1	4,5	3,2
OLBI pacing threshold	1,8	1,9	2,1	1,8
Current drain on OLBI pacing	66,6	68,2	63,0	50,1

We concluded that OLBI system connected with BP CS lead can help to solve the problem of exit block and risk of unsuccessful CS pacing (11,12).

4. Selection of optimal pacing configuration for BiA pacing in individual patient. Intraoperative evaluation of pacing / sensing conditions is very important for selection of optimal pacing configuration and made of connections of lead's. There are not established official criteria but personal experience (13-16) indicates that: DUP (dual UP - leads in series) configuration can be used only in pts with relatively low PTh values in CS (< 1,5 mV) and if impedance of RA lead is higher than CS lead's one. If values of impedance are comparable and PTh values in CS are relatively high we can expect lost of LA capture using this configuration during follow-up (13,15,16). Split BP connection in classical (Daubert's) configuration can be used independently from values of impedance of each of leads but for anodic CS pacing relatively low (<1,5V) values of PTh in CS are required; significantly higher PTh values in CS requires utility of cathodic current for LA pacing and inverted split BP system is preferable (13,15,16). It is necessary to remember that two "high impedance" ("low energy") leads can not be used in split BP configuration but in this situation DUP system is the best solution (13,15,16). Our long term experience indicated additionally that ring of

CS lead can be used for pacing/sensing of LA in place of tip of lead if intraoperative pacing/sensing conditions are significantly better. It is clear that for application of the most effective configuration of leads connection for BiA pacing several different "Y connectors" have to be available during implantation. The figure 3 shows examples of BIOTRONIK's dual BP "Y connector" and inverter for (proximal) ring cathodal pacing.

5. Longer pulse width (PW) programming in split BP BiA pacing system. Split BP configuration (using "Y connector") is the most popular one for permanent BiA pacing. Relatively high CS PTh and high resistance (two resistors in the some circuit) increases energy requirement (13,15,16). During standard follow up in 20 pts. with this pacing system we examined threshold strength parameters using different PW (17).

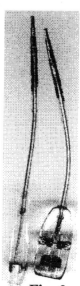

Fig. 3

Pulse width (ms)	Pulse voltage (V)	Pulse current (mA)	Pulse energy (µJ)	Batt. current drain (mA)
	BiA		BiA s-BP	
0,25	7,8	12,0	18,9	32,2
0,50	**5,7**	**11,3**	**25,8**	**32,7**
0,75	5,2	9,2	23,4	36,5
1,0	4,1	6,5	16,0	30,1
1,5	3,3	4,2	12,4	23,4

Table 6. Pulse width and energy cons. in SPB BiA pacing system

The results indicated, that during pacing using SBP configuration - values of impulse intensity are still located nearly "knee" of the strength – duration curve even during 1,0-1,5 ms PW. Lower values of pulse current and pulse energy observed during longer PW seems to confirm this hypothesis. Increase of impedance values is the known effect of prolongation of PW and secondary energy consumption decrease – can explain significant decrease of battery current drain observed by us. Using transformer systems for high amplitude pacing provide to loss of some energy and it explain slight energy saving (battery current drain) if longer PW instead high pulse amplitude is programmed (17). Programming of longer PW enables slight energy saving in pts with SBP BiA pacing systems. Routine PW programming as 0,5 ms seems not to be optimal for pts with splitted atrial leads (17).

CONCLUSIONS: Today LA and BiA pacing are still in infancy but clinical demand for this modes of pacing makes it urgent challenge for biomedical technology. We hope further progress in CS lead constructions (better stability and improvement of effectiveness of pacing); further development will have to make them easy for removal too. Especial BiA pacemaker with additional BP LA designed channel (with increased capacitor) will solve the problems of too high (split BP) or too low (dual UP system) impedance related problems and pro-arrhythmic effect of anodic stimulation. Dual chamber IEGM would be very helpful for proper diagnosis of atrial arrhythmias additionally.

References

1. Gras D., Mabo Ph., Daubert C. Left atrial pacing: technical and clinical conciderations. In: Barold S.S., Mugica J. (ed.): Recent Advances in Cardiac Pacing. Goals for 21st century. Armonk, New York; Futura Publishing Company Inc.1998: 181-202

2. Kutarski A., Poleszak K., Oleszczak K. et al. Biatrial and coronary sinus pacing – long term experience with 246 patients. Progress in Biomedical Research, June 1998, 114-120

3. Daubert C., Leclerq Ch., Le Breton H., et al. Permanent left atrial pacing with a specifically designed coronary sinus lead. PACE, 1997; 20: 2755-2764

4. Kutarski A., Zakliczyński M., Oleszczak K. et al. Coronary sinus (CS) pacing of orthotopic cardiac allograft – a new solution of donnor's right atrium pacing / sensing problems. In: Raviele A. (ed.) Cardiac Arrhythmias 1999/ Proceedings of the 6th International Workshop on Cardiac Arrhtythmias. Venice, 5-8 1999. Springer 1999: 25 (abstr)

5. Moss A., Rivers R. Atrial pacing from the coronary vein. Ten-year experience in 50 patients with implanted prvenous pacemakers. Circulation, 1978;57: 103-106

6. Greenberg P., Castellanet M., Messenger J., Ellestad M. Coronary sinus pacing. Clinical follow-up. Circulation, 1978; 57: 98-103

7. Kutarski A., Oleszczak K., Poleszak K., Koziara D. Coronary sinus. The second standard lead position for permanent atrial pacing. W: Vardas P. Red. Europace. Monduzzi Editore S.p.A. 1997: 405-409

8. Kutarski A., Oleszczak K., Poleszak K. Permanent CS pacing from the ring of standard BP leads. Progr. Biomed. Res. 1998; 4: 184-192

9. Kutarski A., Schaldach M., Oleszczak K. et al. The new BIOTRONIK coronary sinus (CS) designed lead. The first

experience. Proceedings of International meeting Atrial Fibrillation. Bologna, Italy. September 16-17, 1999: 181 (abstr.)

10. Frank R., Petitot J.C., Himbert C. et al. Left atrial pacing with screw-in lead inside the coronary sinus. Arch Mal Coeur Vaiss 1998; 91, 3: 201 (abstr.)

11. Kutarski A., Poleszak K., Oleszczak K. et al. Does the OLBI (TM) configuration solve the problem of exit block during permanent coronary sinus pacing? Progr. Biomed Res. 1999; 3: 208-214

12. Kutarski A., Oleszcak K., Schaldach M. et al. In Adornato E. (ed.) Rhythm Control from Cardiac Evaluation to Treatment. Proceedings of the VI Southern Symposium on Cardiac Pacing. Giardini-Naxos – Taormina. September 9-12 1998 Edizioni Luigi Pozzi S.r.l. 1998. 343-353

13. Kutarski A., Schaldach M., Wójcik M. et al. OLBI stimulation in biatrial pacing? A comparison of acute pacing and sensing conditions for split bipolar and dual cathodal unipolar cionfigurations. Progr Biomed Res. 1999; 3,4: 236-240

14. Kutarski A., Widomska-Czekajska T. et al. Clinical and technical aspecs of permanent BiA pacing using standard DDD pacermaker. Long-term experience in 47 patients. Progr Biomed Res. 4,4: 394-404

15. Kutarski A., Schaldach M., Wójcik M. et al. OLBI stimulation for biatrial (BiA) pacing? A comparison of acute pacing/sensing conitions with slit bipoles (SBP) and dual cathodal unipolar (DUP) configuration. PACE 1999; 22, 6: A12 (abstr)

16. Kutarski A., Oleszczak K., Wójcik M. Split bipoles (SBP) or dual cathodal UP (DUP) configuration for permanent biatrial (BiA) pacing? A comparison of output requirement and sensing conditions. PACE 1999;22, 6: A155 (abstr)

17. Kutarski A., Wójcik M., Oleszczak K. Pulse width programming in patients with biatrial pacing systems. Progr Biomed Res. 1999; 4: 112-116

18. Kutarski A., Oleszczak K., Poleszak K., Koziara D. High energy bipolar coronary sinus pacing - a simple mode of atrial resynchronisation? PACE 1997; 20: 2308 (abstr.)

19. Kutarski A., Poleszak K., Koziara D., Oleszczak K. High energy bipolar coronary sinus (CS) pacing shows some resynchronising and antiarrhythmic effects. Heartweb; 4 (2): p00006. http: //.www.heartweb.org/heartweb/1298/p0006.htm

50.

CARDIAC PACING IN PATIENTS WITH MARKED FIRST-DEGREE AV BLOCK

I. Eli Ovsyshcher, M.D., Ph.D., S. Serge Barold, M.D.

Arrhythmia Service, Cardiology, Soroka University Medical Center & Faculty of Health Sciences, Ben Gurion University of the Negev, BeerSheva, Israel; Cardiac Electrophysiology Service, North Ridge Hospital , Fort Lauderdale, Florida, USA

Introduction

Beyond its goal of reducing mortality and morbidity, pacemaker therapy attempts to restore 3 basic electrophysiological (and resultant mechanical) functions of the heart: normal atrial and ventricular activation sequences[1-5], optimal AV synchronization[5] and rate response to exercise. Even sophisticated systems cannot achieve truly physiological pacing and may produce variable deterioration of mechanical function. Changing parameters to improve one of the aforementioned electrophysiological functions may sometimes adversely affect another. Consequently in symptomatic patients from a long PR interval (LPRI) as an isolated abnormality the clinician must establish that the benefit of optimizing AV synchrony with a shorter AV delay outweighs the loss of left ventricular (LV) function produced by pacing induced aberrant ventricular depolarization[1-6]. This determination can sometimes be made clinically and noninvasively, but a hemodynamic study with temporary pacing may be required (Figure 1, see next page).

Significance of Mitral Regurgitation

In patients with LPRI atrial systole with premature and incomplete "atriogenic" closure of the mitral valve causes varying degrees of end-diastolic mitral regurgitation (MR) in mid or late diastole[7-8]. This MR is inconsequential in the normal heart but may be important in patients with severe LV dysfunction[9].

Indications for Pacing

It is now recognized that even isolated marked LPRI can cause symptoms similar to the pacemaker syndrome especially in the presence of normal LV function[10]. A P wave too close to the preceding QRS complex produces basically the same hemodynamic derangement as VVI pacing with retrograde VA conduction[4,11].This is why symptomatic LPRI has been called "pacemaker syndrome without a pacemaker"[12]. The ACC/AHA guidelines for pacemaker implantation now advocate pacing in

From Ovsyshcher IE. *Cardiac Arrythmias and Device Therapy: Results and Perspectives for the New Century.* Armonk, NY: Futura Publishing Company, Inc., © 2000

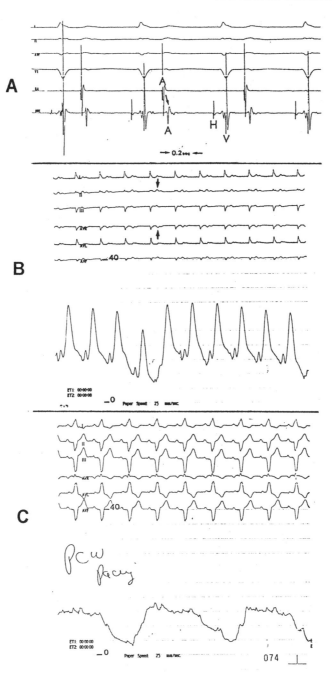

Figure 1. Surface electrocardiogram (ECG) and intracardiac electrogram (IEG) in patient with marked 1° AV block.

A. ECG and IEG recordings. Heart rate (HR)=81bpm. AH and PR intervals are markedly prolonged: AH=440ms. RA - high right atrial IEG and HBE - His bundle recording. Note that the sequence of atrial activation (from RA to HBE) is consistent with sinus rhythm and rules out retrograde atrial activation.

B. Same patient. HR=80bpm, PR=440ms. Pulmonary capillary wedge (PCW) pressure shows giant A waves (20-32 mmHg, mean pressure=20 mmHg) during sinus rhythm (Scale 0-40 mmHg).

C. Same patient. Note the normal PCW pressure (mean=10 mmHg, scale 0-40 mm Hg) after temporary dual chamber pacing with HR=80bpm and AV interval 180ms.

acquired marked 1st degree AV block (>0.30sec.) as a Class IIa indication when patients display "… symptoms suggestive of pacemaker syndrome and documented alleviation of symptoms with temporary AV pacing"[13]. Patients with LPRI may or may not be symptomatic at rest. They are more likely to become symptomatic with mild or moderate exercise when the PR interval does not shorten appropriately and atrial systole shifts progressively closer towards the previous ventricular systole. In some patients symptoms may be subtle. The class IIa recommendation does not apply to patients with LPRI associated with dilated cardiomyopathy, and congestive heart failure (CHF) as discussed later. The necessity and appropriateness of a temporary AV pacing study in LPRI patients are questionable, especially if the PR interval is very long and does not shorten on exercise. During a resting study it may not be possible to demonstrate symptomatic improvement, and the execution of exercise studies with temporary dual-chamber pacemaker in place is difficult. Therefore a permanent pacemaker may be recommended in selected patients without a temporary pacing study that would add unnecessary risk and cost[14].

AV Delay vs Asynchronous Activation
Iliev et al.[15,16] recently compared the AAI and DDD modes in patients with sick sinus syndrome (DDD pacemakers) and native but long AV conduction in otherwise normal hearts. At a pacing rate of 70 ppm at rest, there was no overall difference in cardiac output (CO) during AAI and DDD pacing. However when the patients were divided according to the AV interval (AVI), those with AVI<275ms showed a higher CO during AAI pacing. When the AVI>315ms, CO was higher during DDD pacing. They also established that during DDD pacing that the longer the native AV interval is, the larger the resultant increments in CO. Conversely with a normal or near normal PR interval, a higher CO was found during AAI pacing. At an atrial pacing rate of 90 ppm all the patients had a spontaneous AVI>280 ms and all showed a higher CO during pacing in the DDD mode at that rate[15,16].

Asymptomatic and Mildly Symptomatic Patients
We propose that slightly symptomatic patients with LPRI (>300 ms) but without a clearcut "pacemaker syndrome" be investigated with an exercise test and echo-Doppler examination[8]. A temporary pacing study may then be required to make a decision about permanent pacing. There are no data on the prognosis of asymptomatic patients with LPRI. According to the 1998 ACC/AHA guidelines pacing is not yet indicated in asymptomatic patients with isolated LPRI even with abnormal hemodynamics (decrease of CO and MR). Nevertheless a truly asymptomatic patient with moderately severe

hemodynamic abnormalities probably deserves a pacing study and if it shows good improvement with restoration of optimal AV synchrony, a permanent pacemaker should be considered.

Long PR Interval, Dilated Cardiomyopathy and CHF

Cardiac conduction abnormalities such as 1st degree AV block and left bundle branch block occur frequently in patients with CHF and dilated cardiomyopathy and carry an unfavorable prognosis[8,17-20]. The role of pacing to treat these abnormalities is presently undergoing intensive investigation to determine whether restoration of optimal AV synchrony and/or ventricular resynchronization (requiring LV pacing) can be hemodynamically beneficial[21-23]. Over the last decade long-term studies with conventional DDD pacing and a short AV delay in heterogeneous groups of patients with CHF of various etiologies have generally yielded disappointing results[24]. In patients with 1st degree AV block, conventional DDD pacing abolishes presystolic MR and increases the time for forward flow (diastolic MR also occurs with complete AV block and with severe LV disease even when the PR interval is normal). Elimination of diastolic MR plays as yet an undefined role in the overall hemodynamic benefit of conventional DDD pacing in selected patients with severe LV dysfunction, CHF and 1st degree AV block. Abolition of diastolic MR may result in more optimal hemodynamic performance because of a lower left atrial pressure and higher LV preload at the onset of systole[9].

Few patients with a long AV interval respond to conventional DDD pacing on a long term-basis. In some patients, atrial mechanical contraction may be poor or absent and in the presence of markedly elevated pulmonary capillary wedge pressure, atrial contribution may be negligible. Glikson et al.[24] emphasized that in some patients with LPRI a long interatrial conduction time already produces appropriately timed mechanical AV synchrony and such patients would not be expected to improve with pacing. In some patients further deterioration of LV function accompanies the abnormal ventricular depolarization related to pacing.

Selection of Patients for Conventional DDD Pacing

Patients with refractory CHF, a long PR interval and QRS >140 ms should be considered for either LV or biventricular DDDR pacing but this approach is still investigational[21,22]. Those with LPRI and no major intraventricular conduction delay are not presently candidates for biventricular or LV pacing but they could conceivably in the future[25]. An acute study should demonstrate improvement. Responders will show an increase in systolic blood pressure and an increase in peak mitral flow velocity reflecting a higher LV systolic pressure and lower left atrial pressure. The study should also show prolonged MR of at least 450ms and a short ventricular filling time <200ms before considering permanent pacing[24,26]. During the last decade clinical research has shown that mitral flow velocity patterns (MFVP) evaluated by echo-Doppler are a strong and nondependent predictor of survival in CHF. Recent studies have shown that among patients with CHF and "restrictive" hemodynamics there is a group of patients with reversible restrictive MFVP[27]. This group of patients (>30% of patients with CHF) has a significantly better survival rate than patients with nonreversible restrictive MFVP[27]. This group of patients might enjoy the most favorable effect from pacing therapy. It should be stressed that favorable MFVP and/or other acute data do not guarantee a beneficial long-term outcome with conventional DDDR devices.

The 1998 ACC/AHA guidelines[13] advocate conventional dual-chamber pacing as a class IIb indication in patients with "symptomatic, drug-refractory dilated cardiomyopathy with prolonged PR interval when acute hemodynamic studies have demonstrated hemodynamic benefit of pacing". Note that neither the degree of acceptable PR prolongation nor the QRS duration is stated. This recommendation is presently highly controversial especially in the absence of a major intraventricular conduction delay.

Restrictive Cardiomyopathy

Patients with restrictive cardiomyopathy also have a high incidence of LPRI and intraventricular conduction defects. LV diastolic dysfunction with normal systolic function is the hallmark of this condition. Consequently these patients are highly dependent on a properly timed atrial contribution so that a long PR interval may aggravate the hemodynamic abnormalities. Preliminary studies suggest that patients with a restrictive process might benefit from DDD pacing with a short AV interval[28]. This concept also makes sense if there is 1st degree AV block but clinical trials are needed to determine the role of pacing in this situation[8].

Pacemaker Technology

The pacing system must prevent migration of the P wave into the postventricular atrial refractory period (PVARP) where it cannot be tracked.

Functional Atrial Undersensing. Bode et al.[29] recently reported the problems associated with pacing patients with 1st degree AV block. They studied 255 patients with Holter recordings and found 9 patients with atrial undersensing despite an adequate atrial signal. The P waves fell continually within the PVARP (PVARP of 276±26ms; no PVARPs functioned with automatic extension in response to ventricular extrasystoles). All 9 patients exhibited substantial delay of spontaneous AV conduction (284±61ms,range 230-410ms). The combination of a relatively fast sinus rate and prolonged AV conduction provides the appropriate setting for the development of functional atrial undersensing during which the ECG shows sinus rhythm, a long PR interval and conducted QRS complexes but no pacemaker stimuli. The conducted QRS complexes activate the ventricle while the P waves remain trapped in the PVARP. The pacemaker itself acts as a "bystander " in that it can initiate the pacemaker syndrome but the ECG then shows no pacemaker activity. Bode et al.[29] also observed that functional atrial undersensing could be initiated and terminated by appropriately timed atrial and ventricular extrasystoles. Barring disruption of the self-perpetuating process by atrial or ventricular extrasystoles, and assuming no change in AV conduction, functional atrial undersensing should theoretically continue indefinitely as long as the atrial rate remains relatively fast and constant. It will however terminate when slowing of the sinus rate produces a P-P interval longer than the sum of the intrinsic PR interval and PVARP.

Heart Rate. Bode et al.[29] recorded a mean sinus rate of 105±3bpm during functional undersensing because a relatively fast atrial rate facilitates displacement of the P wave toward the PVARP. Some patients with functional atrial undersensing develop marked sinus tachycardia probably as a response to the hemodynamic derangement created by the loss of optimal AV synchrony. The tachycardia often subsides quickly upon restoration of a physiologic AV delay by the pacemaker. As a rule a very long PR interval does not shorten significantly in situations causing sinus tachycardia. Therefore with a fixed PR interval sinus tachycardia may create a vicious cycle because it pushes the P wave closer to the preceding ventricular complex and if this arrangement creates a more unfavorable VA relationship, it will in turn aggravate the sinus tachycardia.

Pacemaker Syndrome. During functional atrial undersensing 5 of the 9 patients reported by Bode et al.[29] developed complaints suggestive of the pacemaker syndrome. They prevented functional atrial undersensing in 7 of their 9 patients by shortening the PVARP and AV delay and previously symptomatic patients became asymptomatic. The other 2 patients exhibited less atrial undersensing.

Significance of PVARP Extension. Functional atrial undersensing can occur with a *short* PVARP whenever a ventricular extrasystole activates an automatic PVARP extension[30]. In this situation an unsensed P wave within the extended PVARP gives rise to a conducted QRS complex which the pacemaker interprets as a ventricular extrasystole whereupon it generates another PVARP extension. The extended PVARP is perpetuated from cycle to cycle as long as the pacemaker interprets the conducted QRS as a ventricular extrasystole.

Prevention of Functional Atrial Undersensing. A relatively short PVARP can often be used to prevent functional atrial undersensing because retrograde VA block is common in patients with first-degree AV block. Other measures[31] include: 1. Capability of programming off the automatic PVARP extension after a ventricular extrasystole. 2. Elimination of the PVARP extension whenever the pacemaker detects a P wave within the PVARP immediately before the next sensed ventricular beat. 3. Noncompetitive atrial pacing with the delivery of a premature but appropriately delayed atrial stimulus whenever the pacemaker senses activity in the PVARP. 4. Prolongation of the atrial escape interval after a sensed ventricular extrasystole. 5. Ablation of the AV junction with resultant complete AV block in difficult situations.

References

1. Rosenqvist M, Bergfeldt L, Haga Y, et al. The effect of ventricular activation sequence on cardiac performance during pacing. PACE 1996:19:1279-1286.

2. Leclercq C, Gras D, Le Helloco A et al. Hemodynamic importance of preserving the normal sequence of ventricular activation in permanent cardiac pacing. Am Heart J 1995;129:1133-1141.

3. Vardas PE, Simantirakis EN, Parthenakis FI et al. AAIR versus DDDR pacing in patients with impaired sinus node chronotropy. PACE 1997;20:1762-1768.

4. Ovsyshcher IE. Towards physiologicalpacing: optimization of cardiac hemodynamics by AV delay adjustment. PACE 1997;20:861-865.

5. Ovsyshcher I, Zimlichman R, Bondy C, et al. Measurement of cardiac output by impedance cardiography in pacemaker patients at rest: effects of various AV delay. JACC 1993;21:761-767

6. Prinzen FW, Van Oosterhout MF, Vanagt WY et al. Optimization of ventricular function by improving the activation sequence during ventricular pacing. PACE 1998; 21:2256-2260.

7. Ishikawa T, Sumica S, Kimura K et al. Critical PQ interval for the appearance of diastolic mitral regurgitation and optimal PQ interval in patients implanted with DDD pacemakers. PACE 1994;17:1989-1994.

8. Ovsyshcher IE. Pacing in patients with long atrioventricular interval. In: Santini M, ed. Progress in Clinical Pacing, Futura Media Services, Inc. Armonk, NY, USA. Chapter 11, pp. 75-84

9.Nishimura RA, Hayes DL, Holmes DR Jr, et al. Mechanism of hemodynamic improvement by dual-chamber pacing for severe left ventricular dysfunction; An acute doppler and catheterization hemodynamic study. J Am Coll Cardiol 1995;25:281-288.

10. Barold SS. Indications for permanent pacing in first-degree block. Class I, II, or III ? PACE 1996;19:747-751.

11. Ellenbogen KA, Gilligan DM, Wood MA et al. The pacemaker syndrome. A matter of definition. Am J Cardiol 1997;79:1226-1229.

12. Chirife R, Ortega DF, Salazar AI. "Pacemaker syndrome " without a pacemaker. Deleterious effects of first-degree AV block. (Abstract). RBM 1990;12:22.

13. Gregoratos G, Cheitlin MD, Freedman RA et al. ACC/AHA guidelines for implantation of pacemakers and antiarrhythmia devices. A report of the American College of Cardiology/American Heart Association task force on practice guidelines (Committee on pacemaker implantation). J Am Coll Cardiol 1998; 31:1175-1209.

14. Hayes DL, Barold SS, Camm AJ et al. Evolving indications for permanent cardiac pacing. An appraisal of the 1998 ACC/AHA guidelines. Am J Cardiol 1998; 82:1082-1086.

15. Iliev I, Yamachika S, Muta K et al. DDD pacing with optimal AV delay versus AAI pacing in patients with AV block I degree. (Abstract). J Am Coll Cardiol 1998;31:433A.

16. Iliev I. Personal communication.

17. Dec GW, Fuster V. Idiopathic dilated cardiomyopathy. NEJM 1994;331:1564-1575.

18. Unverferth DV, Magorien RD, Moeschberger ML et al. Factors influencing the one year mortality of dilated cardiomyopathy. Am J Cardiol 1984;54:147-152.

19. Olshausen KV, Stienen U, Schwartz F et al. Long-term prognostic significance of ventricular arrhythmias in idiopathic dilated cardiomyopathy. Am J Cardiol 1988;61:146-151.

20. Xiao HB, Roy C, Fujimoto S et al. Natural history of abnormal conduction and its relation to prognosis in patients with dilated cardiomyopathy. Int J Cardiol 1996;53:163-170.

21. Cazeau S, Ritter P, Lazarus A et al. Multisite pacing for end-stage heart failure. Early experience. PACE 1996:19:1748-1757.

22. Gras D, Mabo P, Tang T, et al. Multisite pacing as a supplemental treatment of congestive heart failure. Preliminary results of the Medtronic Inc. InSync study. PACE 1998;21:2249-2255.

23. Auricchio A, Salo RW, Klein H et al. Problems and pitfalls in evaluating studies for pacing in heart failure. G Ital Cardiol 1997;27:593-599.

24. Glikson M, Hayes DL, Nishimura RA. Newer clinical application of pacing. J Cardiovasc Electrophysiol 1997; 8:1190-1203.

25. Fei L, Wrobleski D, Groh W et al. Effects of multisite ventricular pacing on cardiac output in normal dogs and dogs with heart failure. J Cardiovasc Electrophysiol 1999;10:935-946.

26. Brecker SI, Gibson DG. What is the role of pacing in dilated cardiomyopathy? Eur Heart J 1996;17:819-824.

27. Pozzoli M, traversi E, Cioffi G et al. Loading manipulations improve the prognostic value of doppler evaluation of mitral flow in patients with chronic heart failure. Circ 1997;95:1222-1230.

28. Kass DA, Chen C-H,Talbot MW, et al. Ventricular pacing with premature excitation for treatment of hypertensive-cardiac hypertrophy with cavity obliteration. Circulation 1999; 100:807-812.

29. Bode F, Wiegand U, Katus HA et al. Pacemaker inhibition due to prolonged native AV interval in dual-chamber devices. PACE 1999;22: 425-1431

30. Wilson JH, Lattner S. Undersensing of P waves in the presence of adequate P wave due to automatic postventricular atrial refractory period extension. PACE 1989;10:1729-1732.

31. Barold SS. Optimal pacing in first-degree AV block. PACE 1999;22:1423-1424

Author Index

ALONSO, C...385

ALTAMURA, G...145

AVIRAM, I...29

ANDERSEN, HR...323

AVITALL, B...119

BAROLD, S.S...307, 349, 409

BAROLD, H.S...307, 349, 409

BATUR, M.K...23

BELHASSEN, B...47

BERUL, CI...217

BHARATI, S...131, 257

CAZEAU, S...385

CHRIST, T...315

CONNOLLY, S.J...333

COURTEMANCHE, M...87

CRYSTAL, E...29, 41, 373

DAUBERT J.C...155, 385

D'ALLONNES, G.R...155

DOCUMACI, B...73

ECTOR, H...95

EL-SHERIF, N...273

FLEIDERVISH, I.A...9, 41

FILIPECKI, A..79

FISHEL, R.S...307, 349

FRIEDMAN, M...29

FRIEDMAN, P...73, 241, 393

FURMAN, S...295

GELVAN, D...373

GLASS, L..87

GROSS, J.N..211

GLIKSON, M..241

GULKO, N..29

HAYES, D.L...365, 393

HERWIG, S...107

HEIDBUCHEL, H...95

HUBMAN, M..315

JUNG, W...107

KANAGARTNAM, P...3

KANOUPAKIS, E.M..137

KARGUL, W..79

KIM, S..101

KONARSKA-KUSZEWSKA, E...79

KRISTENSEN, L...323

KROL, R.B..101

KUTARSKI, A...167, 401

KUSNIEC, J..115

LECLERCQ, C..385

LEVINE, P.A..339

LINDEMANS, F.W...35, 223

LUDERITZ, B..107

LURIA, D..73

MABO, P..155

MALIK, M...35

MALINOWSKI K...315

MANIOS, E.G..137, 175

MICHALAK, Z..79

MILLARD, S.C...119

MOND, H.G..357

MOSS, A.J..55, 285

NEMEC, J...73

NIELSEN, J.C..323

NISAM, S...191

OTO, A..23

OVSYSHCHER, I.E...v, 29, 41, 373, 409

PANDOZI, C..145

PASTORE, J.M..11

PAVIN, D...155

PHILIP, G...101

PETERS, N.S...3

PRAKASH, A...101

PRUSKI, M..79

PRYSTOWSKY, E.N..iii

RABINOVITCH, A...29

RICCI, R...145

ROBBE, H.W.J..223

ROBINSON, J.L...55

RODEN, D.M..249

ROSENBAUM, D.S..11

ROSENHECK, S..229

SANTINI, M...145

SAKSENA, S...101

SCHALDACH, M...315, 401

SCHEINMAN, M.M..63, 263

SCHIER, M..315

SCIANARO, M.C...145

SIMANTIRAKIS, E.N...175

SMITS, K. F.A.A..35

SPURRELL, P...181

STANTON, M.S..201

STRASBERG, B..115

SULKE, N..181

SZYDLO, K..79

TOSCANO, S..145

TRUSZ-GLUZA, M..79

TURITTO, G..273

URBONAS, A..119

VARDAS, P.E...137, 175

WEINER, S..211

WILLEMS, R..95

WILLENBRING, J.E..201

ZAJAC, T...79

ZABARSKY, R..15

ZAREBA, W...55